DAVID HOFFMANN

The Herbal Handbook

A User's Guide to Medical Herbalism

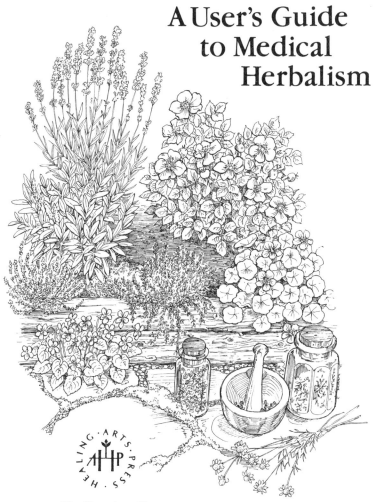

Healing Arts Press
Rochester, Vermont

Healing Arts Press
One Park Street
Rochester, Vermont 05767

*Note to the reader: This book is intended as an infor-
mational guide. The remedies, approaches, and techniques described herein are meant to supplement, and not
to be a substitute for, professional medical care or treatment. They should not be used to treat a serious ailment
without prior consultation with a qualified healthcare
professional.*

**Library of Congress Cataloging-in-Publication
Data**

Hoffmann, David, 1951–
   The herbal handbook: a user's guide to medical
     herbalism / David Hoffmann.
     p. cm.
     Rev. ed. of: The herb user's guide, 1987.
     Bibliography: p.
     Includes index.
     ISBN 0-89281-275-3
     1. Herbs—Therapeutic use. 2. Medicinal plants.
     I. Hoffmann, David, 1951– Herb user's guide.
     II Title.
RM666.H33H64 1989
615'.321—dc19
                          88-23534
                          CIP

Printed and bound in the United States

10 9 8

Healing Arts Press is a division of Inner Traditions
International, Ltd.

Distributed to the book trade in the United States by
American International Distribution Corporation
(AIDC)

Distributed to the book trade in Canada by Publishers
Group West (PGW), Montreal West, Quebec

Distributed to the health food trade in Canada by Alive
Books, Toronto and Vancouver

The Herbal Handbook

By the same author:

Successful Stress Control
The Holistic Herbal

CONTENTS

___ HOW TO USE THE BOOK ___

The HERB USER' GUIDE is offered as an introduction to the fascinating study of Herbalism. It is a field of human endeavour that is at once healing, life enhancing, transformative and fun.

Actions are used here as a primary 'road map' for exploring this vast field. Individual herbs are described under their main action or in a chapter on the body system for which they are most commonly used. To find the main entry on a herb, please use the index.

Each action is explained in a way that ensures an understanding of what it is and how it works. Specific herbal remedies are then given that use this action well.

A unique feature is an overview of a range of remedies that can act in the way described, but also have affinity for the various bodily systems. Each section on an action ends with this information. In this way the book provides the basis for logical and holistic prescribing as described in the chapters on bodily systems.

As an example we can consider a possible herbal prescription to reduce high blood pressure. It might contain:

HAWTHORN BERRIES

LIME BLOSSOM
YARROW

All of these herbs have a reputation for being HYPOTENSIVE, that is a remedy that reduces elevated blood pressure. However, you will see after studying these herbs that we have the following actions represented:

CARDIOVASCULAR TONIC
DIURETIC
NERVINE RELAXANT

With a grasp of some of the physiology that underlies this condition the role of these actions becomes evident. In the section on the systems it is just such an approach that is taken.

No knowledge of physiology is assumed or needed. The processes involved are explained as the book unfolds.

The first step is to gain an overview of the general possibilities in herbal remedies though the actions rather than setting out to learn all the herbs piecemeal.

It is a dilemma to try to structure a way through the wealth of herbal knowledge without creating artificial divides. I hope my attempts to do this are useful and that you enjoy this book.

1
WHAT IS A HERB?

He causeth the grass to grow for the cattle, and herb for the service of man.

Psalm 104:12

Herbs are different things to different people, from weeds, to culinary flavourings, to medicines. The definition depends on the discipline from which you look at it. Take medicine as an example. To a North American Indian, medicine is energy and power, and it is an expression of The Great Spirit. To a member of the American Medical Association, medicine is about illness, pathology and high technological cures for body faults. So the same word has very different interpretations.

Herbs are defined in different ways depending on the discipline in which they are used. In botany they are non-woody plants that are under 30cm high. In ecology the herb layer describes a horizontal level in environments such as forests and woods. To a gardener herbs are ornamental plants used in herbaceous borders, while to a chef they are the aromatic culinary plants.

Strictly speaking, a herb to a medical herbalist is any plant material that can be used in medicine and health care. Thus not only are botanical herbs used (*White Hore-hound*), but flowers (*Marigold*), heart wood of trees (*Guaiacum*), seeds (*Chasteberry*), and bark (*Willow Bark*). In fact, all anatomical parts of plants are used in some form or another. The flowering plants are used as well as ferns, mosses, lichen, seaweed and fungi.

From a broader perspective it can be said that herbalism is the study and practice of the interaction between plants and humanity. This is a definition that covers a vast range of human life. It would include agriculture, horticulture, medicine, forestry, carpentry, construction, clothing materials and their usage, dyeing and natural colours etc. In fact as coal is geologically preserved wood we could push the definition and include much of modern industry in the realms of herbalism.

In this book, you'll be glad to know, we shall limit ourselves to the practical use of medicinal, culinary and dye plants. The broader social and philosophical implications of herbalism and holistic medicine will only be hinted at in passing.

The book is presented in a form that can provide
• A self-training guide for those who would like to gain a foundation in medical herbalism.
• A reference work and source of references for further study, and
• A practical guide to basic skills.

I hope you enjoy this book and welcome you to the growing band of herbalists in Britain. This may be the well-trained professional or the person who thinks it's simply a good idea – we are all working in form or idea with the plants of which the psalmist wrote.

2
_ APPROACHES TO HERBALISM _

...and the fruit thereof shall be for meat, and the leaf thereof for medicine.
Ezekiel 47:12

The use of herbs as a source of healing remedies is inherent in all cultures in all historical times. It is only recently in the scientific, empirical western-influenced countries that such knowledge has been ignored or ridiculed. At least we are starting to remember and recognize the value of the weeds and the hedgerows, the gardens and the window boxes. For some the Bible as an authority is enough, for others different justifications are needed.

There are a number of ways in which to use herbs in health and healing. Nothing inherent in the plant defines its use and so they must be used within some sort of pattern. A number of quite different approaches can be identified:

1. Traditional knowledge.
2. Pharmacology of active ingredients.
3. Within the framework of a philosophical system.
4. Within a new holistic framework.

None of these approaches is better or worse than the others, just different. Plants used in these different ways and contexts can have quite marked differences in effect. This shows that healing is much more than the impact of drug or herb; it is a much broader and deeper phenomenon that involves all of what we are. This will be explored more below. Now let's look at these approaches in more depth.

1. Traditional Knowledge

This is the way most people first come in contact with herbalism. For example, there are snippets of information passed between people, reading popular books on herbal remedies. These books are usually written by journalists who have culled the information from much older books. All of this is fine and good, but it is inherently limited.

It is from tradition that we in the 'scientific' west have received most of our knowledge about what each remedy can do, which illnesses it may be used for and its actions. The knowledge will have its roots in a time when herbs were extensively used in the healing arts of that time, but now such knowledge is nothing more than 'organic drug therapy' if used as it is. Simply using remedies for symptomatic relief or to treat a named disease ignores all the insights of holistic medicine and the other philosphical system.

However, it is a valid way to start. It is worth considering a couple of the sources of these traditions and why we have only handed-down information left to us. In addition to the cultures considered below, we must remember that many healers and herbalists were branded as witches and burnt right up to the eighteenth century. From one perspective, the loss of living herbalism in Europe parallels a history of destruction and oppression of old ways. It is a sorry story indeed. There is a growing perception, however, of the value of traditional knowledge. This is being actively explored and developed by the World Health Organisation, as described below.

The Physicians of Myddfai

An example of modern traditions with vital roots in the past is in Wales. In rural areas there are still many people who know of one or two recipes for quite specific conditions; for example, an ointment for shingles or eczema. These are effective, but the person using them does not know why or often know any other herbal information. The origins of these mixtures lies in the mediaeval physicians of Myddfai from the courts of the Princes of Wales. A deep and profound knowledge of herbs and the healing process was possessed by these people, way in advance of what was available in England and the rest of non-islamic Europe at the time.

However, when the English invaded and conquered Wales, and the court was destroyed, the knowledge and wisdom of the physicians was dispersed throughout the population. In an attempt not to lose it completely, it would appear that certain families were given specific remedies to keep secret and pass down the generations. The recipes and information were never given to anyone outside the family, but the medicine was given freely to any who needed it. Some of this seeded wisdom is still thriving in the hills and valleys of North and West Wales.

Native American Herbal Traditions

The Native American tradition of medicine means living in harmony with nature. Nature's harmony itself is medicine. To Native Americans, health and healing are part of a way of relating to the entire world. American Indian healers feel that they are responsible for the welfare of the Earth and all her creatures. The Indians call the Earth's creator the Great Spirit. They call creation Great Mother, or Grandmother Earth.

This Native American view of the interdependence between human beings and all of Earth's creatures parallels the principles of ecology in modern science. Their tradition of medicine is not as theoretical a science, however. Rather, it is based on direct perceptions, and the knowledge that the medicine man or woman accumulates.

The Native American healer gathers herbs with a genuine feeling of exchange from one aspect of Creation to another. There is a two way flow within the greater whole of the Earth. The Medicine healer perceives plants not merely as chemical combinations that help the human body but also as part of the whole of creation. They are infused with the same spirit, power, and life-forces that animate and flow through all the universe. Believing this, the healer regards plants as relatives, calling them 'medicine people'.

This is indeed a wonderful, ecologically integrated world view that can be related to the philosphical systems described on p.15.

Native American herbalists had established a vast pharmacopoeia of indigenous medicinal plants. Some of the more common ones are *Bearberry, Beech, Birch, Butternut, Corn, Echinacea, False Unicorn Root, Ginseng, Golden Seal, Gravel Root, Oregon Grape, Poplar, Squaw Vine.* Many of the herbs used now as uterine tonics were introduced into Britain from America and traditional use. In addition, virtually every herb introduced from Europe was quickly adopted by the Native American healers.

However, again we have a situation where herbal wisdom has been partially lost through conquest and oppression. The Europeans have a lot to answer for!

The World Health Organisation

Since 1977 the WHO has had an active programme of promotion and development of traditional medicine. At the Thirtieth World Health Assembly a resolution was adopted that urged governments to give 'adequate importance to the utilization of their traditional systems of medicine, with appropriate regulations as to their national health systems.'

This has led to much interest from the scientific and health care community around the world in traditional therapeutics, which are predominantly based on herbal medicines. Some of these traditional approaches are well developed whole health systems, such as the Chinese, but the programme is as interested in small-scale use of plants in local areas.

The theme of promotion and development of traditional medicine is being explored in a number of ways that include:

- Traditional medicine in health care,
- Reasons for the promotion of traditional medicine,
- Patterns of utilization of both traditional and modern medicine,
- The integration of traditional and modern medicine,
- Manpower development for traditional medicine,
- Research and development in traditional medicine.

This world-wide programme of activity raises many vital questions of relevance to western health care. Inherent is the recognition that there is value in traditional approaches to health, both in the plants used and the attitudes and techniques of the healers. References are given in the Bibliography to enable a comprehensive exploration of the vast range of work being promoted by the World Health Organisation, but simplifying for brevity's sake we can identify three broad areas of current work:

1. The evaluation of tradition plant materia medicas and the practices used by the healers. This is leading to the discovery of new drugs but, far more importantly, is showing indigenous plants that may be used in a way that reduces the need to import foreign drugs or become dependent on multinational pharmaceutical companies. The whole pattern of traditional health care is being looked at, because the plants are used in a social and belief system that can be as therapeutic as the plants. This is an insight largely lost in the urbanized west.

2. Integrating traditional medicine into newly developing systems of national health care. Perhaps the best example of this at work is in China, where traditional herbal and acupuncture techniques are used alongside western allopathic medicines. Such developments are being supported throughout the Third World. It is a pity that we in Britain have not yet seen the value of such integration.

3. The training of traditional and modern conventional health workers to an equivalent standard. This promotes co-

operation and respect, while increasing the health care infrastructure of the country concerned.

This is a fascinating development in the history of herbalism and promises much for the future.

2. Pharmacology of Active Ingredients

It is not realized by many that herbs are the foundation of much of modern medicine. This is the result of many years of scientific research into the active ingredients of plant remedies. A wide range of potent drugs have been produced in this way. To name a few: aspirin came from _Willow Bark,_ digoxin for heart failure from the _Foxglove,_ steroids from the _Wild Yam,_ the anti-leukemia drugs vinblastine and vincristine from the _Madagascan Periwinkle._ The list is so long that 70 per cent of the drugs in the British Pharmacopoeia have their origins in plants.

The search for active ingredients in plants has been most successful but is limited by the very nature of the perceptions behind it. Using plants as sources of drugs limits their healing power to that of the context within which they are used. That is pathology-based medicine, focused on illness and the disease process rather than on health and wholeness. In this way the herbs are used to provide drugs in the fight against pathological processes, ignoring their potential for augmenting the inherent wholeness of the life within us.

This approach is part of a philosophically reductionist approach to life and humanity which is so all-pervading in our science-based society that it is rarely acknowledged or even perceived.

The pros and cons of active ingredients or whole plants will be discussed in the chapter on plant constitutents.

Herbalism is crippled when seen as a precursor of modern medicine, of drugs, or of potent active ingredients. Potentially in plants we have not only medicines for illness but augmentors for health. More importantly we have a way in which one aspect of our lives can be re-tuned to nature, to the world that we are part of yet hurt and damage so much.

It is worth pointing out that drug therapy and modern medicine are not the complete saviour they often are made out to be. Drawing on public health statistics from England and Wales in the last three centuries, McKeown has demonstrated that medical advances generally coincided with, rather than caused, improvements in the health of the population. His meticulous researches show that only 10 per cent of the improvement in mortality from infectious disease can be traced to individual medical intervention – including the dramatic and sometimes lifesaving use of antibiotics.

According to McKeown, our better health can largely be attributed to factors unrelated to medicine. These include improvements in nutrition (secondary to better food sources and methods of cultivation), in the environment (especially the treatment and regulation of food and water), and in our behavior (particularly the change in reproductive patterns that limited the size of the population).

3. Used Within a Philosophical System

The use described above is herbalism within a rational, reductionist, scientific 'philosophy', but this is rarely expressed as a philosophy of life. In this present section the approaches to herbalism I mean are profound and all-encompassing philosophical/spiritual world views that provide a model for health as well as guidelines for life. The two most significant systems still thriving today are Indian Ayurvedic medicine and Chinese traditional medicine. In addition to such approaches we must also recognize the philosophical integration of herbal medicine into healing techniques that use astrology and the whole anthroposophical vision of Rudolf Steiner. It is beyond the realms of a book such as this to give these profound systems adequate expression; references can be found in the Bibliography.

As an example, however, we shall look at the Chinese system in some degree. The Ayurvedic system, like the Chinese, works to maintain health and prevent disease through a balance of diet, exercise, thought and environment. It holds the expansive view that nothing exists in the realm of thought that cannot be used as a medicine. Herbs provide a basis for their therapeutics, which also include mental and physical practices intended to help the person concerned develop positive qualities. In the west we are familiar with hatha yoga, but yoga techniques include far more than the body positions. It is thus a whole system within a whole system of the Hindu world view and path of spirituality.

Chinese Healing: The Medicine of Harmony

The whole focus of this tradition is the creation and expression of harmony, a wonderful basis for health care. China's knowledge of herbs goes back to very ancient times. This time-tested practice of polypharmacy in Chinese herbalism is one of its most distinguishing features. Almost all Chinese herbs are used in formulas that combine four to twelve or even more ingredients.

The range of herbs and other substances used in Chinese medicine is another characteristic. The most recent Chinese pharmacopoeia contains over 5,700 entries that include common and uncommon herbs as well as medicinal minerals and animal parts. Today, there are more than 500 herbal formulas in use in Chinese medicine, of which about 200 are the most commonly used.

In the Chinese system herbs are differentiated according to their use as superior, general, or inferior drugs. Superior drugs are those tonics and herbs (_Ginseng_) that can be taken for a long time with no ill side effects. General herbs (_Ephedra_) are used to treat diseases, and their use is discontinued with remission of the disease. Inferior drugs (_Aconite_) are actually poisons that are used in a medicinal way only for brief periods of time, and in small amounts. These guidelines – superior, general, and inferior – contribute to the inherent safety of Chinese herbalism. By categorizing medicines in this way, generations of Chinese herbalists have determined the proper amounts of ingredients to use in their formulae.

Adaptations of the Chinese method of using herbs for health care and prevention of disease can be found in many other eastern countries. One reason it is so popular is because of its emphasis on prevention as a healing method, an approach that stems from an ancient cultural view. Chinese herbalism applies the principle of prevention by emphasizing the use of tonics and adaptogens, or herbs that strengthen the whole body. In particular, the Chinese healers pay special attention to herbs that strengthen or regulate the body's immune system.

To Chinese philosophers/physicians, nature itself is the model, the unifying principle, and the source of understanding. This source is called 'Tao'. The concept of Tao probably has been present in Chinese culture for many thousands of years, and certainly for at least 2,500 years. It is itself a way of being, a way of preserving life and health by living in harmony with nature's principles. But Tao is more than achieving a naturally healthy life through harmony. Tao is the harmony of life itself.

Chinese physicians use five diagnostic methods in order to find a patient's pattern of 'disharmony'. These include observation, listening (to the voice, coughs, etc), smelling body odours, questioning the patient's medical history, and wrist palpation or pulse diagnosis. A comprehensive exploration of this system is beyond the range of a book such as this.

The Tao of Yin and Yang

As a basis for understanding the Chinese use of herbs, the determination of harmony based on the universal theory of yin and yang must be explored. Originally, the Chinese character for yang meant the sunny side of a mountain. Its qualities are associated with heat, stimulation, movement, activity, excitement, vigour, and light. The original character for yin meant the shaded side of a mountain. Yin's qualities are associated with cold, passivity, inaction, darkness, and responsiveness.

In medicine there are five basic principles at work:

● All things are composed of both yin and yang.
● The yin and yang aspects can each be further divided into yin and yang.
● Yin and yang are polar pairs that cannot exist without each other.
● Yin and yang control or balance each other.
● Yin and yang change or transform into each other.

A balance of yin and yang shows a healthy environment. In people, a balance of these two forces represents a state of health. The Chinese healer learns many aspects of yin and yang as shown in seasonal cycles, properties of food and medicine, variations in the constitutions of patients, types and

stages of sickness, and techniques of treatment. Each subject mentioned above is complex and elaborate, as one might suspect from examining these five principles of yin and yang.

There are some basic principles of yin/yang that can be easily applied to any form of natural healing. For example, the functions of toning and eliminating can be related to conditions of yin or yang. A person who is too yin is made more yang with a toning therapy. A person who is too yang is made more yin with an eliminating therapy. Herbs that are hot, warm, sharp, sweet, bland, light, or of weak fragrance are considered yang. They are used to balance a yin condition. Herbs that are cold, cool, sour, bitter, salty, strong, heavy and strongly fragrant are yin, and they are used to balance a yang condition. A herb can also contain both yin and yang characteristics. For example, *Liquorice root* tastes sweet at first, but after a few moments it also tastes bitter. *Ginseng root* is a very yang herb, but it also has a slight bitter taste, while the *Ginseng leaf* has a yin quality; it is used to decrease fire energy, which is yang. In general, roots are considered the most yang part of the plant, while fruits and flowers are the most yin. Compared to its root, a plant's leaves are yin; but compared to its flowers, they are yang.

There is also yin and yang relationship between plants (and people) and their environment. A yin environment often produces more yang herbs, and a yang environment creates more yin herbs. We can take *Ginseng* as an example again. It naturally grows in damp, cold shady places, often high in the mountains on northern slopes. These are all yin conditions which attract their opposite, yang, in the *Ginseng* root. In the tropics there is a much greater yang force due to a greater amount of solar radiation. This great yang power produces plants which are more yin. Tropical plants are generally larger, leafier, juicier, and more fragrant than plants native to cooler climates. Even cactus plants are yin; growing as they do in hot, dry environments, they are full of water. Because of these ecological factors of yin and yang, the foods and herbs that grow in one's own region are considered the best medicine. They are thought to be naturally balanced to the local harmonies of yin and yang that affect people as well.

Other factors affect the degree of yin or yang in herbal medicines. Fresh herbs are considered more yin than dried herbs. A herb can be made more yang by drying it in the sun or more yin by drying it in the shade. The degree of heat used in preparing a herbal infusion also has a relative yin or yang influence. Sun tea, for example, which is simply steeped in a glass jar in the sun, is a yin method of preparation because it is passive. Correspondingly, sun tea is usually made in the summer to balance that season's yang quality. Boiling herbs in water for a short period of time and making an infusion are also yin methods, but they are more yang than making sun tea. Simmering herbs for a long time is an even more yang method, and it is applied most often to roots. Drinking a herb tea that has cooled maximizes its yin quality, while drinking it hot is more 'yang-izing'. Alcohol extraction produces a very yang product; the yin alcohol attracts the yang qualities of the herbs.

Generally, Chinese methods of preparation aim at maximizing the herb's basic qualities. A yang herb is simmered a long time to bring out its yang qualities, which are then used to balance a person's yin condition. Yin herbs (such as volatile oils), are prepared to maintain their yin qualities and are usually given as an infusion. Enhancing the yin in yin herbs is supposed to make them more effective in treating a yang condition. In formulas, though, herbs which embody a strong emphasis of yin or yang are most often balanced with herbs having only a slight emphasis of the opposite value. This reflects the emphasis on harmony, which is so highly valued in Chinese medicine.

In order to make their herbal remedies even more harmonious, Chinese physicians recommend taking them at varying times of the day, depending on the part of the body being treated. If the sickness is in the upper part of the body, teas or medicines are taken one hour after eating. If the tea is for the arms or legs, it is taken one hour before breakfast. Medicines for the bones are taken one hour after dinner or before sleep. Tonics and supplements are taken on an empty stomach, and the patient is advised to remain calm and move slowly afterwards.

From this brief overview of the herbal aspects of Chinese medicine we can get a hint at the complexity but also the integrated wholeness of the system. For a more detailed look at this system either consult a translation of Chinese works or see _The Healing Herbs_ by Gaea and Shandor Weiss (pub. Rodale Press).

4. Within a Holistic Framework

There is a growing awareness that the perspectives of scientific medicine do not provide us with an adequate framework for health. There can be no doubt that drug therapy and surgical technology have provided us with miracles of treatment. Much suffering has been relieved and countless lives saved. This cannot be denied and I would not want to belittle the value within high tech medicine. The limits of treating illness are fast being reached, however. There is a need to focus on prevention and, even more importantly, on health.

The World Health Organisation defines health as:

... more than simply the absence of illness. It is the active state of physical, emotional, mental and social well-being.

It is this kind of health that holistic medicine addresses itself to, and it potentially goes well beyond the confines of a pathology book! It is an appreciation of patients as mental and emotional, social and spiritual, as well as physical beings. It respects their capacity for healing themselves and regards them as active partners in, rather than passive recipients of, health care.

Such an approach has always been an integral part of the healer's heritage. It is named and emphasized now to correct our tendencies to equate medicine and health care with the treatment of disease entity.

The holistic context does not define the techniques used within it. A doctor can be holistically orientated, as can a herbalist or homoeopath. The main point is that the whole person is considered, their inner health as well as mental state, relationships and life in the world.

Holism in medicine can allow a framework within which all these various therapies, or orthodox and 'alternative' medicine, can work together in an integrated whole. There is a wonderful opportunity ahead of turning our National Health Service into a truly Holistic Health Service. This is a worthy vision to hold while that wonderful institution goes through its present period of trauma.

Let's consider some of the implications of such an approach. It is often called the paradigm of Holistic Medicine, paradigm being the Greek word for pattern. This recognizes that a whole new pattern of thought, assumptions and perceptions is arising.

The Paradigm of Holistic Medicine

- Holistic medicine addresses itself to the physical, mental, and spiritual aspects of those who come for care.
- Holistic medicine emphasizes each person's genetic, biological, and psychosocial uniqueness as well as the importance of tailoring treatment to meet each individual's needs.
- A holistic approach to medicine and health care includes understanding and treating people in the context of their culture, their family, and their community.
- Holistic medicine views health as a positive state, not as the absence of disease.
- Holistic medicine emphasizes the promotion of health and the prevention of disease.
- Holistic medicine emphasizes the responsibility of each individual for their own health.
- Holistic medicine uses therapeutic approaches that mobilize the individual's innate capacity for self-healing.
- While not denying the occasional necessity for swift and authoritative medical or surgical intervention, the emphasis in holistic medicine is on helping people to understand and to help themselves, on education and self-care rather than treatment and dependence.
- Holistic medicine makes use of a variety of diagnostic methods and systems in addition to and sometimes in place of the standard laboratory examinations.
- Good health depends on good nutrition and regular exercise.
- Holistic medicine views illness as an opportunity for discovery as well as a misfortune.
- Holism includes an appreciation of the quality of life in each of its stages and an interest in improving it as well as knowledge of the illnesses that are common to it.
- Holistic medicine emphasizes the potential therapeutic value of the setting in

which health care takes place.
- An understanding of and a commitment to change those social and economic conditions that perpetuate ill health are as much a part of holistic medicine as its emphasis on individual responsibility.
- Holistic medicine transforms its practitioners as well as its patients.

These broad outlines, suggested by Dr James Gordon M.D., provide the beginnings of a framework within which any therapy can be placed and so turned into a tool for personal health and transformation.

How can herbal medicine be used in this context?

Herbs and Holism

As will become apparent throughout this book, herbal medicine is a healing technique that is inherently in tune with nature. It may be described as ecological healing as it is due to our shared ecological and evolutionary heritage with the plant kingdom that herbal remedies work.

Through evolutionary time the complex interactions between animals and plants have produced an inherently integrated biological matrix of life. The needs of all within the biosphere are met in it. If this was not the case then species would die out. For humanity, our needs have been met by nature; if they had not we would not be here now. Our health needs were supplied by our environment – in other words, herbs. So on one level we need look no further than natural history to find a context within which to use herbs. The evidence for this degree of integration is shown in the 'active ingredients' and how they work.

At the moment much thought is going into marrying herbalism and holism. On a simple level it is easy because of the inherent integration, but humanity tends to develop clear ideas and patterns of explanation and approach. In the west a number of

guidelines are becoming clear. Most of this book deals with using the approach of 'actions' as an indicator of use. Before exploring them in depth, let's look at another context, one within which the use of actions can take place.

This approach recognizes three broad areas of influence; Challengers, Normalizers and Eliminators. Using this model it also becomes possible to relate western herbal usage to the Eastern traditions.

1. CHALLENGING HERBS WHICH PROVOKE BODILY PROTECTIVE RESPONSES.
These are usually due to specific chemical components in the plants. Examples would be the demulcent mucilage in *Marshmallow* for aiding the stomach. The astringents with their tannin content have a specific effect on tissue which is described in Chapter 3. The purgatives work through their specific chemicals, for example the anthraquinones in *Senna*. These trigger a specific response. The same can be said for expectorants, diuretics and bitters. Again, they are explored in Chapter 3.

These strong and challenging herbs are the basis of herbal use in western medicine, but are the least used in Chinese medicine where the emphasis is on prevention and maintenance of health.

2. NORMALIZERS ACTING BIDIRECTIONALLY
These herbs have a normalizing, supportive action on organs or tissues, acting almost like foods rather than medicines. In chemical terms they would appear to be of no real value, but in holistic and natural medicine terms they provide the core of any real treatment.

Here we have remedies that enable stress or diseased tissue to respond in a way that returns it to normal. Thus we have *Hawthorn Berries* that will lower raised blood pressure and raise low blood pressure, but always returning it to the norm for that person. There are many other examples with nature providing remedies for each organ and function that work in this way.

3. ELIMINATORS

These help the body's eliminatory processes by increasing activity of the eliminatory organs. These are the bowels, kidneys, skin and lungs. In classical naturopathic terms this leads to cleansing, increased nourishment as well as drainage of tissue and specific organs.

Throughout this book it is hoped that the holistic perspectives inherent in herbalism will become clear and usable. The focus will be on how to use practically our understanding of a plant's *actions* and use these properties in releasing our innate self-healing powers.

3
ACTIONS

One of the most comprehensible ways of coming to terms with the vast range of herbal remedies available is to consider them in terms of their actions on the body. It is possible, and in time desirable, to know each plant well, how to use and prepare it for what conditions and which types of people. However, this is a bit much to ask of beginners. It is something that herbalists aim for by their sixties!

This chapter considers the main actions, giving examples and their mode of activity where known. There is a strange state of affairs where part of our knowledge is science based and partially historical and folk wisdom. There is no contradiction here, just a recognition that our remedies work and that science has not caught up with them yet.

Many terms have been coined in the past, and older books have some rather unusual expressions in them. Here we will limit ourselves to those in current usage by professional medical herbalists.

ADAPTOGEN

What is an Adaptogen?

This is a relatively new concept to western medicine and herbalism. However, in China and the East such ideas are the very basis of their preventative approach to health and well being. This is an action that improves the body's adaptability. In other words an adaptogen enables it to avoid reaching a point of collapse or over-stress because it can adapt 'around' the problem.

How Adaptogens Work

There is now much research into these potentially astounding remedies. The core of their action appears to be in helping the body deal with stress. As we shall see in the section on the nervous system in Chapter 6, an inability to cope with the external pressures leads to many internal repercussions. Thus much illness can develop in very diverse forms. *Adaptogens* seem to increase the threshold of resistance to damage via support of adrenal gland and possibly pituitary gland function.

By stretching the meaning of the word it can come to mean what in the past was called a *tonic*. This is especially when a herb can have a normalizing effect; that is, contradictory actions depending on the body's needs. This restorative quality is a common and unique feature of herbal medicines and will be highlighted throughout the book.

Examples

The examples given are two of the herbs given most publicity in recent years. There are a number of Chinese remedies that could be included here, such as *Dong Quai*.

GINSENG   *Panax ginseng*
Part used: Root.
Collection: Ginseng is cultivated in China, Korea and N.E. America.
Constituents: Steroidal glycosides called panaxosides; sterols; vitamins of the D group.
Actions: Adaptogen, Anti-depressive, increases resistance and improves both physical and mental performance.
Indications: Ginseng has an ancient history and as such has accumulated much folklore about its actions and uses. Many of the claims that surround it are inflated but it is clear that this is a unique plant. It has the power to move a person to their physical peak, generally increasing vitality and physical performance. Specifically it will raise lowered blood pressure to a normal level. It affects depression, especially where this is due to debility and exhaustion. It can be used in general for exhaustion states and weakness. It has a reputation as an aphrodisiac. Occasionally the use of this herb may produce headaches.
Preparation and dosage: The root is often chewed or a decoction may be made. Put ½

teaspoonful of the powdered root in a cup of water, bring to the boil and simmer gently for 10 minutes. This should be drunk three times a day.

SIBERIAN GINSENG
                    Eleutherococcus senticosus
Part used: The root of a N.E. Asian shrub.
Constituents: The research so far indicates the pharmacologically important group to be triterpenoid saponins called eleutherosides.
Actions: Adaptogen, a circulatory stimulant, vasodilator.
Indications: This herb may be safely used to increase stamina in the face of undue demands and stress. These may be physical or mental – they are one to the body. Thus it is used for debility, exhaustion and depression, except where these are due to a specific medical reason that calls for defined treatment. It has a growing reputation for increasing all kinds of body resistance. However, the claims may be over-enthusiastic. The claims for circulatory effects come from excellent Russian research, which has not yet been verified in Britain.
Combinations: It is best used by itself, or with herbs that are specifically indicated for a person.
Preparation and dosage: This herb is usually available as tablet or powder, the dosage of which should be between 0.2 – 1g three times a day, over a period of time.

Adaptogens for Different Parts of the Body

Here we are considering a normalizing effect rather than a general beneficial response. Strictly speaking we can mention:
Circulatory system: for the heart *Hawthorn*, for circulation *Lime Blossom* and *Garlic*.
Respiratory system: *Mullein* and *Lobelia* for

the lungs, *Ground Ivy* for the upper respiratory tract.

Digestive system: the bitters as a group can work this way for the liver and pancreas, while the aperients work for the intestines.

Reproductive system: False Unicorn Root and *Chasteberry* for hormonal function and *Blue Cohosh* and *Life Root* for the womb itself.

Nervous system: The nervine tonics can work this way, especially *Oats.*

ALTERATIVE

What is an Alterative?

Alteratives are herbs that will gradually restore the proper function of the body and increase health and vitality. They were at one time known as 'blood cleansers'.

This sounds very unclear, and their mode of action on the body is not understood, but their value in holistic health care cannot be doubted. In broad terms they act to alter the body's processes of metabolism so that tissues can best deal with the range of functions from nutrition to elimination. Many of the herbs with this action improve the body's ability to eliminate waste from the body through the kidneys, liver, lungs or skin. Others work by stimulating digestive function or are anti-microbial, whilst others just work!

The idea of a blood cleanser, while hinting at much says little at all. If the blood was indeed in need of cleansing then there would be a major medical emergency afoot.

Alteratives can be used safely in many diverse conditions as supportive remedies, but should be thought of first where chronic inflammatory or degenerative conditions exist. These would include the skin diseases, various types of arthritis and the wide category of auto-immune problems.

Examples

There are many herbs that have an *alterative* action on the body. Because of the generally life-enhancing nature of herbal remedies many plants could be described as *alterative,* but this would be secondary to their main action and usage. The *diuretic* and *hepatic* remedies could easily be seen as *alterative* but this stretches the point. Here we shall look at three of the main *alterative* herbs in some detail and then briefly review a range.

BURDOCK   *Arctium lappa*
Part used: Roots and rhizome.
Collection: The roots and rhizome should be unearthed in September or October.
Constituents: Flavonoid glycosides, bitter glycosides, alkaloid, anti-microbial substance, inulin.
Actions: Alterative, diuretic, bitter.
Indications: Burdock is one of the best known remedies for the treatment of skin conditions which result in dry and scaly skin. It can be effective for the alleviation of psoriasis if used over a long period of time. Similarly, all types of eczema (though primarily the dry kinds) may be treated effectively if it is used over a period of time. As part of a broad treatment, it will be useful for rheumatic complaints, especially where they are associated with psoriasis. Part of the action of this herb is through the bitter stimulation of the digestive juices and especially of bile secretion. As is shown in the section on bitters, this will aid digestion and appetite. It has been used in anorexia nervosa and similar conditions, also to aid kidney function and to heal cystitis. In

23

general, Burdock will move the body to a state of integration and health, removing such indicators of systemic imbalance as skin problems and dandruff. Externally it makes a good compress or poultice to speed up the healing of wounds and ulcers. Eczema and psoriasis may also be treated this way externally, but it must be remembered that such skin problems can only be healed from within and with the aid of internal remedies.

Combinations: For skin problems, combine with *Yellow Dock, Red Clover* or *Cleavers.*

Preparation and dosage: Decoction: put 1 teaspoonful of the root into a cup of water, bring to the boil and simmer for 10 – 15 minutes. This should be drunk three times a day. For external use see further information in the section on the skin in Chapter 6.

Tincture: Take 2 – 4ml of the tincture three times a day.

CLEAVERS   *Galium aparine*

Common names: Goosegrass, clivers.

Part used: Dried aerial parts and the fresh expressed juice.

Collection: The plant should be gathered before flowering and dried in the shade.

Constituents: Glycoside asperuloside, gallotannic acid, citric acid.

Actions: Diuretic, alterative, anti-inflammatory, tonic, astringent, anti-neoplastic.

Indications: This is a remedy with a long tradition of folk usage. Much of the 'old wives' wisdom has a good solid foundation in herbal therapy. It is a very valuable plant, being perhaps the best tonic to the lymphatic system available. As a lymphatic tonic with alterative and diuretic actions it may be used safely in a wide range of problems where the lymphatic system is involved. These include swollen glands (lymphadenitis) anywhere in the body and especially in tonsillitis and in adenoid trouble. It is helpful in a wide variety of skin conditions, especially in the dry kind such as psoriasis. It is helpful in the treatment of cystitis and other urinary conditions where there·is pain and may be combined with urinary demulcents for this. There is a long tradition for the use of Cleavers in the treatment of ulcers and tumours. This may have its basis in the lymphatic drainage, which helps detoxify tissue. Cleavers also makes an excellent vegetable.

Combinations: for the lymphatic system it will work well with *Poke Root, Echinacea* and *Marigold.* For skin conditions it is best combined with *Yellow Dock* and *Burdock.*

Preparation and dosage: Infusion: pour a cup of boiling water onto 2 – 3 teaspoonsful of the dried herb and leave to infuse for 10 – 15 minutes. This should be drunk three times a day.

Tincture: Take 2 – 4 ml of the tincture three times a day.

NETTLES   *Urtica dioica*

Part used: Aerial parts.

Collection: The herb should be collected just before the small flowers bloom.

Constituents: Histamine, formic acid, chlorophyll, glucoquinine, iron, vitamin C.

Actions: Astringent, diuretic, tonic.

Indications: Nettles are one of the most widely applicable plants we have. They strengthen and support the whole body. They are specific in cases of childhood eczema and beneficial in all the varieties of this condition, especially in nervous eczema. As an astringent Nettles can be used for nose bleeds or to relieve the symptoms wherever there is haemorrhage in the body, for example in uterine haemorrhage.

Combinations: They will combine well with *Figwort* and *Burdock* in the treatment of eczema.

Preparation and dosage: Infusion: pour a cup of boiling water onto 1 – 3 teaspoonsful of the dried herb and leave to infuse for 10 – 15 minutes. This should be drunk three times a day.

Tincture: take 1 – 4 ml of the tincture three times a day.

Alteratives for Different Parts of the Body

Each system of the body has plants that are particularly suited to it, some of which are alteratives. Here we shall see which remedies act as primary alteratives for each of these systems. Other remedies can have such an action as has already been pointed out, but we shall limit ourselves to those most often indicated. How they can be used will be considered in the sections on each system.

Circulatory system: Alterative action is not one that is specifically for this system, but by the nature of this group of herbs, they will aid circulation by helping the whole body to work at its peak. The Lymphatic aspect of this system is aided by *Cleavers, Poke Root* and *Echinacea.*

Respiratory system: The main alteratives for the lungs and respiratory system as a whole are *Mullein, Blood Root, Liquorice* and *Golden Seal.*

Digestive system: All the alteratives that work on the liver, pancreas and other organs of the digestive system are of great importance in the whole of herbal medicine. A small selection would include *Blue Flag, Burdock, Bogbean, Fringetree, Garlic, Golden Seal, Nettles, Sarsaparilla* and *Yellow Dock.*

Urinary system: Many of what herbalists call diuretics could be more accurately described as urinary alteratives. These would include *Buchu, Cleavers,* and *Bearberry.*

Reproductive system: The general alteratives are always of value here but specifics could be *Black Cohosh, Blue Cohosh, False Unicorn Root, Golden Seal, Raspberry Leaves* and *Saw Palmetto.*

Muscles and skeleton: This is explored in more depth in the appropriate section, but alteratives here include *Bogbean, Bladderwrack,* and *Burdock.*

Nervous system: By helping the body to be whole, all alteratives aid the strained nervous system, but *Pasque Flower* and *Red Clover* are especially helpful as alteratives with a nervine action.

Skin: The list could include all those mentioned plus many more. This is the system where alteratives are most often used. It is important to remember that in holistic herbalism there are rarely specific plants that are indicated, rather the need to aid and support the whole body in its return to health. Alteratives often used for the skin are *Burdock, Cleavers, Echinacea, Figwort, Fumitory, Mountain Grape, Red Clover, Sarsaparilla* and *Yellow Dock.*

ANTHELMINTIC

Anthelmintics will destroy or expel worms from the digestive system. Unfortunately, many of the most effective anthelmintics are no longer available since the new Medicines Act was introduced as they can be toxic in high dosage; therefore, those are not listed here. This term is synonymous with Vermifuge and Anti-Parasitic. Of the remedies we are still allowed we can mention *Aloe, Garlic, Pomegranate, Tansy, Thuja, Wormwood,* and *Rue.*

ANTI-BILIOUS

What is an Anti-bilious herb?

The anti-bilious herbs help the body to remove excess bile and can thus aid in cases of biliary and jaundice conditions. Compare with Cholagogues and Hepatics, with whom they are often synonymous.

How Anti-bilious Herbs Work

The mode of action is described in the sections on Cholagogues and Hepatics.

Examples
Here is a list of the main remedies that have this action: *Balmony, Barberry, Dandelion, Fringetree, Golden Seal, Mugwort, Vervain, Wild Yam, Wormwood.*

ANTI-CATARRHAL

What is an Anti-catarrhal?

The anti-catarrhal herbs help the body to remove excess catarrhal build-ups, whether in the sinus area or other parts of the body. They are used mainly in ear, nose and throat infections, but have an essential role to play in many broader based treatments throughout the body.

How Anti-catarrhals Work

Mucous and catarrh is not of itself a problem. It is an essential body product, but when too much is being produced it is usually in response to an infection, helping the body remove the problematic organism, or as a way of the body removing excess carbohydrate from the body. In such cases a low mucous-forming diet is called for, as described in Chapter 6.

Some of the remedies work by producing a more watery mucous secretion, enabling the body to remove it, others reduce the secretion directly. This is not as desirable as it sounds as it may cause a build-up of waste that cannot be cleared from the sinuses.

The astringent action of tannins seems to be common to many of the herbs in this group, as is some volatile oil and flavonoids, but the mode of action is difficult to explain in specific terms, though it undoubtedly works.

Examples
Nature is rich in herbs that have this action on the body. Here we shall look at three of the main anti-catarrhal herbs in some detail and then briefly review a range.

GOLDEN ROD *Solidago virgauria*
Part used: Dried aerial parts.
Collection: Gather stalks at the time of flowering, which is between July and October, preferably from plants not yet

blooming. Dry in the shade or not above a temperature of 40°C.

Constituents: Saponins, essential oil, bitter principle, tannins, flavonoids.

Actions: Anti-catarrhal, anti-inflammatory, antiseptic, diaphoretic, carminative, diuretic.

Indications: One of the best plant remedies we have for catarral states, especially for upper respiratory catarrh, whether acute or chronic. It may be used in combination with other herbs in the treatment of influenza. The carminative properties give it a role in the treatment of flatulent dyspepsia. As an anti-inflammatory urinary antiseptic, *Golden Rod* may be used in cystitis, urethritis and the like. Recent research has suggested a role in lowering blood pressure. It can be used to promote the healing of wounds. As a gargle it can be used in laryngitis and pharyngitis.

Combinations: For upper respiratory catarrh it may be used with *Cudweed, Echinacea, Elderflower* and *Wild Indigo.*

Preparation and dosage: Infusion: pour a cup of boiling water onto 2 – 3 teaspoonsful of the dried herb and leave to infuse for 10 – 15 minutes. This should be drunk three times a day.

Tincture: take 2 – 4 ml of the tincture three times a day.

ELDER   *Sambucus nigra*
Part used: bark, flowers, berries, leaves.
Collection: The flowers are collected in spring and early summer and dried as rapidly as possible in the shade. The bark and berries are best collected in August and September.
Constituents: Flowers: Flavonoids including rutin, isoquercitfrine and kampherol; the hydrocyanic glycoside sambunigrine; tannins; essential oil; mucilage.
Berries: invert sugar; fruit acids; tannin; vitamin C and P; anthrocyanic pigments; traces of essential oil.

Actions: Bark: purgative, emetic, diuretic.
Leaves: externally emollient and vulnerary, internally as purgative, expectorant, diuretic and diaphoretic.
Flowers: Diaphoretic, anti-catarrhal.
Berries: Diaphoretic, diuretic, laxative.

Indications: The Elder tree is a veritable medicine chest by itself. The leaves are used primarily for bruises, sprains, wounds and chilblains. It has been reported that Elder leaves may be useful in an ointment for tumours. Elder flowers are ideal for the treatment of colds and influenza. They may be used quite safely in any catarrhal inflammation of the upper respiratory tract such as hayfever and sinusitis. Catarrhal deafness responds well to Elder flowers. Elder berries have similar properties to the flowers with the addition of their usefulness in rheumatism.

Combinations: For colds and fevers it may be used with *Peppermint, Yarrow* or *Hyssop.* For influenza combine it with *Boneset.* For catarrhal states mix it with *Golden Rod* and *Wild Indigo.*

Preparation and dosage: Infusion: pour a cup of boiling water onto 2 teaspoonsful of the dried or fresh blossoms and leave to infuse for 10 minutes. This should be drunk hot three times a day. Juice: boil fresh berries in water for 2 – 3 minutes, then express the juice. To preserve, bring the juice to the boil with 1 part honey to 10 parts of juice. Take 1 glass diluted with hot water twice a day. Ointment: take 3 parts of fresh Elder leaves and heat them with 6 parts of melted vaseline until the leaves are crisp. Strain and store.

PEPPERMINT   *Mentha piperita*
Part used: Aerial parts.
Collection: The aerial parts are collected just before the flowers open.
Constituents: Up to 2 per cent volatile oil

containing menthol, menthone and jasmone; tannins, bitter principle.

Actions: Carminative, anti-spasmodic, aromatic, diaphoretic, anti-emetic, nervine, antiseptic, analgesic.

Indications: A well known herb that will inhibit mucous secretion temporarily because of its menthol component. It can be used widely wherever there is excess mucous being secreted, helping also with its antispasmodic and carminative actions. Peppermint is one of the best carminative agents available. It has a relaxing effect on the visceral muscles, anti-flatulent properties and stimulates bile and digestive juice secretion, all of which help to explain its value in relieving intestinal colic, flatulent dyspepsia and other associated conditions. The volatile oil acts as a mild anaesthetic to the stomach wall, which allays feelings of nausea and the desire to vomit. It helps to relieve the vomiting of pregnancy and travel sickness. Peppermint plays a role in the treatment of ulcerative colitis and Crohn's disease. The treatment of fevers and especially colds and influenza benefits from its use. As an inhalant it can be used as a temporary treatment of nasal catarrh. Where migraine headaches are associated with the digestion, this herb may be used. As a nervine it acts as a tonic, easing anxiety, tension, hysteria etc. In painful periods it relieves the pain and eases associated tension. Externally it may be used to relieve itching and inflammations.

Combinations: For nasal catarrh, colds and influenza it may be used with *Boneset, Elder flowers* and *Yarrow.*

Preparation and dosage: Infusion: pour a cup of boiling water onto a heaped teaspoonful of the dried herb and leave to infuse for 10 minutes. This may be drunk as often as desired.

Tincture: take 1 – 2 ml of the tincture three times a day.

Anti-catarrhals for Different Parts of the Body

It is not easy to separate this group of herbs into those most suited for different systems. Here is a list of remedies that have this as part of their broad actions. You will see that some are considered to be more appropriate for some systems than others: *Bearberry, Boneset, Cayenne, Coltsfoot, Cranesbill, Echinacea, Elder, Elecampane, Eyebright, Garlic, Golden Seal, Golden Rod, Hyssop, Iceland moss, Irish moss, Marshmallow, Mullein, Peppermint, Sage, Thyme, Wild Indigo, Yarrow.*

_____ ANTI-DEPRESSIVE _____

This is a term that is similar in use to Thymoleptic, and both tend to be synonous with Nervine tonics.

_____ ANTI-EMETIC _____

What is an Anti-emetic?

The anti-emetics can reduce a feeling of nausea and can help to relieve or to prevent vomiting.

How Anti-emetics Work

There are two distinct ways to reduce feelings of nausea and vomiting. First, the

Carminative and Stomachic herbs will settle the digestive processes of the stomach and the Hepatics will aid digestion and so reduce nausea. Secondly, herbs can help by reducing the vomiting reflex of the hindbrain. *Black Horehound* is the most important here.

Examples

As already pointed out, a number of different actions could reduce nausea and vomiting, so here we shall limit ourselves to the directly ANTI-EMETIC remedies. Here we will consider two of the main ANTI-EMETICS in some detail and then briefly review a range.

BLACK HOREHOUND   *Ballota nigra*
Part used: Dried aerial parts.
Collection: The herb should be gathered just as it begins to bloom in July.
Constituents: Flavonoids.
Actions: Anti-emetic, sedative, mild astringent, emmenagogue, expectorant.
Indications: Black Horehound – which should not be confused with *White Horehound* – is an excellent remedy for the settling of nausea and vomiting where the cause lies within the nervous system rather than in the stomach. It may be used with safety in motion sickness for example, where the nausea is triggered through the inner ear and the central nervous system. This herb will also be of value in helping the vomiting of pregnancy or nausea and vomiting due to nervousness. This remedy has a reputation as a normalizer of menstrual function and also as a mild expectorant.
Combinations: For the relief of nausea and vomiting it may be combined with *Meadowsweet* and *Chamomile*.
Preparation and dosage: Infusion: pour a cup of boiling water onto 1 – 2 teaspoonsful of the dried herb and leave to infuse for 10 – 15 minutes. This should be drunk three times a day or as needed.
Tincture: take 1 – 2 ml of the tincture three times a day.

BALM   *Melissa officinalis*
Part used: Dried aerial parts.
Collection: The leaves may be harvested two or three times a year between June and September. They are gathered by cutting off the young shoots when they are approximately 30 cm long. They should be dried in the shade at a temperature not above 35°C.
Constituents: Rich in essential oil containing citral, citronellol, geraniol and linalol; bitter principles; flavones; resin.
Actions: Carminative, anti-spasmodic, anti-depressive, diaphoretic, hypotensive.
Indications: This carminative herb relieves spasms in the digestive tract and settles the whole of the system. It may be used safely in nausea and vomiting due to stomach problems. Of course, the nature of the problem must be identified before treating symptoms. Balm is often used to ease flatulent dyspepsia. Because of its anti-depressive properties, it is primarily indicated where there is dyspepsia associated with anxiety or depression, as the gently sedative oils relieve tension and stress reactions, thus acting to lighten depression. Balm has a tonic effect on the heart and circulatory system causing mild vasodilation of the peripheral vessels, thus lowering blood pressure. It can be used in feverish conditions such as influenza.
Combinations: In digestive troubles it may be combined with *Hops, Chamomile* or *Meadowsweet*. For stress and tension it will combine with *Lavender* and *Lime blossom*.
Preparation and dosage: Infusion: pour a cup of boiling water onto 2 – 3 teaspoonsful of the dried herb and leave to infuse for 10 – 15 minutes. A cup of this tea should be drunk in the morning and the evening, or when needed.

Tincture: take 2 – 6 ml of the tincture three times a day.

A more extensive list on anti-emetic remedies would include many carmin- atives, bitters, and hepatics. Ones that specifically come to mind are: *Balm, Black Horehound, Cayenne, Cloves, Dill, Fennel, Lavender, Meadowsweet, Peach leaves, Ginger.*

ANTI-HAEMORRHAGIC

This is used synonymously with Astringent.

ANTI-INFLAMMATORY

What is an Anti-inflammatory?

The Anti-inflammatory herbs help the body to combat inflammations. Herbs mentioned under demulcents, emollients and vulneraries will often act in this way, especially when they are applied externally. Orthodox medicine places much emphasis on chemicals that work in an anti-inflammatory way to reduce symptoms and ease suffering in many diseases. This symptomatic alleviation is not the way herbal anti-inflammatories should be used, or in fact how they appear to work.

How Anti-inflammatories Work

From research done into this action it seems that herbs can reduce inflammation in a number of different ways. An important point, however, is that they rarely inhibit the natural inflammatory reaction as such, rather they support and encourage the cleansing work the body is doing. An inflammation is a normal and healthy body response to infection or problems of some sort. Through the local natural chemical changes, the heat produced and broader eliminative and immune system responses, the inflammatory reaction will often bring about the changes necessary to heal the focus of disease and restore health. The process is extremely complex chemically and localized inflammations are responded to and supported by the whole body. It is a mistake and even potentially dangerous to inhibit this response unless it is a life-threatening situation. There is no doubt that the introduction of the steroids as powerful anti-inflammatory drugs has saved lives, but it has also brought with it many side-effects and deeper degenerative problems in the body. We have become conditioned into seeing inflammations as something to suppress and smother, rather than work with and help. Herbal remedies offer us this possibility, but as in all health matters there is a balance to achieve. Here it is the need to know when an inflammation is one to encourage with herbs or one to suppress with drugs.

Herbal anti-inflammatories can be broadly placed in three groups according to the way they work. Within the complex of plant biochemistry which works on the human body as a whole, there have been identified specific constituents that have an anti-inflammatory effect. It cannot be over-emphasized that the action of any plant is always more than the action of any specific constituent chemical. Keeping this holistic perspective in mind let us look at the three groups:

1. A large range of plants contain natural aspirin-type chemicals called salicylates. Those with significant quantities have a marked effect, without the dangers to the stomach of aspirin itself. In fact *Meadowsweet*, rich in salicylates, can be used to staunch mild stomach haemorrhage even though the salicylates can cause such problems. The whole aspirin group of drugs were originally isolated from plant sources. Other plants rich in such constituents include *Willow Bark, Wintergreen, Birch,* many of the *Poplars* and *Black Haw.*

2. The steroids themselves were first isolated from plant material and some herbs contain safe-to-use steroidal compounds that will aid in reducing some kinds of inflammation. These include *Liquorice, Wild Yam* and *Ginseng.*

3. As is usual with herbal remedies there are many valuable anti-inflammatories that have no clear-cut chemical basis for their action. This in no way negates their value, rather it shows there is much more to health and well being than pharmaceutical chemistry! Of the many remedies in this group we can mention *Guaiacum, Bogbean, Devil's Claw, Marigold flowers, St John's Wort* and *Black Cohosh.* Many of the aromatic herbs with their wonderful essential oils have this action, one of the best being *German Chamomile.*

Many other 'officially' non-anti-inflammatory remedies or treatments may well have such an action. This is only to be expected from a holistic perspective as any toning or support of the body with herbal remedies will enable the whole body to function well. One of the ways this may be seen is in reduction of rheumatic inflammation when a stomach problem is treated. There is no direct relationship necessarily between the herbs for the stomach and the joints, but still a general improvement in health brings about a reduction in swelling and pain.

Examples

Of the many herbs that have this action, we shall look at three in some depth.

CHAMOMILE GERMAN
Matricaria chamomilla
Part used: The flowers.
Collection: The flowers should be gathered between May and August when they are not wet with dew or rain. They should be dried with care at not too high a temperature.
Constituents: Volatile oil which includes chamazulene and isadol; mucilage; coumarin; flavone glycosides.
Actions: Anti-spasmodic, carminative, anti-inflammatory, analgesic, antiseptic, vulnerary.
Indications: This is one of the best known and widely used of all herbal remedies. In Europe it is used as a tea that can be obtained in most restaurants. The apparently endless list of conditions it can help all fall into areas that the relaxing, carminative and anti-inflammatory actions can aid. The anti-inflammatory action is especially useful in the digestive system where an infused tea will have released much of the soothing oils ready for action on the lining of the gut. It has a specific value in diverticulitis as well as colon trouble in general. It is an excellent, gentle sedative, useful and safe for use with children. It will contribute its relaxing actions in any combination and is thus used in anxiety and insomnia. Indigestion and inflammations such as gastritis are often eased with Chamomile. Similarly, it can be

used as a mouthwash for inflammations of the mouth such as gingivitis and for bathing inflamed and sore eyes. As a gargle it will help sore throats. As an inhalation over a steam bath, it will speed recovery from nasal catarrh. Externally it will speed wound healing and reduce the swelling due to inflammation. As a carminative with relaxing properties it will ease flatulence and dyspeptic pain.

Preparation and dosage: Infusion: pour a cup of boiling water onto 2 teaspoonsful of the dried leaves and let it infuse for 5 – 10 minutes. For digestive problems, this tea should be drunk after meals. A stronger infusion should be used as a mouthwash for conditions such as gingivitis. Half a cup of flowers boiled in 2 litres of water make a steam bath. Cover your head with a towel and inhale the steam.

Tincture: take 2 – 4 ml of the tincture three times a day.

WILD YAM   *Dioscorea villosa*
Part used: Dried underground parts.
Collection: This tropical plant is uprooted in the autumn, most stocks coming from west Africa.
Constituents: Steroidal saponins including dioscine; phytosterols; alkaloids; tannin; much starch.
Actions: Anti-spasmodic, anti-inflammatory, anti-rheumatic, cholagogue.
Indications: At one time this herb was the sole source of the chemicals that were used as the raw materials for contraceptive hormone manufacture. In herbal medicine Wild Yam is a valuable herb that can be used to relieve intestinal colic and to soothe the pain and discomfort of various colon problems such as colitis and diverticulitis, ease painful period cramps and other ovarian and uterine pains. It is of great use in the treatment of rheumatoid arthritis, especially the acute phase where there is intense inflammation.
Combinations: To relieve intestinal colic it

may be combined with *Calamus, Chamomile* and *Ginger*. For rheumatoid arthritis it may be used with *Black Cohosh*. For period pains use with *Cramp Bark* and possibly *Valerian*.
Preparation and dosage: Decoction: put 1 – 2 teaspoonsful of the herb in a cup of water, bring to the boil and simmer gently for 10 – 15 minutes. This should be drunk three times a day.
Tincture: take 2 – 4 ml of the tincture three times a day.

WILLOW BARK   *Salix nigra*
Part used: Bark.
Collection: The bark is collected in the spring when new growth starts.
Constituents: Salicin, tannin.
Actions: Anti-inflammatory, anti-pyretic, analgesic, antiseptic, astringent.
Indications: Black Willow is a safe natural source of the aspirin-like salicylates which helps partially explain its reputation in the treatment of rheumatism and arthritis where there is much associated pain and inflammation. It should always be used as part of a deeper treatment for any connective tissue inflammation anywhere in the body, but it is especially useful in rheumatoid arthritis. It may also be used in fevers such as influenza.
Combinations: It may be used with *Black Cohosh, Celery seed, Guaiacum* and *Bogbean* in the treatment of rheumatoid arthritis.
Preparation and dosage: Decoction: pour a cup of water onto 1 – 2 teaspoonsful of the bark, bring to the boil and simmer for 10 minutes. This should be drunk three times a day.
Tincture: take 2 – 4 ml of the tincture three times a day.

Anti-inflammatories for Different Parts of the Body

Each system of the body has plants that are

particularly suited to it, some of which are anti-inflammatory. Here we shall see which remedies may act in this way for each system. How they can be used will be considered in the sections on each system.

Circulatory system: These herbs may be of use for reducing inflammation in blood vessels; *Lime, Hawthorn berries, Horse Chestnut leaves* and *Yarrow.*

Respiratory system: Strictly speaking there are few anti-inflammatory herbs for this system. However, the anti-septic and demulcent remedies will have such an effect.

Digestive system: These would include *Chamomile, Wild Yam, Liquorice, Golden Seal, Marigold, Peppermint* and *St John's Wort.*

Urinary system: The urinary demulcents and anti-septic remedies will have an anti-inflammatory action, as will those to help with stones. A specific kidney anti-inflammatory is *Golden Rod.*

Reproductive system: The tonics and other specific reproductive remedies will often act in this way. *Ladies Mantle* is a good example.

Muscles and skeleton: The salicylate-containing remedies come into their own here with *Willow Bark, Meadowsweet, White Poplar* and *Birch* being high on the list. Others to consider are *Bogbean, Devil's Claw, Black Cohosh, Feverfew* and *Wild Yam.*

Nervous system: The only true anti-inflammatory for the nerves is *St John's Wort.* However many of the nervines will help, such as *Oats* and *Valerian.*

Skin: There is an abundance of remedies to reduce inflammation on the skin. This is only to be expected if nature does provide us with what we need, considering all the nettles and brambles. Some of the remedies are *Marigold, St John's Wort, Myrrh, Golden Seal, Arnica, Chickweed, Woundwort* and *Plantain.*

ANTI-LITHIC

What is an Anti-lithic?

The anti-lithic herbs prevent the formation of stones or gravel in the urinary system and can help the body in the removal of those already formed. These remedies were far more necessary in past times when the diet was not as healthy and balanced as it is today.

How Anti-lithics Work

There is much discussion amongst herbalists and researchers as to whether these anti-lithics work by 'dissolving' stones or by helping the body to remove those capable of being passed by promoting urine flow and thus flushing of the kidneys and tubes. So yet again we are in the position of knowing a herb does a certain thing without knowing how. Let us not make the mistake of interpreting lack of evidence as meaning they don't work.

Examples

As is shown in the appropriate section, the anti-lithics should always be used with demulcents and possibly anti-microbial herbs such as *Corn Silk* and *Bearberry.* Details of three valuable anti-lithics are given below.

PELLITORY OF THE WALL
Parietaria diffusa
Part used: Aerial parts.

Collection: The parts above ground are collected between June and September.
Constituents: Bitter principle, tannin.
Actions: Diuretic, anti-lithic, demulcent.
Indications: Pellitory of the Wall may be used in the treatment of any inflammation of the urinary system and especially where soothing is needed. It can safely be used with benefit in cystitis and pyelitis. It is a good general diuretic which is used to relieve water retention where it is due to kidney-based causes. Pellitory of the Wall has its main use in the treatment of kidney stone or gravel.
Combinations: It combines well with *Parsley Piert, Buchu, Bearberry* or *Juniper.*
Preparation and dosage: Infusion: pour a cup of boiling water onto 1 teaspoonful of the herbs and infuse for 10 – 15 minutes. This should be drunk three times a day.
Tincture: take 2 – 4 ml of the tincture three times a day.

HYDRANGEA   *Hydrangea arborescens*
Part used: Dried roots and rhizome.
Collection: The roots should be unearthed in the autumn. Clean and slice while still fresh as they become very hard on drying.
Constituents: Glycosides, saponins, resins.
Actions: Diuretic, anti-lithic.
Indications: Hydrangea's greatest use is in the treatment of inflamed or enlarged prostate glands. It may also be used for urinary stones or gravel associated with infections such as cystitis.
Combinations: In kidney stones it is often combined with *Parsley Piert, Bearberry* and

Gravel Root. In prostate problems it combines well with *Horsetail.*
Preparation and dosage: Decoction: put 2 teaspoonsful of the root in a cup of water, bring to the boil and simmer for 10 – 15 minutes. This should be drunk three times a day.
Tincture: take 2 – 4 ml of the tincture three times a day.

PARSLEY PIERT   *Aphanes arvensis*
Part used: The aerial parts.
Collection: This rather small plant should be collected in the summer when in flower.
Constituents: Tannins.
Actions: Diuretic, anti-lithic, demulcent.
Indications: One of our most widely applicable remedies for conditions related to kidney stones or gravel. It will soothe any pain that occurs when passing water, although this symptom must be diagnosed properly. Water retention will be lessened by taking *Parsley Piert.* It is quite safe to take it freely.
Combinations: It will combine well with any of the above remedies.
Preparation and dosage: For an infusion pour a cup of boiling water onto 1 – 2 teaspoonsful of the dried herb and leave to infuse for 10 – 15 minutes. Drink this three times a day.
Tincture: 2 – 4 ml three times a day.
Other useful herbs in this group include *Bearberry, Buchu, Corn Silk, Couchgrass, Gravel Root, Sea Holly, Stone Root,* and *Wild Carrot.*

ANTI-MICROBIAL

What is an Anti-microbial?

The anti-microbial herbs can help the body to destroy or resist pathogenic micro-organisms. In all forms of natural medicine it would be a mistake to talk about remedies being 'anti-biotic' as this literally means anti-life. With herbal remedies there is the possibility to help the body strengthen its own resistance to infective organisms and throw off the illness. While some of our plant remedies contain chemicals which are strongly anti-septic or specific poisons to certain organisms, in general we are talking about herbs that aid the natural immune processes.

Many of the plants with this action are also anti-inflammatory and could be divided into those that are anti-bacterial, anti-fungal, anti-viral, anti-parasitic etc. This has to be seen as an attribute of the general action of the herb which in most cases will be to augment the integrity of the individual's own defence system. There will be times when the use of anti-biotic drugs is essential and life saving; however, this is not as often as we have become accustomed to. The body can benefit from supportive and preventative help that bypasses the need for chemical intervention in an emergency. However, when an emergency arises, let us be thankful for the existence of the anti-biotics.

How Anti-microbials Work

Some research work has been done on these anti-microbial remedies and in such cases an 'active ingredient' has occasionally been found. An example is the German research into the excellent remedy *Echinacea* where a chemical with anti-bacterial properties has been discovered. It is called Echinacein. There is also a volatile oil that is anti-staphylococcal, an amide of the echinacein that is insecticidal, others that are anti-fungal and a depside that attacks bacteria. It also has action against viruses, apparently by inhibiting an enzyme used by viruses to break down cell walls.

This impressive list of actions has been researched from one herb. All too often the lack of research is interpreted as a lack of value: a great mistake!

Other ways in which herbs can work to remove infection is by direct or indirect stimulation of the body's own immune system. *Myrrh* is an example of this. Herbs rich in volatile oils are often directly effective by killing the micro-organism. Examples would be *Garlic, Thyme* and *Eucalyptus.*

Examples

Here we shall look at three of the main anti-microbial herbs in some detail and then briefly review a range.

ECHINACEA   *Echinacea angustifolia*
Part used: Cone flower.
Collection: The roots should be unearthed in the autumn. It is suggested that the fresh extract is more effective than the dried root.
Constituents: Volatile   oil,   glycoside, echinaceine, depside, phenolics.
Actions: Anti-microbial, alterative.
Indications: Echinacea   is   the   prime remedy to help the body rid itself of microbial infections. It is effective against both bacterial and viral attacks, not so much by killing these organisms but by supporting the body's own immunity. It may be used in conditions such as boils, septicaemia and other infections of that sort. In conjunction with other herbs it may be used for any infection anywhere in the body. For example, in combination with *Yarrow* or *Bearberry* it will effectively stop cystitis. It is especially useful for infections of the upper respiratory tract such as laryngitis, tonsillitis, and for catarrhal conditions of the nose and sinus. In general it can be used widely and safely. The tincture or decoction may be used as a mouthwash in the treatment of pyorrhoea and gingivitis. As an external lotion it will speed the healing of septic sores and cuts.
Combinations: This useful herb may be combined with many different plants.
Preparation and dosage: Decoction: put

1 - 2 teaspoonsful of the root in one cup of water and bring it slowly to the boil. Let it simmer for 10 - 15 minutes. This should be drunk three times a day.

Tincture: take 1 - 4 ml of the tincture three times a day.

WILD INDIGO   *Baptisia tinctoria*

Part used: Root.

Collection: The root is unearthed in the autumn after flowering has stopped. Clean the root and cut, dry well.

Constituents: Alkaloids, glycosides, oleo-resin.

Actions: Anti-microbial, anti-catarrhal, febrifuge.

Indications: Wild Indigo is a herb to be considered wherever there is a focus of infection. This is another remedy that supports and stimulates the body's own immune response to infection. It is especially useful in the treatment of infections and catarrh in the ear, nose and throat. It may be used for laryngitis, tonsillitis, pharyngitis and catarrhal infections of the nose and sinus. Taken both internally and as a mouthwash it will heal mouth ulcers, gingivitis and help in the control of pyorrhoea.Used internally it may be helpful in the treatment of enlarged and inflamed lymph glands and also to reduce fevers. Externally an ointment will help infected ulcers and ease sore nipples. A douche of the decoction will help leucorrhoea.

Combinations: For the treatment of infections it may be used with *Echinacea* and *Myrrh*. For lymphatic problems it can be combined with *Cleavers* and *Poke Root*.

Preparation and dosage: Decoction: put ½ - 1 teaspoonful of the root in a cup of water, bring to the boil and simmer for 10 - 15 minutes. This should be drunk three times a day.

Tincture: take 1 - 2 ml of the tincture three times a day.

MYRRH   *Commiphora molmol*

Part used: Gum resin.

Collection: The gum resin is collected from the bushes that secrete it in the arid regions of East Africa and Arabia.

Constituents: Up to 17 per cent essential oil, up to 40 per cent resin, gums.

Actions: Anti-microbial, astringent, carminative, anti-catarrhal, expectorant, vulnerary.

Indications: Myrrh is an effective anti-microbial agent that works in two complementary ways. Primarily it stimulates the production of white blood corpuscles (with their anti-pathogenic actions) and secondarily it has a direct anti-microbial effect. In this way it will aid and support the natural process of defence and immunity. This is a vital job as so much treatment today is done through the use of antibiotic drugs that do the work for the body. At times this is essential, but not to the degree to which we have become accustomed. Myrrh may be used in a wide range of conditions where an anti-microbial agent is needed. It finds specific use in the treatment of infections in the mouth such as mouth ulcers, gingivitis, pyorrhoea, as well as the catarrhal problems of pharyngitis and sinusitis. It may also help with laryngitis and respiratory complaints. Systematically it is of value in the treatment of boils and similar conditions as well as glandular fever and brucellosis. It is often used as part of an approach to the treatment of the common cold. Externally it will be healing and antiseptic for wounds and abrasions.

Combinations: It will combine well with *Echinacea* for infections and as a mouthwash for ulcers and similar problems. For external use it should be combined with distilled *Witch Hazel*.

Preparation and dosage: Infusion: as the resin dissolves in water only with difficulty, it should be powdered well to make an infusion. Pour a cup of boiling water onto 1 - 2 teaspoonsful of the powder and leave to infuse for 10 – 15 minutes. This should be drunk three times a day.

Tincture: as the resin dissolves much easier in alcohol, the tincture is preferable and easily obtainable. Take 1 – 4 ml of the tincture three times a day.

Anti-microbials for Different Parts of the Body

Each system of the body has plants that are particularly suited to it, some of which are anti-microbial. Here we shall see which remedies may be best suited for each of these systems. By the nature of infection and the body's response to it, a general systemic treatment is always appropriate even if done in conjunction with specific local remedies. How they can be used will be considered in the sections on each system.

A partial list of anti-microbial remedies could include:

Aniseed, Balsam of Peru, Bearberry, Caraway Oil, Cayenne, Clove, Coriander, Echinacea, Elecampane, Eucalyptus, Garlic, Gentian, Juniper, Marigold, Marjoram, Myrrh, Olive, Peppermint, Plantain, Rosemary, Rue, Sage, Southernwood, Thyme, Wild Indigo, Wormwood.

Circulatory system: Garlic is always appropriate here because of its value for the circulatory system in general.

Respiratory system: In addition to the main remedies mentioned, i.e. *Echinacea, Wild Indigo* and *Myrrh,* we can add *Aniseed, Balsam of Peru, Clove, Elecampane* and *Thyme.*

Digestive system: Many of the aromatic remedies and some digestive bitters have an anti-microbial effect in the gut. Ones to consider are *Echinacea, Garlic, Gentian, Sage, Marigold, Myrrh* amongst others.

Urinary system: Some of the urinary antiseptic remedies can be too strong if there is any suggestion of kidney disease. Effective remedies are *Bearberry, Juniper berries, Eucalyptus, Yarrow, Echinacea.*

Reproductive system: Here you could use *Echinacea, Garlic, Southernwood, Nasturtium* amongst others.

Muscles and skeleton: The three main oils will help internally and externally.

Nervous system: St John's Wort or *Pasque Flower* in combination with nervines and other anti-microbials can help.

Skin: There are many anti-septic herbs that can be used on the skin. A wash of *Thyme, Rosemary, Marjoram* or *Garlic* can be most effective. *Myrrh* is one of the strongest external remedies. Skin infections must be treated in a broader way however, as is described in the section on the skin in Chapter 6.

ANTI-PARASITIC

Often used as a synonym for Anthelmintic.

ANTI-PYRETIC

A synonym for Febrifuge.

ANTI-SPASMODIC

What is an Anti-spasmodic?

The anti-spasmodics can prevent or ease spasms or cramps in the muscles of the body. They will reduce tension in the body, and, as many of the anti-spasmodics are also nervines, they will sometimes ease psychological tension as well. Many of the herbal remedies that are described as nervines, sedatives or hypnotics also act as anti-spasmodics. The term is synonymous with spasmolytic.

How Anti-spasmodics Work

There are general anti-spasmodics that reduce muscle spasming throughout the body, and there are those that specifically work on certain organs or systems. When this action is needed in the gut, the carminative herbs will often do exceedingly well.

Examples

Nature is rich in herbs that have an anti-spasmodic action on the body. Here we shall look at two of the main herbs in this group in some detail and then briefly review a range.

CRAMP BARK   *Viburnum opulus*
Part used: Dried bark.
Collection: The bark is collected in April and May, cut into pieces and dried.
Constituents: A bitter called viburnin, valerianic acid, salicosides, resin, tannin.
Actions: Anti-spasmodic, sedative, astringent.
Indications: Cramp Bark shows by its name the richly deserved reputation it has

as a relaxer of muscular tension and spasm. It has two main areas of use – first, in muscular cramps and, secondly, in ovarian and uterine muscle problems. Cramp Bark will relax the uterus and so relieve painful cramps associated with periods (dys-menorrhoea). In a similar way it may be used to protect from threatened miscarriage. Because of its astringency it will also help in the treatment of excessive blood loss in periods and especially bleeding associated with the menopause.
Combinations: For the relief of cramp it may be combined with *Prickly Ash* and *Wild Yam*. For uterine and ovarian pains or threatened miscarriage it may be used with *Black Haw* and *Valerian*.
Preparation and dosage: Decoction: put 2 teaspoonsful of the dried bark into a cup of water and bring to the boil. Simmer gently for 10 – 15 minutes. This should be drunk hot three times a day.
Tincture: take 4 – 8 ml of the tincture three times a day.

BLACK HAW   *Viburnum prunifolium*
Part used: Dried bark of root or stem.
Collection: . The bark from the roots and the trunk is collected in the autumn. The shrubs should be dug out and the bark stripped from roots and trunk. The bark from branches should be collected in spring and summer. In both cases the bark should be dried in the shade.
Constituents: Triterpenoids, coumarins, bitter principle, valerianic acid, salicosides, tannin.
Actions: Anti-spasmodic, sedative, hypotensive, astringent.
Indications: Black Haw has a very similar use to *Cramp Bark*, to which it is closely related. It is a powerful relaxant of the

uterus and is used for dysmenorrhoea (uterine cramps) and false labour pains. It may prove useful in threatened miscarriage as well. Its relaxant and sedative actions explain its power in reducing blood pressure, which happens through a relaxation of the peripheral blood vessels. It has been used as an anti-spasmodic in the treatment of asthma.

Combinations: For threatened miscarriage it will combine well with _False Unicorn Root_ and _Cramp Bark._ Other combinations would be similar to those of _Cramp Bark._

Preparation and dosage: Decoction: put 2 teaspoonsful of the dried bark in a cup of water, bring to the boil and simmer for 10 minutes. This should be drunk three times a day.

Tincture: take 5 – 10 ml of the tincture three times a day.

Anti-spasmodics for Different Parts of the Body

Each system of the body has plants that are particularly suited to it, some of which are anti-spasmodic. Here we shall detail which plants are uniquely suited as anti-spasmodics for each system. There is a lot of overlap, as muscle is very similar everywhere! The way they should be used is described in the appropriate section in Chapter 6.

Circulatory system: Mistletoe, Motherwort, Cramp Bark, Black Cohosh, Balm, Lavender, Ladies Slipper and Valerian are important here.

Respiratory system: A range of anti-spasmodics are useful for the respiratory system and include Wild Lettuce, Wild Cherry, Lobelia, Grindelia, Pill Bearing Spurge, Elecampane, Thyme, Aniseed, Angelica Root, Oregano and Garlic.

Digestive System: All the carminative remedies will tend to act in this way in the gut, and hepatics can have such an action in gallbladder problems. Specific herbs to consider are Chamomile, Cramp Bark, Valerian, Hops, Peppermint, Sage, Thyme, Dill, Fennel, Barberry, Sweet Woodruff and Wild Yam.

Urinary system: Here we can think of Cramp Bark, Black Haw, Madder, Sea Holly and Wild Carrot.

Reproductive system: Here Cramp Bark and Black Haw come into their own. In addition the nervine anti-spasmodics such as Pasque Flower, Valerian, Ladies Slipper and Skullcap can help.

Muscles and skeleton: The main muscle relaxant remedies include Cramp Bark, Black Haw, Valerian and Skullcap. Externally Lobelia can be most helpful.

Nervous system: Consult the section on nervines for more information.

Skin: Anti-spasmodics are not directly relevant here.

APERIENT

What is an Aperient?

It is a mild and gentle form of laxative. Aperients work in such a way that only the natural bowel movements and functions are promoted. In this way treatment of constipation can avoid any of the griping pains that often accompanies stronger remedies.

How Aperients Work

There appear to be two ways in which aperients do their work. First, by acting as bulk laxatives for the bowel – dietary fibre is the best source of such bulk. The bulk seeds of herbs such as _Psyllium_ and _Linseed_ can help. Mucilaginous material such as _Agar-Agar_ or the other seaweed gums can also be used. They provide bulk by absorbing water through osmosis and so increase in volume.

The other way aperients work is by a gentle stimulating action on the digestive process. This occurs primarily through the liver, but also through other parts of the whole digestive system.

Examples

Many herbal remedies will have a gentle action on the eliminative processes of the body. It is this very action that makes them so potentially valuable in dealing with deep seated problems.

RHUBARB ROOT   _Rheum palmatum_
Part used: Rhizome of _Rheum palmatum_ and other species, not the garden rhubarb.
Collection: This root is collected in China and Turkey.
Constituents: Anthraquinones, tannins, bitter aromatic principle.
Actions: Bitter stomachic, mild purgative, astringent.
Indications: Rhubarb root has a purgative action for use in the treatment of constipation, but also has an astringent effect following this. It therefore has a truly cleansing action upon the gut, removing debris and then astringing with antiseptic properties as well.
Note: Rhubarb root may colour the urine yellow or red.
Combinations: It should be combined with carminative herbs to relieve any griping that may occur.
Preparation and dosage: Decoction: put ½ – 1 teaspoonful of the root in a cup of water, bring to the boil and simmer gently for 10 minutes. This should be drunk morning and evening.

Tincture: take 1 – 2 ml of the tincture three times a day.

YELLOW DOCK   _Rumex crispus_
Part used: Root.
Collection: The roots should be unearthed in late summer and autumn, between August and October. Clean well and split lengthways before drying.
Constituents: Anthraquinone glycosides, tannins.
Actions: Alterative, purgative, cholagogue.
Indications: Yellow Dock is used extensively in the treatment of chronic skin complaints such as psoriasis. The anthraquinones present have a markedly cathartic action on the bowel, but in this herb they act in a mild way, possibly tempered by the tannin content. Thus it makes a valuable remedy for constipation, working as it does in a much wider way than simply stimulating the gut muscles. It promotes the flow of bile and has that somewhat obscure action of being a 'blood cleanser'. The action on the gall-bladder gives it a role in the treatment of jaundice when this is due to congestion.
Combinations: It will combine well with _Dandelion Root, Burdock_ and _Cleavers._
Preparation and dosage: Decoction: put 1 – 2 teaspoonsful of the root in a cup of water, bring to the boil and simmer gently for 10 – 15 minutes. This should be drunk three times a day.
Tincture: take 1 – 4 ml of the tincture three times a day.

Aperients for Different Parts of the Body

By the very nature of this action it will work only on the bowels. The secondary actions may suggest wider uses, for example with _Yellow Dock_. The real value of this action is that it helps cleanse the body and so has a role in broader treatments of many systems and conditions.

AROMATIC

What is an Aromatic?

The aromatic herbs have a strong and often pleasant odour. This oil-based aroma can stimulate the digestive system. They are often used to add a pleasant aroma and taste to other medicines. The oils are the basis of aromatherapy.

They have much in common with the carminative remedies, so their mode of action is described there.

Examples

Nature is rich in herbs that are aromatic. The smell of newly-mown hay, to the wonderful and uplifting smells of an English garden, can all be described as herbal aromaticity.

Many aromatic herbs are included in other actions with this as a secondary action. It is best to study each of the aromatic and carminative herbs to discover their different uses, using the general structure given for other herbs. We shall look at *Aniseed* as an example and note its wide range of uses.

ANISEED   *Pimpinella anisum*
Part used: Dried fruit.
Collection: The ripe dry fruits should be gathered between July and September.
Constituents: Up to 6 per cent volatile oils which include anethole, 30 per cent fatty oils, choline.
Actions: Expectorant, anti-spasmodic, carminative, parasiticide, aromatic.

Indications: It is the volatile oil in Aniseed that provides the basis for its internal use to ease griping pains, intestinal colic and flatulence. It also has useful expectorant and anti-spasmodic actions which make it useful in bronchitis and where there is persistent irritable coughing, and in whooping cough. Externally, the oil may be used in an ointment base for the treatment of scabies. The oil by itself will help in the control and eradication of lice. It is the oil that provides the unique flavour of aniseed and gives it its power in flavouring unpleasant remedies.

Combinations: For flatulent colic and indigestion mix Aniseed with equal amounts of *Fennel* and *Caraway*. For bronchitis it combines well with *Coltsfoot, White Horehound* and *Lobelia*.

Preparation and dosage: Infusion: the seeds should be gently crushed just before use to release the volatile oils. Pour one cup of boiling water over 1 – 2 teaspoonsful of the seeds and let it stand covered for 5 – 10 minutes. Take one cup three times daily. To treat flatulence, the tea should be drunk slowly before meals.

Oil: one drop of the oil may be taken internally by mixing it into half a teaspoonful of honey.

Of the other aromatics the following should be mentioned: *Angelica, Balm, Basil, Caraway, Cardamon, Celery, Chamomile, Cinnamon, Cloves, Coriander, Dill, Fennel, Hyssop, Ginger, Meadowsweet, Peppermint, Rosemary, Sage, Valerian,* and *Wood Betony*.

ASTRINGENT

What is an Astringent?

If you have ever had a stewed cup of ordinary tea then you have experienced astringency! The tightening of the tissue of the mouth is the astringent action of the tea plant at work. Astringents are remedies that contain constituents that have a binding action on mucous membranes, skin and other exposed tissue. Astringents are sometimes called styptics when used to stop external bleeding or anti-haemorrhagics for internal bleeding.

How Astringents Work

This is usually due to a group of complex chemicals called tannins. They get their name from the use they were put to in the tanning industry. They have the effect of precipitating, or curdling, protein molecules. This is how animal skin is turned to leather, and what happens with the stewed tea. In other words they produce a sort of leather coat on the surface of the tissue in question. This brings about a number of therapeutic benefits:

- A reduction of irritation on the surface of tissues due to a form of numbing,
- A reduction in surface inflammation,
- A barrier against infection is created which is of great help in wounds and burns.

Astringents have a role in a wide range of problems in many parts of the body, but are of great import in wound healing and conditions of the digestive system. In the gut they reduce inflammation and inhibit diarrhoea and are widely used in the various diseases of digestion. Long-term use as medicine or too much tea in the diet can be deleterious to health as there may be an eventual inhibition of proper food absorption across the gut wall.

Examples

Nature is rich in herbs that have an astringent action. Here we shall look at

three of the main ones in some detail and then briefly review a range. Astringent herbs range from the strong such as *Oak Bark* and *Bistort* to much gentler ones such as *Comfrey* and *Periwinkle*. Part of the skill of the herbalist is to know which to use where and when. This skill cannot truly be learnt via books but through experience – a long job!

AGRIMONY   *Agrimonia eupatoria*
Part used: Dried aerial parts.
Collection: The whole of the plant above ground should be collected when the flowers are just blooming. It should be dried in the shade and not above 40° C.
Constituents: Tannins, glycosidal bitters, nicotinic acid, silicic acid, iron, vitamins B and K, essential oil.
Actions: Astringent, tonic, diuretic, vulnerary, cholagogue.
Indications: The combinations of astringency and of bitter tonic properties makes Agrimony a valuable remedy, particularly when an astringent action on the digestive system is needed, as its tonic action is due to the bitter stimulation of digestive and liver secretions. It is a specific in diarrhoea in children and is often useful in colon trouble such as mucous colitis. Agrimony is the herb of choice in appendicitis. It may be used quite freely in indigestion. There is a long tradition of its use as a spring tonic where the bitter digestive stimulation will wake the system up. It may be used in urinary incontinence and cystitis. As a gargle it will relieve sore throats and laryngitis. As an ointment it will aid the healing of wounds and bruises.
Combinations: It is often used with carminatives for digestive problems.
Preparation and dosage: Infusion: pour a cup of boiling water onto 1 – 2 teaspoonsful of the dried herb and leave to infuse for 10 – 15 minutes. This should be drunk three times a day.

Tincture: take 1 – 3 ml of the tincture three times a day.

OAK BARK   *Quercus robur*
Part used: The bark.
Collection: The young bark is carefully pared from the trunk or from branches which are not more than 10 cm thick. Take care to take off only patches, never a whole ring around the trunk, which would kill the tree. The bark is collected in April or May. It must be smooth and free from blemishes.
Constituents: Up to 20 per cent tannin, gallic acid, ellagitannin.
Actions: Astringent, anti-inflammatory, antiseptic.
Indications: Oak Bark may be used wherever an effective astringent is called for. Examples would be diarrhoea, dysentery or haemorrhoids. As a gargle, the decoction can be used in tonsillitis, pharyngitis and laryngitis. It can be used as an enema for the treatment of haemorrhoids and as a douche for leucorrhoea. It is primarily indicated for use in acute diarrhoea, taken in frequent small doses.
Combinations: It is often given with *Ginger* before meals. The addition of *Ginger* adds a carminative action that helps if there is digestive trouble present.
Preparation and dosage: Decoction: put 1 teaspoonful of the bark in a cup of water, bring to the boil and simmer gently for 10 – 15 minutes. This can be drunk three times a day.
Tincture: take 1 – 2 ml of the tincture three times a day.

CRANESBILL, AMERICAN
                    Geranium maculatum
Part used: The rhizome.
Collection: The rhizome is unearthed in September and October, cut into pieces and dried.
Actions: Astringent, anti-haemorrhagic, anti-inflammatory, vulnerary.

Indications: American Cranesbill is an effective, gentle and widely applicable astringent. When bleeding accompanies duodenal or gastric ulceration, this remedy is used in combination with other healing and demulcent herbs. Where blood is lost in the faeces, this herb will help, though careful diagnosis is vital. It is of great use where excessive blood loss occurs during menstruation or a uterine haemorrhage occurs. Of course, skilled gynaecological aid should be called for. As a douche it can be used in leucorrhoea.
Combinations: In peptic ulcers it may be used with *Meadowsweet, Comfrey, Marshmallow* or *Agrimony.* In gynaecological problems it should be combined with uterine tonics and possible other astringents such as *Periwinkle.* In leucorrhoea it can be combined with *Beth Root.*
Preparation and dosage: Decoction: put 1 – 2 teaspoonsful of the rhizome in a cup of cold water and bring to the boil. Let simmer for 10 – 15 minutes. This should be drunk three times a day.
Tincture: take 2 – 4 ml of the tincture three times a day.

Astringents for Different Parts of the Body

Each system of the body has plants that are particularly suited to it, some of which are astringents. Here we shall see which remedies act in this way for each of these systems. How they can be used will be considered in the sections of each system in Chapter 6.
Circulatory system: Astringents are rarely needed internally for this system, although they are used externally for bruises etc. as seen under skin. However, certain cardiovascular remedies are also astringents: *Yarrow, Broom* and *Melilot.*

Respiratory system: The anti-catarrhal remedies can have an apparent astringent action. *Yarrow, Sheppard's Purse, Mouse-ear, Golden Seal, Eyebright* and *Plantain.*

Digestive system: These are just some of the possible herbs: *Oak, Catechu, Bistort, Tormentil, Witch Hazel, Cranesbill, Comfrey, Meadowsweet, Agrimony, Golden Seal, Sheppard's Purse* and *Sage.*

Urinary system: Many of the astringents already mentioned are useful here but specifics are *Horsetail, Couchgrass* and *Yarrow.*

Reproductive system: Here we can mention *Cranesbill, Periwinkle, Ladies Mantle, Golden Seal* and *Beth Root.*

Muscles and skeleton: Astringency is not often relevant in this system.

Nervous system: The same goes for the nervous system.

Skin: Of the many external astringents, or styptics, we can mention *Oak, Witch Hazel, Horsetail, Plantain, Sheppard's Purse, Wood Avens, Yarrow, Arnica* and just about all the astringents mentioned above.

BITTER

What is a Bitter?

These are the 'proof' of nasty tasting medicine being good for you!. The Bitters are herbs that have a predominantly bitter taste. They can range from quite mildly bitter remedies such as *Yarrow* and *Dandelion leaf,* to the profoundly distasteful such as *Rue* and *Wormwood.* It is, of course, because of the taste of these last two plants that they are used in the Bible and still are in our language as symbols of extreme distress and woe. I don't think they taste quite that bad!

It is becoming increasingly apparent that these remedies have a major role in holistic herbal treatment and especially herbal preventative medicine. Because of their wide effect on the body's physiology they help enormously in treating the body as an integrated whole.

How Bitters Work

Much research has gone into this question, revealing some answers but, as usual, raising many more questions! In most herbal bitters, there is a chemical present that is called a 'bitter principle'. This is often a volatile oil, an alkaloid or sesquiterpene. In this case they appear to work in a similar way by triggering a sensory response in the mouth. The sensation of bitterness, and no doubt many subtleties of which we are consciously unaware, is directed by the nerves to the central nervous system. From here a message goes to the gut giving rise to the digestive hormone gastrin. This leads to a whole range of ramifications, all of value to the digestive process and general bodily health:

(i)   there will be a stimulation of the appetite, this will help in convalescence and problems where there is a reduction in appetite. This could range from convalescence to depression. Of course, a stimulation of appetite is not always desirable!

(ii)   there is a general stimulation of the flow of digestive juices from the pancreas, duodenum and liver. This will aid a great range of problems that have their basis in inefficient or allergy distorted digestion.

(iii) the bitters also aid the liver in its detoxification work and increase the flow of bile. The possibilities here are great as many health problems have their roots in an over-worked liver. This is the apparent value of such after-food bitters as coffee and liqueurs like Chartreuse.

(iv) there is a regulatory effect upon the secretion by the pancreas of the hormones that regulate blood sugar, insulin and glucagon. This leads to the need for diabetics to take care when taking bitters for any reason as they may upset their blood sugar balance. On the other hand, in the hands of a skilled practitioner there is some relevance for the use of such remedies in the treatment of late-onset diabetes.

(v) The bitters help the gut wall repair damage through stimulating the self-repair mechanisms.

All of this from a nasty taste in the mouth! Much of these benefits do not occur if the bitter herb is given in a capsule to remove the taste. A pity, but the body knows best here. There is much apparent overlap in practice between the bitters and tonic remedies. The mechanism of action is not always clear, but it is evident that these herbs act to promote health and increase self-healing and resistance in an individual – yet another wonderful gift of nature.

Examples

With Nature being so abundant in herbal bitters, we have many to choose from to describe. Here we shall look at three of the main strong bitters in some detail. You will notice from the review of bitters in Chapter 6 that many of the remedies described elsewhere have a bitter action as well.

WORMWOOD   _Artemisia absinthum_
Part used: Leaves or flowering tops.

Collection: The leaves and flowering tops are gathered at the end of the flowering period between July and September.

Constituents: Rich in essential oils including absinthol, thujol, isovaleric acid; bitter sesquiterpenes; flavonoid glycosides.

Actions: Bitter tonic, carminative, anthelmintic, anti-inflammatory.

Indications: Wormwood has been used in a wide range of conditions, most of which have been vindicated by analysis of the herb. The apparent 'cure-all' nature of this herb can largely be explained in the fundamental impact that its bitter action has on the body. This is explained above. It is primarily used as a bitter and therefore has the effect of stimulating and envigorating the whole of the digestive process. It is often used where there is indigestion. Indigestion is a word that covers many different things and recurrent symptoms need skilled diagnosis. It is an especially powerful remedy in the treatment of worm infestations, particularly roundworm and pinworm. It may also be used to help the body deal with fever and infections. Due to the general tonic action it will be of benefit in many diverse conditions because it benefits the body in general.

Preparation and dosage: Infusion: pour a cup of boiling water onto 1 – 2 teaspoonsful of the dried herb and leave to infuse for 10 – 15 minutes. This should be drunk three times a day.

Pill: the powdered herb may be used to get rid of worms in the form of pills, thus avoiding the extreme bitter taste.

Tincture: take 1 – 4 ml of the tincture three times a day.

RUE   _Ruta graveolens_
Part used: Dried aerial parts.
Collection: The herb should be collected before the flowers open in the summer, and dried in the shade.

Constituents: Essential oil, rutin, furano-coumarins, alkaloids, tannins.

Actions: Anti-spasmodic, emmenagogue, anti-tussive, aborifacient.

Indications: Rue is a herb with an ancient history. The genus name 'Ruta' comes from the Greek work 'reuo', to set free, showing its reputation as a freer from disease. Its main use is the regulation of menstrual periods, where it is used to bring on suppressed menses. The oil of rue is a powerful and potentially dangerous aborti-facient, therefore the plant is best avoided during pregnancy. The other area of usage is due to the plant's anti-spasmodic action. It may be used to relax smooth muscles, especially in the digestive system where it will ease griping and bowel tension. The easing of spasm gives it a role in the stopping of spasmodic coughs. It also in-creases peripheral circulation and lowers elevated blood pressure. If the fresh leaf is chewed, it will help to relieve tension head-aches, ease palpitations and other anxiety problems.

CAUTION: *Avoid during pregnancy*

Combinations: For the use in the regula-tion of periods it will combine well with *False Unicorn Root* and *Life Root*.

Preparation and dosage: Infusion: pour a cup of boiling water onto 1 – 2 teaspoonsful of the dried herb and leave to infuse for 10 – 15 minutes. This should be drunk three times a day.

Tincture: take 1 – 4 ml of the tincture three times a day.

GENTIAN ROOT   *Gentiana lutea*

Part used: The dried rhizome and root.

Collection: The underground parts are dug up in the autumn, sliced and dried slowly. It is during the drying process that the odour, colour and taste develop.

Constituents: Bitter principles, including gentiopicrin and amarogentine; pectin; tannin; mucilage; sugar.

Actions: Bitter, gastric stimulant, siala-gogue, cholagogue.

Indications: Gentian is a wonderful bitter which, as with all bitters, stimulates the appetite and digestion via a general stimula-tion of the digestive juices. Thus it pro-motes production of saliva, gastric juices and bile. It also accelerates the emptying of the stomach. It is indicated wherever there is a lack of appetite and sluggishness of the digestive system. It may thus be used where the symptoms of sluggish digestion appear, these being dyspepsia and flatulence. Through the stimulation of the digestion it has a generally fortifying effect.

Combinations: Gentian is often used with other digestives such as *Ginger* and *Cardamon*.

Preparation and dosage: Decoction: Put ½ teaspoonful of the shredded root in a cup of water and boil for 5 minutes. This should be drunk warm about 15 – 30 minutes before meals, or at any time when acute stomach pains result from a feeling of fullness.

Tincture: Take 1 – 4 ml of the tincture three times a day according to the above guide-lines.

Bitters for Different Parts of the Body

Each system of the body has plants that are particularly suited to it, some of which are bitters. By the nature of 'bitterness', they are widely applicable in a tonic sense, but also equally limited.

Circulatory system: Anything that helps the digestion and reduced wind will take pressure off the heart. The relaxing bitters such as *Hops* and *Valerian,* may have a specific role.

Respiratory system: Certain bitters have expectorant actions as well. In the case of *White Horehound* we have an excellent remedy for all chest problems combined with the value of a potent bitter.

Digestive system: A wide range of plants can be listed here, remembering that the liver and pancreas are included as organs of the digestive system: _Gentian, Wormwood, Rue, Greater Celandine, Barberry, Balmony, Boldo, Golden Seal, Centaury, Chicory, Hops, Mugwort, Blessed Thistle._

Urinary system: The bitters are not directly involved here.

Reproductive system: Many of the bitter remedies have the power of initiating delayed periods. They may, however, cause some cramping and must not be used during pregnancy. The following are the most relevant: _Southernwood, Wormwood,_ _Mugwort, Rue,_ and to a lesser degree because of its mild bitterness, _Yarrow._

Muscles and skeleton: Anything that aids digestion and assimilation of food will be of benefit to the musculoskeletal system. There are two gentle bitters that are very useful in this system: _Bogbean_ and _Willow Bark._

Nervous system: Through the stimulation of healthy body processes, bitters can aid the nervous system in depression and general nervous debility. Any can do it, but those most often used are _Gentian, Wormwood_ and _Mugwort._

Skin: The skin will benefit from bitter herbs by an alterative-type cleansing of the system.

CARDIAC TONIC

What is a Cardiac Tonic?

This is a general term for herbal remedies that have a beneficial action on the heart. Some of the remedies in this group are powerful cardio-active agents such as _Foxglove,_ while others are gentler and safer, such as _Hawthorn_ and _Motherwort._ As the treatment of heart problems is for skilled hands, we shall discuss these remedies in a broad way only. Qualified herbalists need to be consulted if herbal medication is desired for heart treatments. However, this in no way belittles the great good that can be done by the use of _appropriate_ self-help, whether it be herbal remedies, exercise or change of lifestyle.

How Cardiac Tonics Work

The strong and effective cardio-active remedies owe their power to the presence of the cardiac glycoside group of plant consti-tuents. These have the effect of increasing the efficiency of the muscles of the heart _without_ increasing their need for oxygen. This enables the heart to pump enough blood around the body and ensure there is not a build-up of fluid in the lungs or extremities. That sounds wonderful, as indeed it is, but there is always the possibility of accruing too much of the glycosides in the body as the removal rates tend to be low. This is the main drawback of _Foxglove_ and why it is potentially poisonous, unless used with skill and knowledge. Herbalists these days use _Lily of the Valley_ in preference to _Foxglove_ as there is less chance of such problems developing. This is explored in more depth in the section on the Circulatory system in Chapter 6. Other plants that contain cardiac glycosides include _Broom, Squills_ and _Figwort._

Another group of remedies have an observably beneficial action on heart and blood vessels but how they work is either completely obscure or an area of great pharmacological debate. These remedies are herbs such as *Hawthorn, Lime* and *Motherwort.*

Examples

Here we shall look at three examples of the cardiac tonics, but for a more detailed review of herbs and the circulatory system, please refer to Chapter 6.

LILY OF THE VALLEY
Convallaria majalis

Part used: Dried leaves.

Collection: The leaves are gathered at the time of flowering in May and June.

Constituents: Cardiac glycosides including convallatoxin and convallatoxol; saponins including convallarin and convallaric acid; asparagin; flavonoids; essential oil with farnesol.

Actions: Cardio-active, diuretic.

Indications: Lily of the Valley is perhaps the most valuable heart remedy that the medicinal herbalist uses today. This herb has an activity equivalent to *Foxglove,* but without many of its potentially toxic effects. Lily of the Valley may be used in the treatment of heart failure and water retention (dropsy) where this is associated with the heart. It will aid the body where there is difficulty with breathing due to congestive conditions of the heart.

Combinations: It combines well with *Motherwort* and *Hawthorn.*

Preparation and dosage: Lily of the Valley should be used only under qualified supervision.

HAWTHORN BERRIES
Crataegus oxyacanthoides

Part used: The ripe fruits.

Collection: The berries are collected in September and October.

Constituents: Saponins, glycosides, flavonoids, acids including ascorbic acid, tannin.

Actions: Cardiac tonic, hypotensive.

Indications: This remedy provides us with one of the best tonic remedies for the whole of the heart and circulatory system. They act in a normalizing way upon the heart by either stimulating or depressing its activity depending upon the need. In other words, Hawthorn Berries will help the heart return to normal functioning in a gentle way. As a long-term treatment they may safely be used in heart failure or weakness. They can similarly be used in cases of palpitations. As a tonic for the circulatory system they find an important use in the treatment of high blood pressure, arteriosclerosis and angina pectoris. While they can be very effective in the aiding of these conditions, qualified attention is essential. They will play a role in any treatment of vessel problems including varicose veins or even varicose ulcers.

Combinations: For the treatment of high blood pressure and the circulatory system they can be combined beneficially with *Lime Blossom, Mistletoe,* and *Yarrow.*

Preparation and dosage: Infusion: pour a cup of boiling water onto 2 teaspoonsful of the berries and leave to infuse for 20 minutes. This should be drunk three times a day over a long period.

Tincture: take 2 – 4 ml of the tincture three times a day.

MOTHERWORT
Leonurus cardiaca

Part used: Aerial parts.

Collection: The stalks should be gathered at the time of flowering, which is between June and September.

Constituents: Bitter glycosides including leonurin and leonuridine; alkaloids including leonuinine and stachydrene; volatile oil; tannin.

Actions: Sedative, emmenagogue, antispasmodic, cardiac tonic.

Indications: The very names of this valuable remedy give a guide to its range of uses. 'Motherwort' shows its relevance to menstrual and uterine conditions while 'cardiaca' indicates its use in heart and circulation treatments. It is valuable in the stimulation of delayed or suppressed menstruation, especially where there is anxiety or tension involved. It is a useful relaxing tonic for aiding in menopausal changes. It may be used to ease false labour pains. It is an excellent tonic for the heart, strengthening without being straining. It is a specific for over-rapid heart beat, or palpitations, especially where it is brought about by anxiety and other such causes. It may be used in all heart conditions that are associated with anxiety and tension.

Preparation and dosage: Infusion: pour a cup of boiling water onto 1 – 2 teaspoonsful of the dried herb and leave to infuse for 10 – 15 minutes. This should be drunk three times a day.

Tincture: take 1 – 4 ml of the tincture three times a day.

Cardiac Tonics for Different Parts of the Body

By the very nature of such a specific action, it is not usually directly relevant to all the body systems. Many of the cardiac tonics will have other actions on the body, however, and it is this range we shall explore here.

Circulatory system: The primarily cardioactive remedies include *Lily of the Valley, Foxglove, Broom, Squill, Figwort* and *Bugleweed,* while the more tonic remedies include *Hawthorn, Motherwort, Rosemary, Balm, Yarrow* and *Mistletoe.* There are remedies that specifically benefit the vessels of the circulatory system and these include *Hawthorn, Lime Blossom, Horse Chestnut, Garlic* and *Yarrow.*

Respiratory system: Any problem with the action of the heart might have an effect on lung congestion via a 'backlog' of blood waiting to be pumped. So the cardiac tonics may benefit the lungs by helping the heart rather than directly helping the chest itself. *Garlic* is renowned for its anti-microbial and generally beneficial action on the lungs, and *Angelica* is another gentle cardiac tonic that will help lung problems.

Digestive system: A number of the 'heart' herbs will aid digestion or support the system in a number of different ways. These include *Rosemary, Lime, Motherwort, Yarrow, Garlic, Angelica* and *Balm.*

Urinary system: Most of the herbs that have a direct impact in aiding the heart's action will increase the amount of blood passing through the kidney and so act as diuretics. *Yarrow* is a herb that is used in urinary problems, as is *Broom.* Thus their cardiac tonic action must be taken into account, especially with *Broom.*

Reproductive system: The cardiac tonics are not directly involved in the functioning of this system. *Yarrow* may play a dual role here, but only very slightly.

Muscles and skeleton: Herbs that act as circulatory stimulants and in this way act on the whole system, play an important role in the musculoskeletal system by increasing peripheral blood flow. This may reduce swelling and ease stiffness. Such herbs include *Cayenne, Ginger, Prickly Ash, Mustard* and *Horse Radish.*

Nervous system: *Motherwort, Lime Blossom, Balm* and *Rosemary* all have a relaxing effect on the nervous system. As we shall see, many nervines help the circulatory system by relaxing the mind and body as a whole.

Skin: The only directly applicable remedy here is *Figwort.* However, where the skin problem is due to varicosity in veins, then cardiac tonics are very important, for example, *Hawthorn, Horse Chestnut, Yarrow* and *Lime Blossom.*

CARMINATIVE

What is a Carminative?

Carminatives are herbal remedies that are rich in volatile oils. Through their activity the digestive system is stimulated to work properly and with ease. The main action is to soothe and settle the gut wall, thereby easing griping pains and helping the removal of gas from the digestive tract. Many of the aromatic herbal remedies have a carminative effect on the body.

How Carminatives Work

To a large extent, the mode of action of the carminative herbs is the result of the complex of oils they contain. These oils and their activity are discussed in the section on plant constituents.

Examples

Nature is rich in herbs that have a carminative action on the digestive system. Here we shall look in some detail at three of the main herbs with this action and then briefly review a range.

Many of the herbs described as having other primary actions are also carminatives. For example, *Peppermint* and *Aniseed* are described under different actions. It is a dilemma for me to try to structure a way through the wealth of herbal knowledge without creating artificial divides.

FENNEL   *Foeniculum vulgare*
Part used: The seeds.
Collection: The seeds should be harvested when ripe and split in the autumn. The brown umbel should be cut off. Comb the seeds to clean them. Dry slightly in the shade.

Constituents: Up to 6 per cent volatile oil which includes anethole and fenchone; fatty oil 10 per cent.
Actions: Carminative, aromatic, anti-spasmodic, stimulant, galactogogue, rubefacient, expectorant.
Indications: Fennel is a good stomach and intestinal remedy which relieves flatulence and colic while also stimulating the digestion and appetite. It is similar to *Aniseed* in its calming effect on bronchitis and coughs. It may be used to flavour cough remedies. Fennel will increase the flow of milk in nursing mothers. Externally the oil eases muscular and rheumatic pains. The infusion may be used to treat conjunctivitis and inflammation of the eyelids as a compress.
Preparation and dosage: Infusion: pour a cup of boiling water onto 1 – 2 teaspoonsful of slightly crushed seeds and leave to infuse for 10 minutes. This should be drunk three times a day. To ease flatulence, take a cup half an hour before meals.
Tincture: Take 2 – 4 ml of the tincture three times a day.

GINGER   *Zingiber officinale*
Part used: The rootstock.
Collection: The rootstock is dug up when the leaves have dried. The remains of the stem and root fibres should be removed. Wash throughly and dry in the sun.
Constituents: Rich in volatile oil which includes zingiberene, zingiberole, phellandrene, borneol, cineole, citral, starch, mucilage, resin.
Actions: Stimulant, carminative, rubefacient, diaphoretic.
Indications: Ginger may be used as a stimulant of the peripheral circulation in

cases of bad circulation, chilblains and cramp. In feverish conditions, Ginger acts as a useful diaphoretic, promoting perspiration. As a carminative it promotes gastric secretion and is used in dyspepsia, flatulence and colic. As a gargle it may be effective in the relief of sore throats. Externally it is the base of many fibrositis and muscle sprain treatments.

Preparation and dosage: Infusion: pour a cup of boiling water onto 1 teaspoonful of the fresh root and let it infuse for 5 minutes. Drink whenever needed.

Decoction: if you are using the dried root in powdered or finely chopped form, make a decoction by putting 1½ teaspoonsful to a cup of water. Bring it to the boil and simmer for 5 – 10 minutes. This can be drunk whenever needed.

Tincture: the tincture comes in two forms, Weak Tincture BP which should be taken in a dose of 1.5 – 3 ml three times a day and the Strong Tincture BP which should be taken in a dose of 0.25 – 0.5 ml three times a day.

CARAWAY   _Carum carvi_

Part used: Seeds.

Collection: The flowering heads (umbels) are collected in July and left to ripen. The seeds are then easily collected as they can be shaken off.

Constituents: Up to 6 per cent volatile oil including carvone and limonene; fatty oil and tannin.

Actions: Carminative, anti-spasmodic, expectorant, emmenagogue, galactagogue, astringent, aromatic.

Indications: Caraway is used as a calming herb to ease flatulent dyspepsia and intestinal colic, especially in children. It will stimulate the appetite. Its astringency will help in the treatment of diarrhoea as well as in laryngitis as a gargle. It can be used in bronchitis and bronchial asthma. Its anti-spasmodic actions help in the relief of period pains. It has been used to increase milk flow in nursing mothers.

Combinations: For flatulence and colic Caraway combines well with _Chamomile_ and _Calamus,_ in diarrhoea with _Agrimony_ and _Bayberry_ and in bronchitis with _White Horehound._

Preparation and dosage: Infusion: pour a cup of boiling water onto 1 teaspoonful of freshly crushed seeds and leave to infuse for 10 – 15 minutes. This should be drunk three times a day.

Tincture: take 1 – 4 ml of the tincture three times a day.

Carminatives for Different Parts of the Body

By the nature of this action, it works on the gut and so has a more generalized effect on other systems of the body. As the action owes much of its efficacy to the volatile oil component, it should be remembered that some of these oils have quite specific effects themselves.

Circulatory system: Carminatives may ease apparent cardiac symptoms through removing the pressure of flatulence and digestive pain. This is only an apparent effect, however, as most of the carminatives have no action on this system at all. The following herbs do have an effect through their oils on the cardiovascular system: _Balm, Chamomile, Garlic, Motherwort,_ and _Ginger._

Respiratory system: Many of these herbs will help this system through an anti-microbial, anti-spasmodic or anti- catarrhal effect. These include _Peppermint, Aniseed, Angelica, Eucalyptus, Garlic, Mustard, Sage_ and _Thyme._

Digestive system: The list here could be extremely large. This is a small selection; _Aniseed, Caraway, Cardamon, Cinnamon,_

Chamomile, Dill, Fennel, Ginger, Juniper, Mustard, Parsley, Peppermint, Sage, Thyme, Valerian, Wormwood.

Urinary system: Because of the oils, some of the carminatives can be irritating to the kidney and have the effect of removing water from the body (diuresis). Prime examples are *Juniper* and *Eucalyptus.*

Reproductive system: Again some of the oils can have an effect upon the female reproductive system. The most important one is *Pennyroyal.* This is explored in more depth in the section on the reproductive system.

Muscles and skeleton: *Celery Seed* is a carminative that is also specifically anti-inflammatory for this system. Others include *Angelica* and *Wintergreen.*

Nervous system: Many volatile oil-containing remedies will soothe the nervous system. These include *Valerian, Hops, Ladies Slipper, Chamomile* and *Balm.*

Skin: Carminatives may be relevant to the skin by helping the digestion and so help body metabolism in general. In some cases the herb is good for the skin because of other effects of the plant or its oils. Such herbs are *Thyme* and *Sassafras.*

CHOLAGOGUE

What is a Cholagogue?

This is an action that has the specific effect of stimulating the flow of bile from the liver. In orthodox pharmacology there is a differentiation between 'direct cholagogues' which actually increase the amount of secreted bile, and 'indirect cholagogues' which simply increase the amount of bile being released by the gallbladder. This differentiation is not very important in holistic herbal practice, especially as we are not going to use purified ox bile!

How Cholagogues Work

Most of the remedies that have the action of bitter or hepatic are also cholagogues so please consult these sections as well. A whole range of plant constituents will have this action on the liver tissue, but without it being forced or damaging. The secretion of bile is of great help to the whole digestive and assimilative process, and as we are what we eat – we are what we digest. The role of bile is partially that of facilitating fat

digestion but also of being a natural laxative, and thus cleansing to the system. Without exploring the vast complexities of liver function, it is worth noting that bile formation and flow are fundamental to it all. Thus these herbs have a much deeper value than 'simply' the release of bile, they help ensure a strong and healthy liver and so enliven the whole being.

Examples

Out of the many possible examples we shall pick three, but please also consider bitters and hepatics as well as the others mentioned below.

BALMONY   *Chelone glabra*
Part used: Dried aerial parts.
Collection: The aerial parts are collected and dried during the flowering period between July and September.
Actions: Cholagogue, anti-emetic, stimulant, laxative.
Indications: Balmony is one of the herbs that has entered British usage from the North American Indians. It has a long and deserved reputation as a curative remedy

for liver and gallbladder problems. Balmony acts as a tonic on the whole digestive and absorptive system. It has a stimulating effect on the secretion of digestive juices, and through this most natural way its laxative properties are produced. Balmony is used in gallstones, inflammation of the gallbladder and in jaundice. It stimulates the appetite, eases colic, dyspepsia and biliousness and is helpful in debility. Externally it has been used in inflamed breasts, painful ulcers and piles. It may be considered a specific in gallstones that lead to congestive jaundice.

Combinations: for the relief of constipation, Balmony may be combined with *Butternut.* For jaundice it will best be used with *Golden Seal,* and for gallbladder problems with *Fringe Tree Bark.*

Preparation and dosage: Infusion: pour a cup of boiling water onto 2 teaspoonsful of the dried herb and let infuse for 10 – 15 minutes. This should be drunk three times a day.

Tincture: take 1 – 2 ml of the tincture three times a day.

FRINGETREE   *Chionanthus virginicus*
Part used: The root bark.
Collection: The roots are unearthed in spring or autumn. Wash carefully and peel the bark. They should be dried with care.
Constituents: Phyllyrin, a lignin glycoside, saponins.
Actions: Hepatic, cholagogue, alterative, diuretic, tonic, anti-emetic, laxative.
Indications: Fringetree bark may be safely used in all liver and gallbladder problems, especially when they have developed into jaundice. It is a specific for the treatment of gallbladder inflammation and a valuable part of treating gallstones. It is a remedy that will aid the liver in general and as such it is often used as part of a wider treatment for the whole body. Through its action of

releasing bile it acts as a gentle and effective laxative.

Combinations: For the treatment of liver and gallbladder conditions it may be used with *Balmony, Wahoo* or *Wild Yam.*

Preparation and dosage: Infusion: pour a cup of boiling water onto 1 – 2 teaspoonsful of the bark and leave to infuse for 10 – 15 minutes. This should be drunk three times a day.

Tincture: take 1 – 2 ml of the tincture three times a day.

GOLDEN SEAL   *Hydrastis canadensis*
Part used: Root and rhizome.
Collection: Unearth root and rhizome from three-year-old plants in the autumn, after the ripening of the seeds. Clean carefully and dry slowly in the air.
Constituents: 5 per cent of the root consists of the alkaloids hydrastine, berberine and canadine; traces of essential oil; resin; fatty oil.
Actions: Tonic, astringent, anti-catarrhal, laxative, muscular stimulant, oxytocic, bitter.
Indications: Golden Seal is one of the most useful herbs in the materia medica. It owes most of its specific uses to the powerful tonic qualities shown towards the mucous membranes of the body. This is why it is of such help in all digestive problems, for example in gastritis, peptic ulceration and colitis. Its bitter stimulation gives it a role in loss of appetite, usually bringing it back. Via the alkaloids present it will stimulate bile production and secretion, bringing with it all the benefits that accrue. All catarrhal states benefit from Golden Seal, especially upper respiratory tract catarrh. The tonic and astringency contribute to its use in uterine conditions such as menorrhagia and haemorrhage. With the additional stimulation of involuntary muscles, it is an excellent aid during childbirth, but for just this reason it should be avoided during

pregnancy. Externally it is used for the treatment of eczema, ringworm, pruritis (itching), earache and conjunctivitis.

CAUTION: As Golden Seal stimulates the involuntary muscles of the uterus, it should be avoided during pregnancy.

Combinations: In stomach conditions it combines well with *Meadowsweet, Marsh-mallow Root* and *Chamomile.* In uterine haemorrhage it is best combined with *Peri-winkle* and *Beth Root.* Externally as a wash for irritation and itching it combines well with distilled *Witch Hazel.* As ear drops it may be combined with *Mullein.*

Preparation and dosage: Infusion: pour a cup of boiling water onto ½ – 1 teaspoons-ful of the powdered herb and leave to infuse for 10 – 15 minutes. This should be drunk three times a day.

Tincture: take 2 – 4 ml of the tincture three times a day.

Cholagogues for Different Parts of the Body

Each system of the body has plants that are particularly suited to it, some of which are cholagogues. However, by the nature of the action it works generally as a body tonic, through being quite specific in its action on the liver. How they can be used will be considered in the sections on each system.

Circulatory system: Their value in this system is through a general improvement of body functioning, not a direct impact. Only where a cholagogue has diuretic action as well can any direct claims be made.

Respiratory system: Certain herbs will be anti-microbial and anti-catarrhal which will benefit the whole system. Also tonics to mucous membranes will help, so we have herbs such as *Boneset, Golden Seal, Rosemary, Sage* and *Wild Indigo.*

Digestive system: Here we have a long list that includes *Artichoke, Balmony, Barberry, Black Root, Blue Flag, Boldo, Butternut, Dandelion Root, Fringetree Bark, Gentian, Greater Celandine, Wahoo, Wild Yam.*

Urinary system: There is only an indirect benefit to this system; however, *Dandelion Root,* although weaker than the leaves is still partially diuretic in action. *Boneset* can be a marked diuretic in feverish conditions.

Reproductive system: Cholagogic remedies such as *Golden Seal* and *Barberry* have a marked action on the muscles of the womb, as shown above. *Rosemary* has a tonic and emmenagogue action while most of the bitters that have been mentioned will stimulate the womb or menstrual activity.

Muscles and skeleton: These herbs help in this system by generally aiding the metabolic activity of the body.

Nervous system: The enlivening 'side-effect' of the cholagogues helping assimilation will help the nervous system. Debility and depression may be actively eased by such remedies. *Rosemary* is a nervine.

Skin: Taken internally these remedies will often aid in the cleansing of the body and so clear skin problems. Examples are *Blue Flag, Dandelion, Fumitory, Golden Seal, Mountain Grape, Yellow Dock, Golden Seal* will also be of use externally in some conditions.

DEMULCENT

What is a Demulcent?

A demulcent herb is rich in mucilage and can soothe and protect irritated or inflamed internal tissue. When they are used on the skin demulcents are called emollients.

How Demulcents Work

As with many other herbal action, the undoubted experience of what these demulcents do cannot always be explained pharmacologically. These herbs contain varying amounts of complex mucilage materials. These gummy, slimy chemicals have a clear and direct action on the lining of the intestines that soothes and reduces irritation by direct contact. However, as we shall see, there are some remedies that have a similar action far from the sight of absorption into the body. This means that they cannot have such a direct action on, say, the urinary system, because the mucilage will have been broken down into its constituent parts, thus losing its unique soothing action. There is no doubt that herbs can act as urinary demulcents or demulcents to the lungs.

Recent research in Germany has suggested that this may be due to some complex reflex response initiated in the gut. The mechanism proposed relates to embryonic development and the early developmental associations of tissues. The complexities are beyond the scope of this book, but it shows that the action of a plant can be subtle and complex.

In general all mucilage containing demulcents have the general properties of:

● Reducing irritation down the whole length of the bowel,
● Reducing the sensitivity of the digestive system to gastric acids (also to digestive bitters),
● Helping to prevent diarrhoea and reducing the digestive muscle spasms which cause colic,
● Easing coughing by a soothing of bronchial tension,
● Relaxing and easing painful spasm in the bladder and urinary system, and sometimes even in the uterus.

Examples
Nature is rich in herbs that have demulcent action on the body. Here we shall look at three of the main demulcent herbs in some detail and then briefly review a range.

COMFREY   *Symphytum officinale*
Part used: Root and rhizome, leaf.
Collection: The roots should be unearthed in the spring or autumn when the allantoin levels are the highest. Split the roots down the middle and dry in moderate temperatures of about 40 – 60° C.
Constituents: Mucilage, gum, allantoin, tannin, alkaloids, resin, volatile oil.
Actions: Vulnerary, demulcent, astringent, expectorant.
Indications: Comfrey is renowned for its impressive wound-healing properties. This is partially due to the presence of allantoin. This chemical stimulates cell proliferation and so augments wound-healing both inside and out. With its high percentage of mucilage as well, Comfrey becomes a powerful healing agent in gastric and duodenal ulcers, hiatus hernia and ulcerative colitis. Its astringency will help haemorrhages wherever they occur, internally or on the skin. In cases of bronchitis and irritable cough, it will soothe and reduce irritation while helping expectoration. Comfrey may be used externally to speed wound-healing and guard against scar tissue developing incorrectly. Care should be taken with very deep wounds, however, as the external application of Comfrey can lead to tissue forming over the wound before it is healed deeper down, possibly leading to abscesses. It may be used for any external ulcer, for wounds and fractures as a compress or poultice.
Combinations: In digestive inflammations and even ulceration, it combines well with

Marshmallow and *Meadowsweet.* For chest and bronchial troubles use it with *Coltsfoot, White Horehound* or *Elecampane.*

Preparation and dosage: Decoction: put 1 – 3 teaspoonsful of the dried herb in a cup of water, bring to the boil and let simmer for 10 – 15 minutes. This should be drunk three times a day. For external applications it can be used as an ointment, poultice or compress, the techniques for which are described elsewhere.

Tincture: take 2 – 4 ml of the tincture three times a day.

MARSHMALLOW   *Althaea officinalis*
Part used: Root and leaf.
Collection: The leaves should be collected in summer after flowering and the root unearthed in late autumn. It is cleaned of root fibres and cork and should be dried immediately.
Constituents: Root: 25 – 35 per cent mucilage; tannins; pectin; asparagine.
Leaf: mucilage; traces of an essential oil.
Actions: Root: demulcent, diuretic, emollient, vulnerary.
Leaf: Demulcent, expectorant, diuretic, emmollient.
Indications: This wonderful demulcent partially owes value to the high mucilage content. Marshmallow is a demulcent that can be used wherever soothing and healing properties are called for. The root is used mainly for digestive problems and on the skin, while the leaf is used for the lungs and the urinary system. This is not a strict differentiation but can be of therapeutic value. In all inflammations of the digestive tract, such as inflammations of the mouth, gastritis, peptic ulcer, enteritis and colitis, the root is strongly advised. For bronchitis, respiratory catarrh and irritating coughs Marshmallow leaf should be considered. In urethritis and urinary gravel, the leaf is very soothing. In fact this herb is very soothing for any mucous membrane irritations any-

where. Externally, the root is often used for varicose veins and ulcers as well as abscesses and boils.
Combinations: In ulcerative conditions, internal or external, it may be used with *Comfrey.* For bronchitis and other chest problems, it may be used with *Liquorice* and *White Horehound.* It is often mixed with *Slippery Elm* to make ointments.
Preparation and dosage: Decoction: the root should be made into a decoction by putting a teaspoonful of the chopped herb into a cup of water and boiling it gently for 10 – 15 minutes. This should be drunk three times a day.
Infusion: for an infusion of the leaf, pour boiling water onto 1 – 2 teaspoonsful of the dried leaf and let infuse for 10 minutes. This should be drunk three times a day also.
Compress: a compress or poultice can be valuably made from this herb.
Tincture: take 1 – 4 ml of the tincture three times a day.

SLIPPERY ELM BARK   *Ulmus fulva*
Part used: Inner bark.
Collection: The bark is stripped from the trunk and large branches in the spring. In commercial use this usually leads to the tree dying, as a large part of the bark is stripped. Ten-year-old bark is recommended.
Constituents: Mucilage, tannin.
Actions: Demulcent, emmolient, nutrient, astringent.
Indications: Slippery Elm Bark is a soothing nutritive demulcent which is perfectly suited for sensitive or inflamed mucous membrane linings in the digestive system. It can be used in gastritis, gastric or duodenal ulcer, enteritis, colitis and the like. It is often used as a food during convalescence as it is gentle and easily assimilated. In diarrhoea it will soothe and astringe at the same time. Externally it makes an excellent poultice for use in cases

of boils, abscesses or ulcers.

Combinations: For digestive problems it may be used with _Marshmallow._

Preparation and dosage: Decoction: use 1 part of the powdered bark to 8 parts of water. Mix the powder in a little water initially to ensure it will mix. Bring to the boil and simmer gently for 10 – 15 minutes. Drink half a cup three times a day.

Poultice: mix the coarse powdered bark with enough boiling water to make a paste.

Demulcents for Different Parts of the Body

Each system of the body has plants that are particularly suited to it, some of which are demulcents. Here we shall see which remedies act as demulcents for each of these systems. How they can be used will be considered in the sections on each system. _Circulatory system:_ The heart and circulation in general does not need demulcency as such. However, _Lime Blossom_ appears to have such an action on the blood vessels. _Respiratory system:_ Many plants will soothe inflamed tissue in the chest, throat and sinuses. These include _Elecampane, Comfrey, Mullein, Coltsfoot, Golden Rod, Marshmallow root, Liquorice, Lungwort. Digestive system:_ Of the many plants that could be used for the whole of the gut we should mention _Comfrey, Marshmallow, Iceland Moss, Irish Moss, Liquorice, Flaxseed_ and _Slippery Elm. Urinary system:_ Excellent kidney and bladder demulcents are _Corn Silk, Couch Grass_ and _Parsley Piert. Reproductive system:_ There are many tonic and anti-inflammatory remedies for this system but no real demulcents. _Muscles and skeleton:_ Vulneraries and anti-inflammatories have a more direct value in this system than demulcency as such. The undoubted value of _Comfrey_ here is due to its healing/vulnerary properties. _Nervous system:_ Demulcents are only of direct value in this system when applied to the skin as in shingles. The tonics that work on this system can be thought of as 'surrogate' demulcents, especially _Oats. Skin:_ The emollient herbs are all demulcent and include, _Comfrey, Marshmallow Root, Plantain, Slippery Elm, Chickweed, Flaxseed._

DEPURATIVE

This is a term that is used in the same sense as alterative.

DIAPHORETIC

What is a Diaphoretic?

This is an action that produces or promotes sweating. This has the value of helping the skin eliminate waste from the body. The skin is one of the major ways in which the body ensures a clean and harmonious inner environment. With diaphoretics we can help this vital function. Some of these remedies produce an actual observable sweat, while others just aid the sub-sensible sweating that goes on all the time. The diaphoretics have been used traditionally to increase sweating during fevers in the belief that this will help the body throw off the problem.

How Diaphoretics Work

Many of the diaphoretics are also remedies that will cause the dilation of the surface capillaries, thus helping poor circulation. It is thought that the stimulation of sweat glands occurs because the blood vessels in the area are dilated. This cannot explain all that is seen to occur but goes part of the way. The deeper value of these remedies comes from the way they can support the work of the kidney by increasing cleansing through the skin. Thus they have a role in a holistic treatment of kidney problems but also any broadly based approach to health.

Examples

Nature is rich in herbs that have a diaphoretic action. Many are also diuretics and others are the peripheral vasodilators described above. A good, strong curry is an example of the last group!

YARROW   *Achillea millefolium*
Part used: Aerial parts.
Collection: The whole of the plant above ground should be gathered when in flower between June and September.
Constituents: Up to 0.5 per cent volatile oil, flavonoids, tannins, a bitter alkaloid.
Actions: Diaphoretic, hypotensive, astringent, diuretic, antiseptic.
Indications: Yarrow is one of the best diaphoretic herbs and is a standard remedy for aiding the body to deal with fevers. It lowers blood pressure due to a dilation of the peripheral vessels. It stimulates the digestion and tones the blood vessels. As a urinary antiseptic it is indicated in infections such as cystitis. Used externally

it will aid in the healing of wounds. It is considered to be specific in thrombotic conditions associated with high blood pressure.
Combinations: For fevers it will combine well with *Elder Flower, Peppermint, Boneset* and with *Cayenne* and *Ginger*. For raised blood pressure it may be used with *Hawthorn, Lime Blossom* and *Mistletoe*.
Preparation and dosage: Infusion: pour a cup of boiling water onto 1 – 2 teaspoonsful of the dried herb and leave to infuse for 10 – 15 minutes. This should be drunk hot three times a day. When feverish it should be drunk hourly.
Tincture: take 2 – 4 ml of the tincture three times a day.

BONESET   *Eupatorium perfoliatum*
Part used: Dried aerial parts.
Collection: Boneset should be collected as soon as the flowers open in August or September.
Constituents: A bitter glycoside called eupatorin, volatile oil, gallic acid, a glucosidal tannin.
Actions: Diaphoretic, aperient, tonic, antispasmodic, relaxes mucous membranes.
Indications: Boneset is one of the best remedies for the relief of the associated symptoms that accompany influenza. It will speedily relieve the aches and pains as well as aid the body in dealing with any fever that is present. Boneset may also be used to help clear the upper respiratory tract of mucous congestion. Its mild aperient activity will help clear the body of any build-up of waste and ease constipation. It can safely be used in any fever and also as a general cleansing agent. It may provide symptomatic aid in the treatment of muscular rheumatism.
Combinations: In the treatment of influenza it may be combined with *Yarrow, Elder Flowers, Cayenne* or *Ginger*.
Preparation and dosage: Infusion: Pour a

cup of boiling water onto 1 – 2 teaspoonful of the dried herb and leave to infuse for 10 – 15 minutes. This should be drunk as hot as possible. During fevers or the flu it should be drunk every half hour.
Tincture: take 2 – 4 ml of the tincture three times a day.

CAYENNE   *Capsicum minimum*
Part used: The fruit.
Collection: The fruit should be harvested when fully ripe and dried in the shade.
Constituents: Capsaicin, carotenoids, flavonoids, essential oil, vitamin C.
Actions: Stimulant, diaphoretic, carminative, tonic, sialagogue, rubefacient, antiseptic.
Indications: Cayenne is the most useful of the stimulating diaphoretics. In American herbalism it is considered almost a cure-all, essential as part of most treatments. This may prove a bit too strong for gentler palates! Its potent diaphoretic qualities make it of wide applicability in most fevers, infections and general body cleansing. It regulates the blood flow, equalizing and strengthening the heart, arteries, capillaries and nerves. It is a general tonic and is specific for the circulatory and digestive system. It may be used in flatulent dyspepsia and colic. If there is insufficient peripheral circulation, leading to cold hands and feet and possibly chilblains, Cayenne can be invaluable. It is used for treating debility and for warding off colds. Externally it is used as a rubefacient in problems such as lumbago and rheumatic pains. As an ointment it helps *unbroken* chilblains, as long as it is used in moderation! As a gargle in laryngitis it combines well with *Myrrh.* This combination is also a good antiseptic wash.
Preparation and dosage: Infusion: pour a cup of boiling water onto ½ – 1 teaspoonful of Cayenne and leave to infuse for 10 minutes. A tablespoonful of this infusion should be mixed with hot water and drunk when needed.
Tincture: take 0.25 – 1 ml of the tincture three times a day or when needed.

Diaphoretics for Different Parts of the Body

Each system of the body has plants that are particularly suited to it, some of which are diaphoretics. Here we shall see which remedies act in this way for each of these systems. How they can be used will be considered in the sections on each system.
Circulatory system: Diaphoretics will often stimulate circulation in general, but examples of herbs that play a role in this system are *Cayenne, Garlic, Ginger, Lime Flowers, Yarrow.*
Respiratory system: Here we can mention *Angelica, Boneset, Elder Flower, Garlic, Ginger, Golden Rod, Peppermint, Pleurisy Root, Thyme, White Horehound.*
Digestive system: The list here could be very long, but selecting we can mention *Angelica, Bayberry, Cayenne, Chamomile, Fennel, Garlic, Ginger, Peppermint, Rosemary.*
Urinary system: The main ones would be *Buchu, Boneset, Gravel Root,* and *Yarrow.*
Reproductive system: Perhaps *Black Cohosh* is the most specific for this system, although all the general ones will help.
Muscles and skeleton: *Guaiacum* is most important as are *Cayenne, Boneset, Ginger* and *Prickly Ash.*
Nervous system: We can mention *Vervain, Chamomile* and *Lime Blossom.*
Skin: All the herbs mentioned will benefit the skin.

DIGESTIVE BITTER

This is a term that is synonymous with bitter.

DIURETIC

What is a Diuretic?

Strictly speaking a diuretic is a remedy that increases the secretion and elimination of urine from the body. In herbal medicine with its ancient traditions, a diuretic tends to mean a herb that has some sort of beneficial action on the urinary system. Thus not only do we mean diuretics as such, but can also include urinary demulcents and anti-inflammatory remedies. They have a vital role in any good treatment of illness as they will help the body eliminate waste and support the whole process of inner cleansing that is needed. Many of the diaphoretics act as diuretics when taken cold.

How Diuretics Work

If we limit ourselves to herbal diuretics in the strict sense of the word, there appears to be two broad groups, those that increase kidney blood flow and those that reduce the water reabsorption in the nephrons of the kidney.

- The first group includes not only diuretics such as *Broom* but all the herbs that are cardio-active and circulatory stimulants. These increase the blood flow in the kidney by effects on the heart or elsewhere in the body. Because there is more blood passing though the kidney, more urine is pro-duced. Caffeine-containing herbs such as *Tea* and *Coffee* also have this effect.

- The second group works via many different means, but they cause the diuresis because some of their constituents are excreted via the kidney. This may change the osmotic balance causing more water to be lost. This appears to be the case with *Dandelion Leaf, Couchgrass* and *Corn Silk*. Others work by irritating the reabsorption mechanism in some way, either through volatile oils, saponins or alkaloids. Herbs for the urinary system listed under Anti-lithic and Demulcents would fit here.

Examples

Nature is rich in diuretics. Many have been discussed under other sections. Important ones to be found elsewhere are *Dandelion Leaf, Corn Silk, Yarrow, Lily of the Valley, Hydrangea* and *Elder, Pellitory of the Wall, Parsley* and *Parsley Piert*. Here we shall look at another three examples.

The most effective diuretic is *Dandelion Leaf*.

BEARBERRY   *Arctostaphylos uva-ursi*
Part used: The leaves.
Collection: The evergreen leaves may be collected throughout the year, but preferably in spring and summer.
Constituents: Glycosides, including arbu-

tin and ericolin. 6 per cent tannin, flavonoids and resin.

Actions: Diuretic, astringent, antiseptic, demulcent.

Indications: This is a herbal diuretic that is still recognized by orthodox medicine, especially on the continent. Apart from its value in removing excess water from the body, Bearberry has a specific antiseptic and astringent effect upon the membranes of the urinary system. It will generally soothe, tone and strengthen them. Specifically it is used where there is gravel or ulceration in either the kidney or bladder. It may be used in the treatment of infections such as pyelitis and cystitis or as part of a holistic approach to more chronic kidney problems. It has a useful role to play in the treatment of gravel or a calculus in the kidney. With its high astringency it is used in some forms of bed wetting. As a douche it may be helpful in vaginal ulceration and infection.

Combinations: Bearberry may be combined with *Couch grass* and *Yarrow* and *Echinacea* for urinary infections. For kidney stones it combines well with *Parsley Piert* and *Pellitory of the Wall.*

Preparation and dosage: Infusion: pour a cup of boiling water onto 1 – 2 teaspoonsful of the dried leaves and let infuse for 10 – 15 minutes. This should be drunk three times a day.
Tincture: take 2 – 4 ml of the tincture three times a day.

COUCH GRASS   *Agropyron repens*
Part used: The rhizome.

Collection: The rhizome should be unearthed in spring or early autumn. Wash it carefully and dry in sun or shade.

Constituents: Triticin, mucilage, silicic acid, potassium, inositol, mannitol, glycoside, an anti-microbial substance.

Actions: Diuretic, demulcent, anti-microbial.

Indications: Couch grass may be used in urinary infections such as cystitis, urethritis and prostatitis. As a broadly applicable and safe diuretic it can be used in most conditions where this action is needed. Its demulcent properties soothe irritation and inflammation. It is of value in the treatment of enlarged prostate glands. It can also be used for easing or removing kidney stones and gravel. As a tonic diuretic, Couch grass has been used with other herbs in the treatment of rheumatism.

Combinations: For cystitis, urethritis and prostatitis it may be used with *Buchu, Bearberry* or *Yarrow.* It can be combined with *Hydrangea* for prostrate problems.

Preparation and dosage: Decoction: put 2 teaspoonsful of the cut rhizome in a cup of water, bring to the boil and let simmer for 10 minutes. This should be drunk three times a day.
Tincture: take 3 – 6 ml of the tincture three times a day.

BUCHU   *Agathosma betulina*
Part used: Leaves.

Collection: The leaves should be collected during the flowering and fruiting stage.

Constituents: Up to 2.5 per cent volatile oils which contain diosphenol, limonene and menthone.

Actions: Diuretic, urinary antiseptic.

Indications: Buchu may be used in any infection of the genito-urinary system, such as cystitis, urethritis and prostatitis. In water retention it can be used quite freely. Its healing and soothing properties indicate its use together with other relevant remedies in any condition of this system. It can be especially useful in painful and burning urination.

Combinations: In cystitis, it may be used with *Yarrow, Bearberry* or *Couchgrass,* in burning urination with *Marshmallow leaf* or *Corn Silk.*

Preparation and dosage: Infusion: pour a cup of boiling water onto 1 – 2 teaspoonsful of the leaves and let infuse for 10 minutes. This should be drunk three times a day.
Tincture: take 2 – 4 ml of the tincture three times a day.

Diuretics for Different Parts of the Body

Each system of the body has plants that are particularly suited to it, some of which are diuretics. Here we shall see which remedies act in this way for each of these systems. How they can be used will be considered in the sections on each system.
Circulatory system: As already pointed out, the cardio-active remedies have a diuretic effect because they increase blood flow through the kidneys. Remedies for this system include _Lily of the Valley, Broom, Dandelion_ and _Yarrow._ All the diuretics that help remove water from the body can be of benefit for the cardiovascular system. Care should be taken to ensure that the right ones are used in the specific condition being treated. _Broom_ should not be used in high blood pressure, for example.
Respiratory system: If chest congestion is occurring due to heart problems, then most of the diuretics will be of value. Remedies that have an affinity for this system include _Boneset, Cleavers, Elder, Yarrow_ and _Eucalyptus._
Digestive system: Some of the laxative herbs act as diuretics as well. Here we can mention _Agrimony, Blue Flag, Boldo, Borage, Celery Seed, Dandelion, Parsley, Pumpkin Seed._
Urinary system: All the remedies mentioned are applicable to this system with the addition of _Sea Holly_ and _Wild Carrot._
Reproductive system: The antiseptic diuretics often work in the same way on the reproductive system. Of especial relevance is _Bearberry, Saw palmetto_ is a mild diuretic.
Muscles and skeleton: Because of their cleansing action, many diuretics help in problems of muscles and bones. _Boneset, Celery Seed, Yarrow_ and _Gravel Root_ are but a few.
Nervous system: _Borage_ and _Bugleweed_ are the only real diuretics to benefit the nervous system directly. However, if there is much tension, using a nervine to relax may allow more urine to be passed.
Skin: All the diuretics potentially help the skin by an inner cleansing process. Especially important are _Cleavers, Couch grass_ and _Dandelion._

EMETIC

What is an Emetic?

Quite simply, these are herbs that cause vomiting. In the so-called 'heroic' age of medicine such an action was used a lot to empty the body, along with cathartic and purgative remedies. Thankfully health is not dependent on such drastic measures these days! The main use of emetics is the first aid treatment of poisoning, where they will empty the stomach content. Comprehensive First Aid kits will usually contain a small bottle of tincture of _Ipecacuanha_ for this purpose.

How Emetics Work

Most emetics work through irritation,

either of the stomach or the nervous system. Some of the expectorant remedies are emetics in high dose, and there is some relationship between the way they work. Please refer to that section (p.65).

Examples

We shall consider one emetic remedy in depth, but also consider *Lobelia, Snake root* and *Squill*. A local name for *Lobelia* in some parts of America is Puke Weed!

IPECACUANHA   *Cephaelis ipecacuanha*
Part used: Root and rhizome.
Collection: The root of this small South American shrub is gathered throughout the year, although the Indians collect it when it is in flower during January and February.
Constituents: Alkaloids including emetine and cephaeline; the glycosidal tannins ipecacuanhic acid and ipecacuanhin; ipecoside; starch; calcium oxalate.
Actions: Expectorant, emetic, sialagogue, anti-protozoal.
Indications: Ipecacuanha is mainly used as an expectorant in bronchitis and conditions such as whooping cough. At higher

doses it is a powerful emetic and as such is used in the treatment of poisoning. Care must be taken in the use of this herb. After an effective emetic dose has been given, large amounts of water should be taken as well. In the same way that ipecacuanha helps expectoration through stimulation of mucous secretion and then its removal, it stimulates the production of saliva. It has been found effective in the treatment of amoebic dysentery.
Combinations: In bronchial conditions Ipecacuanha combines well with *White Horehound, Coltsfoot* and *Grindelia*. In amoebic dysentery it may be used with *American Cranesbill* or *Echinacea*.
Preparation and dosage: Infusion: as this is a very powerful herb, only a small amount should be used. 0.01 – 0.25 grams of the herb are used for an infusion. Pour a cup of boiling water onto a small amount of the herb (equalling the size of a pea) and leave to infuse for 5 minutes. This can be drunk three times a day. If you need to use it as a powerful emetic, 1 – 2 grams should be used, which equals ¼ – ½ teaspoonful when used for an infusion.

EMMENAGOGUE

What is an Emmenagogue?

Strictly speaking these are remedies that stimulate menstrual flow and activity. In most herbals the term is used in the wider sense of a remedy that normalizes and tones the female reproductive system. This broad definition makes it almost meaning-

less. With herbal remedies there is a whole range of distinct treatments that can be used for the reproductive system either directly or indirectly.

Please refer to the section on remedies and actions for the reproductive system where emmenagogues, uterine tonics and hormonal normalizers are considered.

EMOLLIENT

What is an Emollient?

These are remedies that soften, soothe and protect the skin. They are used externally and have a similar role for the skin that demulcents have internally.

How Emollients Work

They usually act beneficially through a mucilage component, an oil or simply bulk. It is worth accepting the handed down wisdom of the ages here. We know which herbs are emollient; perhaps that is enough.

Examples

Nature is abundant in herbs that are emollient on the skin. Here we shall look at three of the commonest herbs in this group, although there are many excellent ones, as listed.

In addition to the examples given, the following should be considered: *Balm of Gilead, Borage, Coltsfoot, Comfrey, Fenugreek, Liquorice, Mallow, Marshmallow, Mullein, Slippery Elm.*

You will notice that most of these are demulcent herbs, and the examples given under that action could as easily been given here.

PLANTAIN, GREATER *Plantago major*
Part used: Leaves or aerial parts.
Collection: Gather during flowering throughout the summer. Dry as fast as possible as the leaves will discolour if dried improperly.
Constituents: Glycosides including aucubin, mucilage, chlorogenic acid and ursolic acid, silicic acid.
Actions: Expectorant, demulcent, astringent, diuretic.

Indications: Both the Greater Plantain and its close relative Ribwort Plantain have valuable healing properties. It acts as a gentle expectorant while also soothing inflamed and sore membranes, making it ideal for coughs and mild bronchitis. Its astringency aids in diarrhoea, haemorrhoids and also in cystitis where there is bleeding.
Preparation and dosage: Infusion: pour a cup of boiling water onto 2 teaspoonsful of the dried herb and leave to infuse for 10 minutes. This should be drunk three times a day.
Ointment: an ointment can be made that will aid the treatment of haemorrhoids and cuts.
Tincture: take 2 – 3 ml of the tincture three times a day.

FLAXSEED *Linum usitatissimum*
Part used: Ripe seeds.
Collection: The seed pods are gathered when fully ripe in September.
Collection: 30 – 40 per cent of fixed oil which includes linoleic, linolenic and oleic acids; mucilage; protein; the glycoside linamarin.
Actions: Demulcent, anti-tussive, laxative, emollient.
Indications: Flax may be used in all chest infections, especially in bronchitis with much catarrh formed. It is often used as a poultice in pleurisy and other pulmonary conditions. As a poultice it can be used for boils and carbuncles, shingles and psoriasis. As a purgative it relieves constipation.
Combinations: As a poultice for the chest it combines well with *Mustard.* For boils, swellings and inflammations it combines with *Marshmallow Root* and *Slippery Elm.*

Preparation and dosage: Infusion: pour a cup of boiling water onto 2 – 3 teaspoonsful of the dried herb and leave to infuse for 10 – 15 minutes. This should be drunk morning and evening

Poultice: For making a poultice see Chapter 8.

Tincture: take 2 – 6 ml of the tincture three times a day.

CHICKWEED   _Stellaria media_
Part used: Aerial parts.
Collection: This very common weed of gardens and fields can be collected all year round, although it is not abundant during the winter.
Constituents: Saponins.
Actions: Anti-rheumatic, vulnerary, emollient.

Indications: Chickweed finds its most common use as an external remedy for cuts, wounds and especially for itching and irritation. If eczema or psoriasis causes this sort of irritation, Chickweed may be used with benefit. Internally it has a reputation as a remedy for rheumatism.

Combinations: Chickweed makes an excellent ointment when combined with _Marshmallow._

Preparation and dosage: Infusion: pour a cup of boiling water onto 2 teaspoonsful of the dried herb and leave to infuse for 5 minutes. This should be drunk three times a day. For external use Chickweed may be made into an ointment or can be used as a poultice. To ease itching, a strong infusion of the fresh plant makes a useful addition to bath water.

EXPECTORANT

What is an Expectorant?

These are herbs that help the body to remove excess mucous from the lungs. However, the word is often used to mean a remedy that is a tonic for the respiratory system. Here we shall use the word in the strict sense.

How Expectorants Work

The working of expectorants has to be seen in the context of how remedies are used for the whole system. Please consult the section on the respiratory system. From what has been said there we can consider the stimulating expectorants and the relaxing expectorants. The first group works by chemically irritating the lining of the bronchioles to stimulate the expulsion of material. They are often also emetics in high dosage. They appear to work by way of a reflex action on the lining of the gut, related to the plant constituents called saponins. In this group we can mention _Balm of Gilead, Blood Root, Daisy, Elecampane, Ipecacuanha, Mouse-Ear, Violet_ and _White Horehound._

This is only a partial list of the stimulating expectorants all of which vary in strength and indications.

The relaxing expectorants would seem to act also by reflex but here it is to soothe bronchial spasm and loosen mucous secretions. This loosening is occasioned by producing a thinner mucous, lifting the stickier stuff up from below. This makes them useful in dry, irritating coughs. You will notice that this action is similar in some respects to the demulcents, and both actions owe a lot to their content of mucilage and occasionally volatile oils. We can mention from the large list: *Aniseed, Coltsfoot, Comfrey, Grindelia, Hyssop, Irish Moss, Liquorice, Lungwort, Marshmallow, Plantain, Skunk Cabbage* and *Sundew.*

A third group can be identified that can work in both ways and are especially valuable in any broader treatment of the lungs. Worthy of mention are *Elderflowers, Lovage, Mullein* and *Garlic.*

Examples

As you can see, Nature is rich in expectorants. Here we shall look at three of the main ones in some detail and then briefly review a range.

WHITE HOREHOUND *Marrubium vulgare*
Part used: Dried leaves and flowering tops.
Collection: White Horehound is gathered while the herb is blossoming between June and September. It is dried in the shade at a temperature not greater than 35° C.
Constituents: Sesquiterpene bitters including marrubin; essential oil; mucilage; tannins.
Actions: Stimulating expectorant, anti-spasmodic, bitter digestive, vulnerary.
Indications: White Horehound is a valuable plant in the treatment of bronchitis where there is a non-productive cough. It combines the action of relaxing the smooth muscles of the bronchioles while promoting mucous production and thus expectoration. It is used with benefit in the treatment of whooping cough. The bitter action stimulates the flow and secretion of bile from the gallbladder and thus aids digestion. White Horehound is used externally to promote the healing of wounds.
Combinations: It combines well with *Coltsfoot, Lobelia* and *Mullein.*
Preparation and dosage: Infusion: pour a cup of boiling water onto ½ – 1 teaspoonful of the dried herb and leave to infuse for

10 – 15 minutes. This should be drunk three times a day.
Tincture: take 1 – 2 ml of the tincture three times a day.

COLTSFOOT *Tussilago farfara*
Part used: Dried flowers and leaves.
Collection: The flowers should be gathered before they have fully bloomed (end of February to April) and dried carefully in the shade. The leaves are best collected between May and June. They should be chopped up before they are dried and stored. The fresh leaves can be used until autumn.
Constituents: Flowers: mucin; flavonoids rutin and carotene; taraxanthin; arnnidiol and faradiol; tannin, essential oil. Leaves: Mucin, abundant tannin; glycosidal bitter principle; inulin; sitosterol; zinc.
Actions: Relaxing expectorant, anti-tussive, demulcent, anti-catarrhal, diuretic.
Indications: Coltsfoot combines its famous soothing expectorant effect with an anti-spasmodic action. There are useful levels of zinc in the leaves. This mineral has been shown to have marked anti-inflammatory effects. Coltsfoot can be used in chronic or acute bronchitis, irritating coughs, whooping coughs and asthma. Its soothing expectorant action gives Coltsfoot a role in most respiratory conditions, including the chronic states of emphysema. When there is a chest infection involved it is most effective when used with an anti-microbial remedy. As a mild diuretic it has been used in cystitis. The fresh bruised leaves can be applied to boils, abscesses and suppurating ulcers.
Combinations: In the treatment of coughs it may be used with *White Horehound* and *Mullein.* For bronchitis use with *Garlic* or *Echinacea.*
Preparation and dosage: Infusion: pour a cup of boiling water onto 1 – 2 teaspoonsful of the dried flowers or leaves and let infuse

for 10 minutes. This should be drunk three times a day, as hot as possible.

Tincture: take 2 – 4 ml of the tincture three times a day.

MULLEIN   *Verbascum thapsus*
Part used: Dried leaves and flowers.
Collection: The leaves should be collected in mid summer before they turn brown. Dry them in the shade. The flowers should be gathered between July and September during dry weather. They should be dried in the shade or with artificial heat not higher than 40°C. The flowers turn brown in the presence of moisture and become ineffective.
Constituents: Mucilage   and   gum; saponins; volatile oil; flavonoids including hesperidin and verbascoside; glycosides including aucubin.
Actions: Expectorant, demulcent, mild diuretic, mild sedative, vulnerary.
Indications: Mullein is a very beneficial respiratory remedy useful in most conditions that effect this vital system. It is an ideal remedy for toning the mucous membranes of the respiratory system, reducing inflammation while stimulating fluid production and thus facilitating expectoration. Mullein can be thought of as one of the best toners and normalizers for the whole chest. It is considered a specific in bronchitis where there is a hard cough with soreness. Its anti-inflammatory and demulcent properties indicate its use in inflammation of the trachea and associated conditions. Externally an extract made in olive oil is excellent in soothing and healing any inflamed surface.
Combinations: In bronchitis it combines well with *White Horehound, Coltsfoot* and *Lobelia.*
Preparation and dosage: Infusion: pour a cup of boiling water onto 1 – 2 teaspoonsful of the dried leaves or flowers and let infuse for 10 – 15 minutes. This should be drunk

three times a day.
Tincture: take 1 – 4 ml of the tincture three times a day.

Expectorants for Different Parts of the Body

Each system of the body has plants that are particularly suited to it, some of which are also expectorants. Here we shall see which expectorants are uniquely applicable for each of these systems. How they can be used will be considered in the sections on each system.

Circulatory system: A congestive problem with the lungs can have a deleterious effect on the heart in time, so by stretching a point we could say that respiratory remedies may help the heart. There are three expectorants that have a direct cardio-vascular action: *Horse Chestnut, Squill* and *Daisy.*

Respiratory system: These are reviewed above.

Digestive system: All the stimulating expectorants may act as emetics if taken in too high a dose (*Ipecacuanha*), while the relaxing expectorants may be either demulcents (*Comfrey*) or carminatives (*Aniseed*). It is worth cross-referring often here.

Urinary system: Some of the expectorants will soothe the urinary system, a good example being *Corn Silk.* However, as they work to aid the excretion of waste from the body, in this case through the lungs, there may well be some effect upon kidney function by way of increasing body cleansing. This could happen with a herb that is 'not meant to be' a diuretic. Healing does not always follow rules that we know about!

Reproductive system: The herbs that are also anti-spasmodic will be helpful in menstrual cramps, for example *Lobelia,* although the alkaloid rich or saponin-containing emetics should be avoided during pregnancy. *Golden Seal,* which can work as an expectorant while helping the mucous membranes of the lungs, will also be of use for the reproductive tract.

Muscles and skeleton: The stimulating remedies can be used in liniments that increase circulation to the muscles and so ease aches and pains. Examples include *Balsam of Peru, Balsam of Tolu* and *Thyme. Lobelia* is a good muscle relaxant.

Nervous system: Cowslip, Vervain, Thyme and *Hyssop* can all have relaxing nervine actions.

Skin: By helping respiration and so the whole of the person's health, these remedies may aid the skin in a broad holistic way. Expectorants that can be used internally or externally for the skin as well include: *Balm of Gilead, Balsam of Tolu, Comfrey, Elder Flowers, Elecampane, Garlic, Golden Seal, Thuja.*

FEBRIFUGE

These are remedies that reduce fevers. The whole issue of treating fevers and the appropriate herbs is discussed in the section on Fevers in Chapter 6.

GALACTAGOGUE

What is a Galactagogue?

These are herbs that will increase the flow of milk in a lactating woman. They do this safely without forcing any hormonal pressure on the body. However they don't always work. There are so many factors involved in controlling the flow of breast milk; if something goes awry it may be difficult to correct herbally. A good wholesome diet, plus the right herbs, in the context of a loving and supportive relationship, will do as much as anything. It is essential for general health to be at its peak for the galactagogues to do their work as well as they can.

How Galactagogues Work

As so little work appears to have been done on these excellent herbs, no one knows how they work, a not unusual situation in modern herbal medicine.

Examples

There are a number that can be safely tried. They include *Goat's Rue, Milk Thistle, Fennel, Aniseed, Fenugreek, Nettles, Vervain* and *Cleavers.*

As you will notice most of these are discussed under other actions, and in various parts of the book but we shall discuss *Goat's Rue* here.

GOAT'S RUE   *Galega officinalis*
Part used: Dried aerial parts.
Collection: The stalks with the leaves and flowers are gathered at the time of flowering, which is between July and August. Dry in the shade.
Constituents: Alkaloids, saponins, flavone glycosides, bitters, tannin.
Actions: Reduces blood sugar, galactagogue, diuretic diaphoretic.

Indications: Goat's Rue is one of many herbal remedies with the action of reducing blood sugar levels. It can be of value in a holistic treatment of diabetis mellitus. This must not replace insulin therapy, however, and should occur under professional supervision. It is also a powerful galactagogue, stimulating the production and flow of milk. It has been shown to increase milk output by up to 50 per cent in some cases. It may also stimulate the development of the mammary glands.

Preparation and dosage: Infusion: pour a cup of boiling water onto 1 teaspoonful of the dried leaves and let infuse for 10 – 15 minutes. This should be drunk twice a day. Tincture: take 1 – 2 ml of the tincture three times a day.

HEPATIC

What is a Hepatic?

Hepatics are herbal remedies which in a wide range of ways aid the work of the liver. They tone, strengthen and in some cases increase the flow of bile. In a broad holistic approach to health they are of great importance because of the fundamental role of the liver in the working of the body.

How Hepatics Work

There is no simple or single answer here. The bitters and cholagogues all act as hepatics, but then so do a range of remedies without such specific actions. Here is the epitome of herbal remedies that do wonders for the body, without us necessarily knowing how. This lack of biochemical knowledge does not stop them working their wonders!

Examples

Nature is rich in hepatics. This is to be expected when their vital health-enhancing properties are taken into account. Here we shall look at three of the main hepatic herbs in some detail and then briefly review a range. Also review the sections on bitters and cholagogues.

DANDELION   *Taraxacum officinale*
Part used: Root or leaf.

Collection: The .oots are best collected between June and August when they are at their most bitter. Split longitudinally before drying. The leaves may be collected at any time.

Constituents: Glycosides, triterpenoids, choline up to 5 per cent potassium.

Actions: Diuretic, cholagogue, anti-rheumatic, laxative, tonic.

Indications: Here is an example of how different parts of a plant can have a markedly different medicinal use. Dandelion leaf is a very powerful diuretic, comparable to the action of the drug 'Frusemide'. The usual consequence of a drug stimulating the kidney function is the loss of vital potassium from the body, which would aggravate any cardio-vascular problem present. With Dandelion however, we have one of the best natural sources of potassium. It thus makes an ideally balanced diuretic that may be safely used wherever such an action is needed, including water retention due to heart problems. The root is one of our most widely applicable, gentle tonics for liver function. As a cholagogue it may be used in inflammation and congestion of liver and gallbladder. It is specific in cases of congestive jaundice. As part of a wider treatment for muscular rheumatism it can be most effective. This herb is a most valuable general tonic and perhaps the best widely applicable diuretic and liver tonic.

Combinations: For liver and gallbladder problems it may be used with _Barberry_ or _Balmony_. For water retention it may be used with _Couch grass_ or _Yarrow_.

Preparation and dosage: Decoction: put 2 – 3 teaspoonsful of the root into one cup of water, bring to the boil and gently simmer for 10 – 15 minutes. This should be drunk three times a day. The leaves may be eaten raw in salads.

Tincture: take 5 – 10 ml of the tincture three times a day.

BOLDO   _Peumus boldo_
Part used: Dried leaves.
Collection: Gather the evergreen leaves at any time. Dry them carefully in shade.
Constituents: 2 per cent volatile oils, the alkaloid boldline, glycosides, resins and tannin.
Actions: Cholagogue, hepatic, diuretic sedative.
Indications: Boldo is an excellent and gentle remedy for the liver, gallbladder and digestion in general. It is a specific for gallbladder problems such as stones or inflammations. It is also used when there is visceral pain due to other problems in the liver or gallbladder. Boldo has mild urinary demulcent and antiseptic properties and so would be used in cystitis.
Combinations: When treating gallbladder or liver problems it combines well with _Fringetree Bark_ and _Dandelion Root_.
Preparation and dosage: Infusion: pour a cup of boiling water onto 1 teaspoonful of the dried leaves and let infuse for 10 – 15 minutes. This should be drunk three times a day.

Tincture: take 1 – 2 ml of the tincture three times a day.

MILK THISTLE   _Silybum marianum_
Part used: The seeds.
Collection: The mature seed heads are cut and stored in a warm dry place. After a few days, tap the heads and collect the seeds.
Constituents: The flavones silybin, silydianin and silychristin; flavonoids; essential oil; bitter principle; mucilage.
Actions: Cholagogue, hepatic, galactagogue, demulcent.
Indications: There are two main areas in which this herb is used. Research has shown that it promotes the regeneration of diseased liver cells and protects them against some poisons. This exciting finding gives Milk Thistle a role in any chronic liver disease and especially those due to alcohol, drug or dietary abuse. It will also aid gallbladder problems. The other use is suggested by the herb's name. It will increase the production of milk and is completely safe to use by all breastfeeding mothers.
Preparation and dosage: Infusion: pour a cup of boiling water onto 1 teaspoonful of the bruised seeds and let infuse for 10 – 15 minutes.

Tincture: take 1 – 4 ml three times a day.

Hepatics for Different Parts of the Body

The same comments go for hepatics as for cholagogues, so please consult that section. A representative list of herbs that would fit into this category include: _Agrimony, Aloe, Balm, Balmony, Barberry, Black Root, Blue Flag, Boldo, Bogbean, Celery, Centaury, Dandelion Root, Fringetree Bark, Fumitory, Gentian, Golden Seal, Horseradish, Montain Grape, Wahoo, Wild Indigo, Wild Yam, Wormwood, Yarrow, Yellow Dock._

HYPNOTIC

What is a Hypnotic?

Hypnotics are herbal remedies that will help to induce a deep and healing state of sleep. They have nothing at all to do with hypnotic trances!

How Hypnotics Work

If you consult the section on the nervous system, it becomes clear there are many ways and degrees of herbal impact upon the nerves. Herbs that help you sleep have modes of action that vary from mild muscle-relaxing properties, through volatile oils that ease psychological tensions, to remedies that contain strong alkaloids that work directly upon the central nervous system and put you to sleep. Some of the most effective plant hypnotics are illegal for the very degree of their effectiveness. This includes the whole range of Opium Poppy derivatives. The remedies mentioned here and elsewhere are entirely safe and contain no addictive properties.

Hypnotic herbs should always be used within the context of an approach to sleep problems involving relaxation, food, and lifestyle in general.

Please refer to the section on the Nervous system for detailed information on the selection of herbs within this group.

Examples

As has already been pointed out, there is a range of hypnotic remedies with varying strength and applicability. Please consult the actions of nervines and sedatives for remedies other than those detailed here.

Mild hypnotics would include: *Chamomile, Lime Blossom, Vervain* and many others of the gentle relaxing nervines. Stronger remedies would include *Cowslip, Hops, Skullcap,* and *Valerian,* leading to quite strong herbs such as *Jamaican Dogwood, Passion Flower, Wild Lettuce* and *Lady's Slipper.*

PASSION FLOWER   *Passiflora incarnata*
Part used: Dried leaves.
Collection: If the foliage alone is to be collected, this should happen just before the flowers bloom, between May and July. The foliage may be collected with the fruit after flowering. It should be dried in the shade.
Constituents: Alkaloids including harmine, harman, harmol and passiflorine; flavone glycosides; sterols.
Actions: Sedative, hypnotic, anti-spasmodic, anodyne.
Indications: Passion Flower is one of the most effective herbs for treating intransigent insomnia. It aids the transition into a restful sleep without any 'narcotic' hangover. It may be used wherever an anti-spasmodic is required, for example in Parkinson's disease, seizures and hysteria. It can be quite effective in nerve pain such as neuralgia and the viral infection of nerves called shingles. It may be used in asthma where there is some associated tension.
Combinations: For insomnia it will combine well with *Valerian, Hops* and *Jamaican Dogwood,* especially if part of a whole approach to the problem. To ease muscular spasm, colic and pain it can be tried either by itself, with the herbs just mentioned, or *Cramp Bark.*
Preparation and dosage: Infusion: pour a cup of boiling water onto 1 teaspoonful of the dried herb and let infuse for 15 minutes. Drink a cup in the evening for sleepless-

ness, and a cup twice a day for the easing of other conditions.

Tincture: take 1 – 4 ml of the tincture and use the same way as the infusion.

JAMAICAN DOGWOOD *Piscidia erythrina*
Part used: Stem bark.
Collection: The bark is collected in vertical strips from trees growing in the Caribbean, Mexico and Texas.
Constituents: Glycosides including piscidin, jamaicin, icthyone; flavonoids including sumatrol, lisetine, piscerythrone, piscidine, rotenone; resin alkaloid.
Actions: Sedative, hypnotic, anodyne.
Indications: Jamaican Dogwood is a powerful sedative, used in its West Indian homeland as a fish poison. While not being poisonous to humans, the given dosage level should not be exceeded. It is a powerful remedy for the treatment of painful conditions such as neuralgia and migraine. It can also be used in the relief of ovarian and uterine pain. Its main use is perhaps in insomnia where this is due to nervous tension or pain.
Combinations: For the easing of insomnia it is best combined with *Hops, Passion Flower* or *Valerian.* For painful periods it may be used with *Black Haw* or *Cramp Bark.* It is difficult to generalize about migraine so I shall avoid committing myself and say it 'depends on the indications'. (Students of herbal medicine get thoroughly annoyed with that expression!)
Preparation and dosage: Decoction: put 1 – 2 teaspoonsful of the root in a cup of water, bring to the boil and simmer gently for 10-15 minutes. This should be drunk when needed.

Tincture: take 1 – 4 ml of the tincture three times a day.

HOPS   *Humulus lupulus*
Part used: Flower inflorescence.

Collection: The Hops cones are gathered before they are fully ripe in August and September. They should be dried with care in the shade.
Constituents: Lupulin,   bitters,   resin, volatile oil, tannin, oestrogenic substance.
Actions: Sedative, hypnotic, antiseptic, astringent.
Indications: Hops is a remedy that has a marked relaxing effect upon the central nervous system. It is used extensively for the treatment of insomnia. It will ease tension and anxiety, and may be used where this tension leads to restlessness, headache and possibly indigestion. As an astringent with these relaxing properties it can be used in conditions such as mucous colitis. It should, however, be avoided where there is a marked degree of depression as this may be accentuated. Externally the antiseptic action is utilized for the treatment of ulcers.
CAUTION: Do not use in cases with marked depression.
Combinations: For insomnia it can be combined with *Valerian* and *Passion Flower,* although the taste of such a mixture has to be experienced to be believed!
Preparation and dosage: Infusion: pour a cup of boiling water onto 1 teaspoonful of the dried flowers and let infuse for 10 – 15 minutes. A cup should be drunk at night to induce sleep. This dose may be strengthened if needed.

Tincture: take 1 – 4 ml of the tincture three times a day.

Hypnotics for Different Parts of the Body

Each system of the body has plants that are particularly suited to it, some of which are hypnotics of varying strength. Here we shall see which remedies are appropriate for each system and hypnotics as well. How they can be used will be considered in the sections on each system.

It is safe to say that all of the hypnotic remedies can help the whole body, in that sleep is such a vital health process.

Circulatory system: Here we can mention *Motherwort, Lime Blossom, Balm.* Notice they are all in the milder group. *Mistletoe* can help but must be used with care.

Respiratory system: All of the hypnotics can help as antispasmodics in conditions such as asthma, if used at the right dose. *Wild Lettuce* eases irritable coughs.

Digestive system: The relaxing nervines and carminatives are important, of which we can mention *Chamomile, Vervain, Balm, Hops* and *Valerian.* The anti-spasmodic herbs will help with intestinal colic, for example *Hops, Jamaican Dogwood, Passion*

Flower and *Valerian.*

Urinary system: Hypnotics are important here when used as muscle relaxants.

Reproductive system: The same remarks hold good.

Muscles and skeleton: All the hypnotics will aid in reducing muscle tension and even the pain associated with problems in this system. They may be used internally or as lotions. Especially important are *Jamaican Dogwood* and *Valerian.*

Nervous system: All these remedies work on the nervous system. Please consult the chapter on that system.

Skin: Chamomile and *Cowslip* are healing, but otherwise the value of hypnotics here is to ensure that the body has a good recuperative rest each night.

_____ LAXATIVE _____

What is a Laxative?

Laxatives are herbs that actively stimulate the bowels to promote movements. This is as opposed to the aperients that gently support the normal bowel processes. There can be no strict demarcation apart from at the extremes of each action. An important point is that stimulating laxatives should not be used long term. If this appears to be necessary then diet, general health and stress should all be closely considered.

How Laxatives Work

There are a number of different modes of action here. The best understood is that due to the presence of plant constituents called anthraquinone glycosides. These are discussed in the section on constituents, but their action here is to stimulate greater contractions of the muscle walls of the large

intestine. This occurs between 8 – 12 hours after taking the remedy. A problem with this is that it might cause griping pain in the abdomen. A list of remedies that contain anthraquinones include *Senna, Alder Buckthorn, Cascara Sagrada* and *Aloes.*

A gentler form of laxative are those that work via an action on the liver as cholagogues. The milder ones are the aperients.

There are much stronger plants that have actions known as purgatives, cathartics and drastic hydrogogues. These are quite violent remedies are should not be used, although some of them are in the official Pharmacopoeia.

Examples

Of the many remedies that can work as laxatives I have chosen three that can be used safely and have avoided drastic remedies altogether.

BUTTERNUT   *Juglans cinerea*
Part used: The bark of the tree is used, which is a native of North America.
Constituents: Juglone (an anthraquinone); tannin; essential oils.
Actions: Laxative, cholagogue.
Indications: This is a good general herb for constipation when dietary changes and exercise have not got things moving! It is especially useful when the problem relates to liver sluggishness as Butternut is a gentle cholagogue as well. Because of this combination of actions it may help skin problems when these have a basis in incomplete cleansing of the body via the bowels.
Combinations: This herb is often best used by itself, or it can be safely combined with any other mixture.
Preparation and dosage: A decoction is made of 1 – 2 teaspoonsful of the dried bark three times a day.

SENNA PODS
             Cassia angustifolia and *C. senna*
Part used: Dried fruit pods.
Collection: The pods are gathered during the winter in Egypt, Sudan, Jordan and India.
Constituents: Anthraquinones.
Actions: Cathartic.
Indications: Senna pods are used as a powerful cathartic in the treatment of constipation. It is vital to recognize, however, that the constipation is a result of something else and not the initial cause and that this has to be sought and dealt with. See the section on the digestive system in Chapter 6 for more information.
Combinations: It is best to combine Senna pods with aromatic, carminative herbs to increase palatability and reduce griping, for instance by using *Cardamom, Ginger* or *Fennel.*
Preparation and dosage: Infusion: the dried pods should be steeped in warm water for 6 – 12 hours. If they are Alexandrian

Senna Pods use three to six in a cup of water; if they are Tinnevelly Senna, use four to twelve pods. These names are given to two different species when sold commercially.
Tincture: take 2 – 7 ml of the tincture three times a day.

BLUE FLAG   *Iris versicola*
Part used: Rizome.
Collection: The rhizome is best collected in the autumn.
Constituents: Oleoresin, salicylic acid, alkaloid, tannin.
Actions: Cholagogue, alterative, laxative, diuretic, anti-inflammatory.
Indications: This useful remedy has a wide application in the treatment of skin diseases, apparently aiding the skin by working through the liver, the main detoxifying organ of the body. It may be used in skin eruptions such as acne, spots and blemishes. For the more chronic skin problems such as eczema and psoriasis, it is valuable as part of a wider treatment. It may be used with value where there is constipation associated with liver problems or biliousness.
Combinations: Blue Flag combines well with *Echinacea* or *Burdock* and *Yellow Dock.*
Preparation and dosage: Decoction: put ½ – 1 teaspoonful of the dried herb into a cup of water and bring to the boil. Let it simmer for 10 – 15 minutes. This should be drunk three times a day.
Tincture: take 2 – 4 ml of the tincture three times a day.

Laxatives for the Body as a Whole

Laxatives will aid every part of the body if used in such a way as to help in the eliminative process, rather than forcing bowel movements. If used with care and discretion they can speed healing in many diverse conditions. If used too liberally, they will replace the body's own gut control and cause what could be called a 'digestive addiction'. In the end a proper bowel move-ment will occur only if the person takes their anthraquinone-containing remedy. This is to be avoided at all costs.

NERVINE

What is a Nervine?

A nervine is a plant remedy that has a beneficial effect upon the nervous system in some way. This makes the word nervine into a bit of a catch-all expression, and to study them properly they must be differentiated into nervine relaxants, nervine stimulants and nervine tonics. It may be superfluous to point this out, but any successful treatment of nervous system problems with herbs will involve treating the whole body and not simply the signs of agitation and worry. Of course, the agitation can be reduced greatly, but the whole system must be strengthened in the face of the storm!

With life being such a stress and problem for humanity today, we shall put more attention on these actions than has been the case up to now.

Nervine Tonics

Perhaps the most important contribution herbal medicine can make in the whole area of stress and anxiety is in strengthening and 'feeding' the nervous system. In cases of shock, stress or nervous debility, the nervine tonics strengthen and restore the tissues directly. This group of remedies are invaluable.

We shall discuss three of the main nervine tonics, but we could also include the representatives of the adaptogens. This term has been coined to describe their undoubted ability to aid the whole of the body and mind to cope with demands made upon it.

Other nervine tonics that have, in addition, a relaxing effect include *Damiana, Skullcap* and *Wood Betony*. Of these 'relaxing nervine tonics', *Skullcap* is often the most effective, particularly for problems related to stress.

OATS   *Avena sativa*
Part used: Seeds and the whole plant.
Collection: The fruit and straw are gathered at harvest time, in August about four weeks after the rye harvest. The stalks are cut and bound together. Leave them upright to dry and then thresh out the fruit. The straw is just the crushed dry stalks.
Constituents: Seeds: 50 per cent starch; alkaloids including trigonelline and avenine; saponins; flavones; sterols; vitamin B.
Plant straw: Rich in silicic acid; mucin; calcium.
Actions: Nervine tonic, anti-depressant, nutritive, demulcent, vulnerary.
Indications: Oats is one of the best remedies for 'feeding' the nervous system, especially when under stress. It is specific in cases of nervous debility and exhaustion, especially when associated with depression. It may be used with most of the other nervines, both relaxant and stimulatory, to strengthen the whole of the nervous system. It is also used in general debility. The high levels of silicic aid in the straw will explain its use as a remedy for skin conditions, especially in external applications.

Combinations: For depression it may be used with _Skullcap, Damiana_ and _Lavender._ For debility and exhaustion it will combine with whatever is indicated in that person.

Preparation and dosage: Oats may most conveniently be taken in the form of porridge or gruel.

Fluid extract: in liquid form it is most often given as a fluid extract. Take 3 – 5 ml three times a day.

Bath: a soothing bath for use in neuralgia and irritated skin conditions can be made: 500 grams of shredded straw is boiled in 2 litres of water for half an hour. The liquid is strained and added to the bath.

ST JOHN'S WORT   _Hypericum perforatum_
Part used: Aerial parts.
Collection: The entire plant above ground should be collected when in flower and dried as quickly as possible.
Constituents: Glycosides including retin; volatile oil; tannin; resin; pectin.
Actions: Nervine tonic, anti-inflammatory, astringent, vulnerary.
Indication: When taken internally it has a sedative, restorative and pain-reducing effect, which gives it a place in the treatment of neuralgia, anxiety, tension and similar problems. With its tonic action on the whole nervous system it may be used freely in nervous debility and stress. It is especially regarded as a herb to use where there are menopausal changes triggering irritability and anxiety. It is recommended, however, that it is not used when there is marked depression. In addition to neuralgic pain, it will ease fibrositis, sciatica and rheumatic pain. Externally it is a valuable healing and anti-inflammatory remedy. As a lotion it will speed the healing of wounds and bruises, varicose veins and mild burns. The oil is especially useful for the healing of sunburn.

Combination: For stress and debility it goes well with _Skullcap_ and many other nervines. For healing the skin it has a well-deserved reputation with _Marigold Petals._

Preparation and dosage: Infusion: pour a cup of boiling water onto 1 – 2 teaspoonfuls of the dried herb and leave to infuse for 10 – 15 minutes. This should be drunk three times a day. External use: see the section on the skin in Chapter 6.

Tincture: take 1 – 4 ml of the tincture three times a day.

VERVAIN   _Verbena officinalis_
Part used: Aerial parts.
Collection: The herb should be collected just before the flowers open, usually in July. Dry quickly.
Constituents: Bitter glycosides called verbenalin; essential oil; mucilage; tannin.
Actions: Nervine tonic, sedative, antispasmodic, disphoretic, possible galactagogue, hepatic.
Indications: Vervain is a herb that will tone and strengthen the whole nervous system while relaxing any tension and stress. It can be used to ease depression and melancholia, especially when this follows illness such as influenza. It has also been used to help in seizure and hysteria. As a diaphoretic, it can be used in the early stages of fevers. As a hepatic remedy it will be found of help in inflammation of the gallbladder and jaundice. It may be used as a mouthwash against caries and gum disease.
Combinations: In the treatment of depression it may be used with _Skullcap, Oats_ and _Damiana._
Peparation and dosage: Infusion: pour a cup of boiling water onto 1–3 teaspoonsful of the dried herb and leave to infuse for 10–15 minutes. This should be drunk three times a day.
Tincture: take 2–4 ml of the tincture three times a day.

Nervine Relaxants

This group of nervine remedies is increasingly appropriate in our times of stress and confusion. In cases of stress and tension, the nervine relaxants can help a lot to alleviate the symptoms. They are the closest natural alternative for the orthododox nerve tranquilizers, but should always be used in a broad holistic way. Too much tranquilizing, even that achieved through herbal medication, can in time deplete and weigh heavily on the whole nervous system.

The following list is far from complete but includes the main nervine relaxant herbs: *Black Cohosh, Chamomile, Jamaican Dogwood, Lime Blossom, Passion Flower, Black Haw, Cramp Bark, Lady's Slipper, Mistletoe, Rosemary, Skullcap, Californian Poppy, Hops, Lavender, Motherwort, St John's Wort, Valerian, Hyssop, Lemon Balm, Pasque Flower.*

As can be seen from this list, many of the relaxants also have other properties and can be selected to aid in related problems. This is one of the great benefits of using herbal remedies to help in stress and anxiety problems. The physical symptoms that can so often accompany the ill-ease of anxiety may well be treated with herbs that work on the anxiety itself.

In addition to the herbs that work directly on the nervous system, the anti-spasmodic herbs – which affect the peripheral nerves and the muscle tissue – can have an indirect relaxing effect on the whole system. When the physical body is at ease, ease in the psyche is promoted. Many of the nervine relaxants have this anti-spasmodic action. Also refer to hypnotics, which in lower dosage will have a relaxing action on mind and body.

A vitally important nervine relaxant described under anti-spasmodics is *Valerian.*

SKULLCAP   *Scutellaria laterifolia*
Part used: Aerial parts.
Collection: The whole of the aerial parts should be collected late in the flowering period during August and September.
Constituents: Flavonoid glycoside including scutellarin and scutellarein; trace of volatile oil; bitter.
Actions: Nerve tonic, sedative, anti-spasmodic.
Indications: Skullcap is perhaps the most widely relevant nervine available to us in the materia medica. It relaxes states of nervous tension while at the same time renewing and revivifying the central nervous system. This makes it of value wherever there is stress, anxiety or tension. A cup of Skullcap at the office instead of coffee would do wonders. It is just a pity it doesn't taste good enough! It has a specific use in the treatment of seizure and hysterical states as well as epilepsy. It may be used with complete safety and confidence in all exhausted or depressed conditions. It is often found to be rapidly effective as well as safe in the easing of pre-menstrual tension.
Combinations: It combines well with *Valerian* for the relief of anxiety and tension symptoms.
Preparation and dosage: Infusion: pour a cup of boiling water onto 1-2 teaspoonsful of the dried herb and leave to infuse for 10-15 minutes. This should be drunk three times a day or when needed.
Tincture: take 2-4 ml of the tincture three times a day.

PASQUE FLOWER   *Anemone pulsatilla*
Part used: Aerial parts.
Collection: The stalks should be gathered at the time of flowering, which is in March or April.
Constituents: Glycosides, saponins, tannins, resin.

_____ THE HERBAL HANDBOOK _____

Actions: Sedative, analgesic, anti-spasmodic, antibacterial.

Indications: Here we have another valuable relaxing remedy that has specific properties as well. Pasque Flower is an excellent relaxing nervine for use in problems relating to nervous tension and spasm in the reproductive system. It may be used with safety in the relief of painful periods (dysmenorrhoea), ovarian pain and painful conditions of the testes. It may be used to reduce tension reaction and headaches associated with them. It will help insomnia and general overactivity. The antibacterial actions give this herb a role in treating infections that affect the skin, especially boils. It is similarly useful in the treatment of respiratory infections and asthma. The oil or tincture may ease earache.

Combinations: For painful periods it will combine well with *Cramp Bark.* For skin conditions it combines with *Echinacea.*

CAUTION: Do not use the fresh plant!

Preparation and dosage: Infusion: pour a cup of boiling water onto ½–1 teaspoonful of the dried herb and leave to infuse for 10–15 minutes. This should be drunk three times a day or when needed.

Tincture: take 1–2 ml of the tincture three times a day.

LAVENDER   *Lavendula officinalis*
Part used: Flowers.
Collection: The flowers should be gathered just before opening between June and September. They should be dried gently at a temperature not above 35°C.
Constituents: The fresh flowers contain up to 0.5 per cent of volatile oil that contains among other constituents linalyl acetate, linalol, geraniol, cineole, limonene and sesquiterpenes.
Actions: Carminative, anti-spasmodic, anti-depressant, rubefacient.
Indications: This beautiful herb has many uses, culinary, cosmetic and medicinal. It is

an effective herb for headaches, especially when they are related to stress. Lavender can be quite effective in the clearing of depression, especially if used in conjunction with other remedies. As a gentle strengthening tonic of the nervous system it may be helpful for nervous debility and exhaustion. It can be used to soothe and promote natural sleep. Externally the oil may be used as a stimulating liniment to help ease the aches and pains of rheumatism. A drop of the pure oil rubbed into the temples may clear a headache.

Combinations: For depression it will combine well with *Rosemary, Kola, Damiana* or *Skullcap.* For headaches it may be used with *Wood Betony* or *Feverfew.*

Preparation and dosage: Infusion: to take internally, pour a cup of boiling water onto 1 teaspoonful of the dried herb and leave to infuse for 10 minutes. This can be drunk three times a day.

External use: the oil should not be taken internally but can be inhaled, rubbed on the skin or used in baths.

Nervine Stimulants

Direct stimulation of the nervous tissue is not very often needed in our times of hyperactivity. In most cases it is more appropriate to stimulate the body's innate vitality with the help of nervine or even digestive tonics, which work by augmenting bodily harmony and thus have a much deeper and longer-lasting effect than nervine stimulants.

In the last century much more emphasis was placed by herbalists upon stimulant herbs. It is, perhaps, a sign of the times that our world is supplying us with more than enough stimulus.

When direct nervine stimulation is indicated, the best herb to use is the *Kola Nut,* although *Coffee, Mate, Tea* and *Black Tea* should also be remembered. A problem

78

with these commonly used stimulants is that they have a number of side-effects and can themselves be involved in causing many minor psychological problems such as anxiety and tension. Like the other nerve stimulants mentioned above, short-term use is appropriate at times. Daily cups of strong coffee causes too many problems to list!

Some of the herbs rich in volatile oils are also valuable stimulants, one of the commonest and best being *Peppermint.*

KOLA   *Cola vera*
Part used: Seed kernel.
Collection: The Kola tree grows in tropical Africa and is cultivated in South America. The seeds are collected when ripe and are initially white, turning the characteristic red upon drying.
Constituents: Alkaloids which include more than 1.25 per cent caffeine and theobromine; tannin; volatile oil.
Actions: Stimulant to central nervous system, anti-depressive, astringent, diuretic.
Indications: Kola has a marked stimulating effect on the human consciousness. It can be used wherever there is a need for direct stimulation, which is less often than is usually thought. Through regaining proper health and therefore right functioning, the nervous system does not need such help. In the short term it may be used for nervous debility, in states of atony and weakness. It can act as a specific in nervous diarrhoea. It will aid in states of depression and may in some people give rise to euphoric states. In some varieties of migraine it can help greatly. Through the stimulation it will be valuable part of the treatment for anorexia. It can be viewed as specific in cases of depression associated with weakness and debility.
Combinations: Kola will go well with *Oats, Damiana* and *Skullcap.*
Preparation and dosage: Decoction: put 1–2 teaspoonsful of the powdered nuts in a cup of water, bring to the boil and simmer gently for 10–15 minutes. This should be drunk when needed.
Tincture: take 1–4 ml of the tincture three times a day.

Nervines for Different Parts of the Body

As you will have seen, there is much to the study of nervines, which makes it difficult to relate them to each body system as we have with different actions. They will be referred to in the sections on the body systems in Chapter 6.

_____ PECTORAL _____

What is a Pectoral?

This is an old, but honourable, word meaning a remedy that is good for the lungs. It finds no place in modern medicine where specific drugs treat specific illnesses. Where the whole person is being aided herbally, however, they come into their own.

How Pectorals Work

Who knows? This might sound flippant, but the point is that they *do* strengthen a weak chest. All the expectorant remedies, whether the stimulating, relaxing or normalizing kind can be described as pectorals. Please refer to p. 65.

Examples

In addition to the examples given under expectorant, the following three herbs are good pectorals.

ELECAMPANE   *Inula helenium*
Part used: Rhizome.
Collection: The rhizome should be unearthed between September and October. The large pieces should be cut before drying in the sun or artificially at a temperature of 50–70°C.
Constituents: 40 per cent inulin, essential oil called helenin, mucilage, triterpenes, bitter principle.
Actions: Expectorant, anti-tussive, diaphoretic, stomachic, anti-bacterial.
Indications: Elecampane is a specific for irritating bronchial coughs, especially in children. This herb, in a similar way to *Mullein,* is generally beneficial and tonic for the whole complex of the lungs. It may be used wherever there is copious catarrh formed, e.g. in bronchitis or emphysema. This remedy shows the complex and integrated ways in which herbs work. The mucilage has a relaxing effect accompanied by the stimulation of the essential oils. In this way expectoration is accompanied by a soothing action which in this herb is combined with an anti-bacterial effect. It may be used in asthma and bronchitic asthma. Elecampane has been used in the treatment of tuberculosis. The bitter principle makes it useful also to stimulate digestion and appetite.
Combinations: Elecampane combines well with *White Horehound, Coltsfoot, Mullein,* and *Yarrow* for respiratory problems. The combination chosen will depend upon whether there is infection, asthma, allergy etc. This is all discussed later.
Preparation and dosage: Infusion: pour a cup of cold water onto 1 teaspoonful of the shredded root. Let stand for 8–10 hours. Heat up and take very hot three times a day.

Tincture: take 1–2 ml of the tincture three times a day.

LOBELIA   *Lobelia inflata*
Part used: Aerial parts.
Collection: The entire plant above ground should be collected at the end of the flowering time, between August and September. The seed pods should be collected as well.
Constituents: Alkaloids including lobeline, lobelidine, lobelanine, isolobelanine; bitter glycosides; bloatile oil; resin; gum.
Actions: Respiratory stimulant, anti-asthmatic, anti-spasmodic, expectorant, emetic.
Indications: Lobelia is one of the most useful systemic relaxants available to us. It has a general depressant action on the central and autonomic nervous system and on neruo-muscular action. It may be used in many conditions in combination with other herbs to further their effectiveness if relaxation is needed. Its primary specific use is in bronchitic asthma and bronchitis. An analysis of the action of the alkaloids present reveal apparently paradoxical effects. Lobeline is a powerful respiratory stimulant, while isolobinine is an emetic and respiratory relaxant, which will stimulate catarrhal secretion and expectoration while relaxing the muscles of the respiratory system. The overall action is a truly holistic combination of stimulation and relaxation!
Combinations: It will combine well with *Cayenne, Grindelia, Pill-bearing Spurge, Sundew* and *Ephedra* in the treatment of asthma.
Preparation and dosage: Infusion: pour a cup of boiling water onto ¼–½ teaspoonful of the dried leaves and let infuse for 10–15 minutes. This should be drunk three times a day.
Tincture: take ½–1 ml of the tincture three times a day.

BLOOD ROOT   *Sanguinaria canadensis*
Part used: Dried rhizome.
Collection: The rhizome is unearthed in early summer (May to June) or in autumn when the leaves have dried. It should be dried carefully in the shade.
Constituents: Alkaloids including sanguinarine, chelerythrine, protopine and homochelidine; red resin, citric acid, malic acids.
Actions: Expectorant, anti-spasmodic, emetic, cathartic, antiseptic, cardio-active, topical irritant.
Indications: Blood Root finds its main use in the treatment of bronchitis in any of its forms. While the stimulating properties show in its power as an emetic and expectorant, it demonstrates relaxing action on the bronchial muscles. It thus has a role in the treatment of asthma, croup and laryngitis. It acts as a stimulant in cases of deficient peripheral circulation. It may be used as a snuff in the treatment of nasal polypi.
Combinations: May be combined with *Lobelia* in bronchitic asthma. In pharyngitis it combines well with *Red Sage* and *Cayenne.*
Preparation and dosage: Decoction: put 1 teaspoonful of the rhizome in a cup of cold water, bring to the boil and leave to infuse for 10 minutes. This should be drunk three times a day.
Tincture: take 2–4 ml of the tincture three times a day.

Pectorals for Different Parts of the Body

Each system of the body has plants that are particularly suited to it, some of which are pectorals. How they can be used will be considered in the sections on each system.
Circulatory system: Both *Blood Root* and

Squill have a direct cardio-active effect; however, all pectoral herbs will help circulation indirectly by improving the tone of the lungs and thus pulmonary circulation.
Respiratory system: All the herbs mentioned here, under expectorants and as respiratory anti-microbials and demulcents, will aid the whole of this system.
Digestive system: Some of the pectorals are demulcent to the gut and include *Comfrey, Liquorice, Lungwort, Marshmallow*. Some will be specific digestive aids such as *Golden Seal, Elder Flower* and *Vervain*. The more aromatic pectorals will be carminative in the gut and include *Aniseed, Elder, Garlic Hyssop* and *Thyme*.
Urinary system: By aiding the lungs to do their job properly, the excretory load on the kidneys is eased to some degree. This may be essential in some kidney problems.
Reproductive system: In a broadly similar way to those already described, many of these herbs help the reproductive system in an indirect way. The demulcent pectorals may be helpful in some cases, such as *Comfrey, Marshmallow* and *Irish Moss*. *Golden Seal* is broadly used in gynaecological conditions involving the membranes.
Muscles and skeleton: Apart from effects due to improving health in general, these herbs will aid the musculature and inflammation, *Angelica, Balsam of Peru, Balsam of Tolu, Comfrey* and *Elder*.
Nervous system: Pectorals with a nervine action as well include *Hyssop, Vervain* and *Wild Cherry Bark*.
Skin: Pectorals can aid skin conditions in the way they aid kidney problems, by taking some of the excretory load off the skin. While they may all work this way indirectly we can mention these as helpful to the skin: *Comfrey, Elder, Elecampane, Garlic, Golden Seal, Thuja* and *Thyme*. The demulcent pectorals can act as emolients if necessary.

RUBEFACIENT

What is a Rubefacient?

Rubifacients are herbs that when applied to the skin, in some form, will cause a gentle and localized increase in surface blood flow (vasodilation). This usually shows as a reddening of the skin. They can vary in potency, and in older medical texts get sub-divided by this power. A vesicant produces actual blistering.

How Rubefacients Work

Their value is based on bringing blood to the area involved. This has two broad benefits. First the increase in flow through will aid in the cleansing and nourishment of the affected part. This mimics the process of inflammation but is less painful as the biochemical basis is different. This is the basis of the stimulating liniment or mustard bath. The other area of use, though less favoured today, is drawing blood from deeper parts of the body into the skin which may relieve visceral pain. By using rubefacients on different parts of the skin, different internal areas may be affected.

They are used mostly today to ease the pain and swelling of arthritic joints; however, their use is best left to a qualified practitioner.

Examples

Many of the stimulant remedies will be rubefacient as well, anything that tastes hot, in fact! Apart from the two listed we can add: *Cayenne, Cloves, Garlic, Ginger, Nettle, Peppermint Oil, Rosemary Oil, Rue.*

MUSTARD   *Brassica alba* and *B. nigra*
Part used: The seeds.

Collection: The ripe seed pods are collected in the late summer. Tap the seeds out and dry in a thin layer.
Constituents: Mucilage, fixed oil, volatile oil, sinigrin.
Actions: Rubefacient, irritant, stimulant, diuretic, emetic.
Indications: This well-known spice has its main use in medicine as a stimulating external application. The rubefacient action causes a mild irritation to the skin, stimulating the circulation to that area and relieving muscular and skeletal pain. Its stimulating, diaphoretic action can be utilized in the way that *Cayenne* and *Ginger* are. For feverishness, colds and influenza, Mustard may be taken as a tea or ground and sprinkled into a bath. The stimulation of circulation will aid chilblains as well as the conditions already mentioned. An infusion or poultice of Mustard will aid in cases of bronchitis.
Preparation and dosage: Poultice: Mustard is most commonly used as a poultice which can be made by mixing 100 grams of freshly ground mustard seeds with warm water (at about 45°C) to form a thick paste. This is spread on a piece of cloth the size of the body area that is to be covered. To stop the paste sticking to the skin, lay a dampened gauze on the skin. Apply the cloth and remove after one minute. The skin may be reddened by this treatment which can be eased by applying olive oil afterwards.
Infusion: pour a cup of boiling water onto 1 teaspoonful of mustard flour and leave to infuse for 5 minutes. This may be drunk three times a day.
Foot bath: make an infusion using 1 tablespoon of bruised seeds to 1 litre of boiling water.

HORSERADISH   *Armoracia rusticana*
Part used: Tap root.
Collection: The roots are collected in the winter and stored in sand.
Constituents: Essential oil that contains mustard oil glycosides; sinigrin.
Actions: Stimulant, carminative, rubefacient, mild laxative, diuretic.
Indications: Horseradish is an old household remedy useful wherever a stimulating herb is called for. It can be used in influenza and fevers as a rough equivalent to *Cayenne*

Pepper. It stimulates the digestive process while easing wind and griping pains. It has been used in cases of urinary infection. Externally it has a stimulating action similar to *Mustard Seed.* It can be used for rheumatism and as a poultice in bronchitis.
Preparation and dosage: The fresh root is often used as a vegetable.
Infusion: pour a cup of boiling water into 1 teaspoonful of the powdered or chopped root. Leave to infuse for 5 minutes when being used to treat influenza or fevers.

SEDATIVE

What is a Sedative?

This is an action that calms the nervous system and reduces stress and nervousness throughout the body. Many different herbs are sedatives, and are described under relaxing nervines, hypnotics and anti-spasmodics. In many respects these terms can be used concurrently. To study comprehensively sedatives and other herbal nerve remedies, please consider these other actions as well.

How Sedatives Work

As has been described in the other sections, sometimes we know they work because of specific chemical constituents, but often not enough research has been done to answer all our chemical questions. An example of this is *Valerian* which contains sedative iridoids called valepotriates. Much is known about the truly potent sedative herbs as they are used by orthodox medicine in vast amounts. Here the best example would be the *Opium Poppy,* where a whole range of alkoloids provides medicine with pain killers and relaxants.

   With the bulk of safe and gently effective plant sedatives while not knowing how they work, thousands of years of experience show that they do. Surely this is enough to know?

Examples

Nature is rich in sedatives. Here we shall look at three of them in some detail and then briefly review a range. Refer to Nervines for *Skullcap, Pasque Flower, Lavender, Verbena, St John's Wort,* to Hypnotics for *Passion Flower, Jamaican Dogwood* and *Hops.*

VALERIAN   *Valeriana officinalis*
Part used: Rhizome and roots.
Collection: The roots are unearthed in the late autumn. Clean thoroughly and dry in the shade.
Constituents: Volatile oil including valerianic acid, isovalerianic acid, borneol, pinene, camphene; bolatile alkaloids.
Actions: Sedative, hypnotic, anti-spasmodic, hypotensive, carminative.
Indications: Valerian is one of the most useful relaxing nervines that is available to us. This fact is recognized by orthodox medicine as is shown by its inclusion in many pharmacopeias as a sedative. It may

safely be used to reduce tension and anxiety, over-excitability and hysterical states. It is an effective aid in insomnia, producing a natural healing sleep. As an anti-spasmodic herb it will aid in the relief of cramp and intestinal colic and will also be useful for the cramps and pain of periods. As a pain reliever it is most indicated where that pain is associated with tension. Valerian can help in migraine and rheumatic pain.

Combinations: For the relief of tension it will combine most effectively with *Skullcap,* amongst other nervines. For insomnia it can be combined with *Passion Flower* and *Hops.* For the treatment of cramps it will work well with *Cramp Bark.*

Preparation and dosage: Infusion: pour a cup of boiling water onto 1–2 teaspoonsful of the root and let it infuse for 10–15 minutes. This should be drunk when needed.

Tincture: take 2–4 ml of the tincture three times a day.

LADY'S SLIPPER   *Cypripedium pubescens*
Part used: The root.
Collection: Lady's Slipper is a protected plant in the United Kingdom and so should never be collected if found wild.
Constituents: Volatile oil, resins, glucosides, tannin.
Actions: Sedative, hypnotic, anti-spasmodic, nervine tonic.
Indications: Lady's Slipper is one of a group of widely applicable nervines. It may be used in all stress reactions, emotional tension and anxiety states. It will help elevate the mood, especially where depression is present. It can help in easing nervous pain, though it is best used in combination with other herbs for this purpose. It is perhaps at its best when treating anxiety and tension that is associated with insomnia.
Combinations: It combines well with *Oats*

and *Skullcap.* For nerve pain it may be used with *Jamaican Dogwood, Passion Flower* and *Valerian.*

Preparation and dosage: Infusion: pour a cup of boiling water onto 1–2 teaspoonsful of the root and let infuse for 10–15 minutes. This should be drunk as required.

Tincture: take 1–4 ml of the tincture three times a day.

WILD LETTUCE   *Lactuca virosa*
Part used: Dried leaves.
Collection: The leaves should be gathered in June and July.
Constituents: Latex containing lactucin, lactucone, lactupicrin, lactucic acid; alkaloids; triterpenes.
Actions: Sedative, anodyne, hypnotic.
Indications: The latex of the Wild Lettuce was at one time sold as 'Lettuce Opium', naming the use of this herb quite well! It is a valuable remedy for use in insomnia, restlessness and over-excitability (especially in children) and other manifestations of an over-active nervous system. As an anti-spasmodic it can be used as part of a holistic treatment of whooping cough and dry irritated coughs in general. It will relieve colic pains in the guts and uterus and so can be used in painful periods. It will ease muscular pains related to rheumatism. It has been used as an aphrodisiac.
Combinations: For irritable coughs it may be used with *Wild Cherry Bark.* For insomnia it combines with *Valerian* and *Passion Flower.* In stress and its related problems this herb could be used with *Skullcap.*
Preparation and dosage: Infusion: pour a cup of boiling water onto 1–2 teaspoonsful of the leaves and let infuse for 10–15 minutes. This should be drunk three times a day.

Tincture: take 2–4 ml of the tincture three times a day.

Sedatives for Different Parts of the Body

Each system of the body has plants that are particularly suited to it, some of which are sedatives. Here we shall see which sedatives have a unique affinity for each of these systems. How they can be used will be considered in the sections on each system.

Circulatory system: _Balm, Lime Blossom, Motherwort,_ while each being mild sedatives, are helpful to the cardio-vascular system. However, most remedies that reduce over-activity in the nervous system will aid the heart and problems such as high blood pressure.

Respiratory system: Most sedatives will help in over-tense chest problems such as asthma, but specifically we can mention _Black Cohosh, Blood Root, Bugleweed, Cowslip, Lobelia, Motherwort, Wild Cherry Bark_ and _Wild Lettuce._

Digestive system: All the anti-spasmodic remedies may be of value here to ease colic, but sedatives that actively aid digestion include _Balm, Chamomile, Lavender._

Urinary system: By relaxing the system there may be an increase in water loss. This, however, does not make the herbs involved diuretics. _Saw Palmetto_ is a gentle sedative that does work on the urinary system.

Reproductive system: _Black Cohosh, Blue Cohosh, Cramp Bark, Motherwort, Saw Palmetto_ and _Wild Lettuce_ all have an affinity for this system.

Muscles and skeleton: All sedative remedies will ease muscular tension and thus pain in this complex system. Remedies to bear in mind are _Black Cohosh, Bladderwrack, Cramp Bark_ and _Wild Yam._

Nervous system: All the remedies mentioned relate here.

Skin: All these remedies may help the skin in an indirect way, but these herbs have a good reputation for the skin: _Red Clover, St John's Wort, Pasque Flower_ and _Black Cohosh._

SPASMOLYTIC

This is a term that is synonymous with antispasmodic.

STIMULANT

What is a Stimulant?

The very name stimulant has different connotations depending upon one's assumptions and conditioning. In herbal medicine it is used to describe an action that quickens and enlivens the physiological activity of the body. This is not necessarily an appropriate thing to do. The needs of the individual and their unique state of health must be taken into account. Debility may be due to too much activity within the body as well as not enough. Here we have a problem of differential diagnosis that calls for skill, knowledge and a certain amount of intuition.

How Stimulants Work

In some cases the specific stimulation is due

to the presence of alkaloids in the plant. Caffeine is perhaps the best known and most widely used of these alkaloids, and is present in herbs such as *Coffee, Tea, Mate, Kola* as well as in chocolate. Other, more perfidious alkaloids are contained in plants such as the *Coca Tree,* the source of cocaine. The chemistry of these specific stimulants is complex and not pertinent here. Whenever safe and legal stimulants of this kind are used they are combined with nervine tonics or relaxants to balance out over-activity.

In herbalism the term stimulant has a broader meaning that does not necessitate potent chemicals. Bitters often act as stimulants in the way defined above.

Examples

The herbs described under rubefacient and diaphoretic can all be used as stimulants. Important ones already described are: *Cayenne, Ginger, Mustard, Wormwood* and *Yarrow.* To these we may add the following two examples that work in a gentler way.

BAYBERRY   *Myrica cerifera*
Part used: Rootbark.
Collection: The root should be unearthed in spring or autumn and its bark pared off and dried.
Constituents: Tannins, resin, volatile oil.
Actions: Astringent, circulatory stimulant, diaphoretic.
Indications: As a circulatory stimulant Bayberry plays a role in many conditions when they are approached in a holistic way. Due to its specific actions it is a valuable astringent in diarrhoea and dysentry. It is indicated in mucous colitis. As a gargle it helps sore throats and as a douche it helps in leuccorrhoea.It may be used in the treatment of colds.
Combinations: As a digestive astringent it may be used with *Comfrey Root* and *Agrimony.*

Preparation and dosage: Decoction: put 1 teaspoonful of the bark into a cup of cold water and bring to the boil. Leave for 10-15 minutes. This should be drunk three times a day.
Tincture: take 1-3 ml of the tincture three times a day.

PRICKLY ASH   *Zanthoxylum americanum*
Part used: The bark and berries.
Collection: The berries are collected in late summer and the bark is stripped from the stems of this shrub in the spring.
Constituents: Alkaloids, volatile oil in the berries.
Actions: Stimulant (especially circulatory), tonic alterative, carminative, diaphoretic.
Indications: Prickly Ash may be used in a way that is similar to *Cayenne,* although it is slower in action and a lot less traumatic to take! It is used in many chronic problems such as rheumatism and skin diseases. Any sign of poor circulation calls for the use of this herb, such as chilblains, cramp in the legs, varicose veins and varicose ulcers. Externally it may be used as a stimulation liniment for rheumatism and fibrositis. Due to its stimulating effect upon the lymphatic system, circulation and mucous membranes, it will have a role in the holistic treatment of many specific conditions.
Preparation and dosage: Infusion: pour a cup of boiling water onto 1-2 teaspoonsful of the bark and let infuse for 10-15 minutes. This should be drunk three times a day.
Tincture: take 2-4 ml of the tincture three times a day.

Stimulants for Different Parts of the Body

Each system of the body has plants that are particularly suited to it, some of which are stimulants. Here we shall see which remedies act in this way. How they can be used will be considered in the sections on each system.

By far the most important and all encompassing are *Cayenne* and *Ginger*. Please study these two to get a better picture of stimulants and their respective uses.

Circulatory system: This action must be used with care in cardio-vascular problems, though stimulation can often aid and support an ailing heart if used with knowledge. The stimulants *Bayberry, Ginseng, Prickly Ash, Rosemary, Rue, Wormwood* and *Yarrow* may affect this system.

Respiratory system: The diaphoretic chest remedies can be considered stimulant in action. Specifics would include *Angelica, Balm of Gilead, Benzoin, Eucalyptus, Garlic, Ground Ivy, Horseradish, Mustard, Peppermint, Sage, White Horehound* and *Yarrow.*

Digestive system: As already pointed out, the bitters may be considered as stimulants. We can mention *Balmony, Bayberry, Caraway, Cardamon, Cinnamon, Coffee, Dandelion Root, Galangal, Garlic, Gentian, Horseradish, Mustard, Peppermint, Rosemary, Rue* and *Wormwood.*

Urinary system: Bearing in mind the wide application of *Cayenne,* we can add *Eucalyptus, Gravel Root, Juniper, Yarrow.*

Reproductive system: Stimulants in this system usually act in the form of emmenagogues and so should be used with care during pregnancy. We can mention *Pennyroyal, Rosemary, Rue, Southernwood, Tansy* and *Wormwood.*

Muscles and skeleton: The vital role of both *Ginger* and *Cayenne* are reinforced here as stimulant to peripheral circulation. We can add *Mustard* and *Horseradish.* The rubifacient remedies are mostly stimulants.

Nervous system: Nervous stimulants include *Cola, Coffee, Tea* and *Mate.* The other plant stimulants of the central nervous system are illegal.

Skin: The rubifacients are stimulants and while being applied to the skin are not for the skin as such but to be absorbed by it. The vulneraries stimulate healing but are not stimulants as such.

STYPTIC

This is a term that is synonymous with an externally used astringent.

THYMOLEPTIC

This means a remedy that raises the mood and counteracts depression. Please refer to the section on the nervous system for more details.

TONIC

What is a Tonic?

These are plant remedies that either strengthen and enliven a specific organ or the whole body. They truly are gifts of Nature to a suffering humanity – whole plants that enliven whole human bodies, gifts of Mother Earth to her children. To ask how they work is to ask how life works. If anyone knows the answer to that one please let me know. . .

Examples

Nature is abundant in herbs that have a tonic action on the body. Thank God! Here we shall look at three tonics chosen almost at random. Most of the herbs mentioned in this book will work as tonics in the right time and place. The possible exception is Senna!

GOLDEN SEAL   *Hydrastis canadensis*
Part used: Root and rhizome.
Collection: Unearth root and rhizome from three-year-old plants in the autumn, after the ripening of the seeds. Clean carefully and dry slowly in the air.
Consituents: 5 per cent of the root consists of the alkaloids hydrastine, berberine and canadine; traces of essential oil; resin; fatty oil.
Actions: Tonic, astringent, anti-catarrhal, laxative, muscular stimulant, oxytoxic, bitter.
Indications: Golden Seal is one of the most useful herbs Nature has given us. It owes most of its specific uses to the powerful tonic qualities shown towards the mucous membranes of the body. Golden Seal will generally do you good. It is much used in all digestive problems, for example in gastritis, peptic ulceration and colitis. Its bitter stimulation gives it a role in loss of appetite. All catarrhal states benefit from Golden Seal, especially upper respiratory tract catarrh. The tonic and astringency contribute to its use in uterine conditions such as menorrhagia (excessive menstruation) and haemorrhage. With the additional stimulation of involuntary muscles, it is an excellent aid during childbirth, but for just this

reason it should be avoided during pregnancy. Externally it is used for the treatment of eczema, ringworm, pruritis (itching), earache and conjuctivitis.
CAUTION: As Golden Seal stimulates the involuntary muscles of the uterus, it should be avoided during pregnancy.
Combinations: In stomach conditions it combines well with *Meadowsweet, Marshmallow* and *Chamomile.* In uterine haemorrhage it is best combined with *Beth Root.* Externally as a wash for irritation and itching it combines well with *Marigold Petals* and distilled *Witch Hazel.* As ear drops it may be combined with *Mullein.*
Preparation and dosage: Infusion: pour a cup of boiling water onto ½–1 teaspoonful of the powdered herb and leave to infuse for 10–15 minutes. This should be drunk three times a day.
Tincture: take 2–4 ml of the tincture three times a day.

BLACK COHOSH   *Cimicifuga racemosa*
Part used: Root and rhizome.
Collection: The roots are unearthed with the rhizome in autumn after the fruits have ripened. They should be cut lengthwise and dried carefully.
Constituents: Resin, bitter glycosides, ranunculin (which changes to anemonin upon drying), salicylic acid, tannin, oestrogenic principle.
Actions: Tonic, emmenagogue, anti-spasmodic, alterative, sedative.
Indications: Black Cohosh is one of the valuable herbs that come to us via the North American Indians. Although widely applicable as a tonic, it has a most powerful action as a relaxant and a normalizer of the female reproductive system. It may be used beneficially in cases of painful or delayed menstruation. Ovarian cramps or cramping pain in the womb will be relieved by Black Cohosh. It has a normalizing action on the

balance of female sex hormones and may safely be used to regain normal hormonal activity. It is very active in the treatment of rheumatic pains, but also in rheumatoid arthritis, osteo-arthritis, in muscular and neurological pain. It finds use in sciatica and neuralgia. As a relaxing nervine it may be used in many situations where such an agent is needed. It will be useful in labour to aid uterine activity while allaying nervousness. Black Cohosh will reduce spasm and so aid in the treatment of pulmonary complaints such as whooping cough. It has been found beneficial in cases of tinnitus.

Combinations: For uterine conditions combine with *Blue Cohosh* and possible *False Unicorn Root.* For rheumatic problems use with *Bogbean* and *Willow Bark.*

Preparation and dosage: Decoction: pour a cup of water onto ½–1 teaspoonful of the dried root and bring to the boil. Let it simmer for 10–15 minutes. This should be drunk three times a day.

CENTAURY   *Centaurium erythraea*
Part used: Dried aerial parts.
Collection: The foliage should be collected at the time of flowering, which is from July to September. Dry it in the sun.
Constituents: Glycosidal bitter principles gentiopicrin and erythrocentaurine; nicotinic acid compounds; traces of essential oil; oleanolic acid and other acids; resin.
Actions: Bitter, tonic, aromatic, mild nervine, gastric stimulant.
Indications: It may be used whenever a digestive and gastric stimulant is required. It is indicated primarily in appetite loss (anorexia) when it is associated with liver weakness. Centaury is a useful herb in dyspepsia and in any condition where a sluggish digestion is involved.
Combinations: In dyspepsia it combines well with *Meadowsweet, Marshmallow Root* and *Chamomile.* In anorexia nervosa it is indicated with *Burdock Root* and *Chamomile.*

Preparation and dosage: Infusion: pour a cup of boiling water onto 1 teaspoonful of the dried herb and leave to infuse for 5–10 minutes. Drink one cup half an hour before meals.
Tincture: take 1–2 ml of the tincture three times a day.

Tonic Herbs for Different Parts of the Body

Each system of the body has plants that are particularly suited to it, some of which are tonics. Here we shall see which remedies act in this way for each of these systems. How they can be used will be considered in the sections on each system. By the nature of tonics we can only talk in general terms of those for each system. Most are interchangeable when it comes to their tonic action. However always take into account the broader picture of the individual herb's range of actions. It needs this breadth of vision to enable a coherent choice to be made.

Circulatory system: Here we can mention *Hawthorn Berries, Horsechestnut, Lime Blossom. Garlic, Ginseng, Mistletoe, Motherwort;*
Respiratory system: *Angelica, Aniseed, Boneset, Cayenne, Coltsfoot, Comfrey, Elecampane, Garlic, Golden Seal, Grindelia, Ground Ivy, Hyssop, Liquorice, Poke Root, Thyme, Yarrow.*
Digestive system: *Agrimony, Angelica, Aniseed, Balmony, Bayberry, Black Root, Boldo, Centaury, Chamomile, Comfrey, Condurango, Cranesbill, Dandelion, Fringetree, Garlic, Gentian, Golden Seal, Mugwort, Rue, Wormwood.*
Urinary system: *Bearberry, Buchu, Cleavers, Couchgrass, Gravel Root, Hydrangea, Parsley, Yarrow.*
Reproductive system: *Beth Root, Black Cohosh, Black Haw, Cranesbill, Damiana, False Unicorn Root, Golden Seal, Raspberry, Squaw Vine.*

Muscles and skeleton: Agrimony, Angelica, Black Cohosh, Bogbean, Boneset, Burdock, Comfrey, Nettles, Sarsaparilla, Wild Yams. *Nervous system:* Balm, Black Cohosh, Bugleweed, Damiana, Ginseng, Lady's Slipper, Lime, Mistletoe, Motherwort, Mug-wort, Oats, Skullcap, Vervain, Wood Betony. *Skin:* Burdock, Cleavers, Comfrey, Echinacea, Dandelion, Fumitory, Garlic, Golden Seal, Marigold, Mountain Grape, Myrrh, Nettles, Poke Root, Red Clover, Sarsaparilla, Yellow Dock.

VULNERARY

What is a Vulnerary?

These are herbal remedies that bring about healing in wounds or inflammation. The term is often used to describe herbs for skin lesions, but the action is just as relevant for wounds such as stomach ulcers. This is one of those actions that overlaps with others, for example, many astringents and demulcents are vulneraries, because of their properties in those actions.

How Vulneraries Work

Sometimes it is because of the presence of tannin producing an impervious layer, under which the natural healing process can occur. With others it is the soothing mucilage. In the case of *Comfrey* there is also a chemical called allantoin that stimulates cell growth and division. This will speed the healing of wounds and even, in some cases, bones.

Examples

As we have evolved within an environment ripe for damaging ourselves, it is only to be expected that Nature is rich in herbs that have a vulnerary action on the body.

Most of the best ones have already been described under different action, so please refer to them there:

Comfrey – demulcent
Chickweed – emollient
Elder – anti-catarrhal
Flax Seed – emollient
Golden Seal – tonic
Marshmallow – demulcent
Mullein – expectorant
Plantain – emollient
St John's Wort – nervine
Yarrow – diaphoretic
Cranesbill – astringent
Oak Bark – astringent
Burdock – alterative
Willow Bark – anti-inflammatory

Of the many others we could mention I shall include in this section a herb that could fit under many actions, *Marigold*.

MARIGOLD　　　　　*Calendula officinalis*
Part used:　Yellow petal (florets).
Collection:　Either the whole flower tops or just the petals are collected between June and September. They should be dried with great care to ensure there is no discolouration.
Constituents:　Saponins, carotenoids, bitter principle, essential oils, sterols, flavonoids, mucilage.
Actions:　Anti-inflammatory, astringent, vulnerary, anti-fungal, cholagogue, emmenagogue.
Indications:　Marigold is one of the best herbs for treating local skin problems. It may be used safely wherever there is an inflammation on the skin, whether due to infection or physical damage. It may be used for any external bleeding or wound, bruising or strains. It will also be of benefit in slow-healing wounds and skin ulcers. It

is ideal for first aid treatment of minor burns and scalds where local treatments may be with a lotion, a poultice or compress, whichever is most appropriate. Internally it acts as a valuable herb for digestive inflammations or ulcers. Thus it may be used in the treatment of gastric and duodenal ulcers. As a cholagogue it will aid in the relief of gallbladder problems and also through this process help in many of the vague digestive complaints that are called indigestion. Marigold has marked anti-fungal activity and may be used both internally and externally to combat such infections. As an emmenagogue it has a reputation of helping delayed menstruation and painful periods. It is in general a normalizer of the menstrual process.

Combinations: For digestive problems it may be used with _Marshmallow Root_ and _American Cranesbill._ As an external soothing application it can be used with _Slippery Elm_ and any other relevant remedy. A useful antiseptic lotion will be produced by combining it with _Golden Seal_ and _Myrrh._

Preparation and dosage: Infusion: pour a cup of boiling water onto 1–2 teaspoonsful of the florets and leave to infuse for 10–15 minutes. This should be drunk three times a day.

External use: See the directions in the section on Skin in Chapter 6.

Tincture: take 1–4 ml of the tincture three times a day.

4
AROMATHERAPY

The fragrance of flowers is one of their most wonderful gifts to humanity, and in recent years the healing value of this aroma has been increasingly acknowledged.

As with the very best of herbal medicine, the oils are beautiful things. Nature provides us with a healing that is aesthetic and uplifting even before you start using it! Whether it is looking at a flower, walking through a meadow or smelling an aromatic oil the subtler aspects of Gaia, of Nature, are at work healing and showing us how whole we really are.

It is plant oils that are the basis of the aroma and are called essential oils. Chemically each plant has an amazing array of different specific oils that combine to produce the unique quality of each type of flower. Research has shown that they have a distinct effect upon the mind as well as their anti-septic and other properties.

Aromatherapy, the use of essential oils, is a vast field and I would point anyone interested in a more in-depth look to see the books recommended in the Bibliography. Here we shall just briefly consider the oils that are commonly used.

The oils may be used for the whole spectrum of ills that befall us, from physical to mental and stress problems. Many oils have strong anti-septic and anti-bacterial properties. The application of *Chamomile* and *Lavender* oils to infected wounds can be as effective as the use of phenol. Eucalyptus sprayed in the air has a role in any sickroom. As examples of essential oils for psychological problems we can consider *Orange Flower* for anxiety, worry or insomnia; *Rose* for stress and depression (it also has a reputation for hangovers!); *Basil, Rosemary* and *Patchouli* can stimulate mental clarity, concentration and memory.

So many actions are represented here, and the oils can be approached in a similar way to that described in the previous chapter. However, they each have quite unique properties and so they are described briefly here.

Essential oils will be most effective if used as part of a whole health programme. The oils should *never* be used internally unless under the guidance of a skilled medical herbalist or aromatherapist.

Here we shall consider a selection of oils used in aromatherapy which are safe and easily available.

Basil: A refreshing and stimulating oil that

is a nerve tonic; it aids concentration and clarifies the mind.

Benzoin: Rich with a vanilla-like aroma. A warming and energizing oil that helps circulation, and may be used as an inhalation for laryngitis and upper respiratory problems.

Bergamot: An anti-depressant and gentle relaxant. As an antiseptic it can be used for acne, ulcers, cold sores and wounds. As an inhalation it helps with lung problems.

Black Pepper: A stimulating oil for muscular aches and bad circulation. It may be used in baths to stop 'flu symptoms developing.

Camphor: A first aid remedy as a cold compress for bruises and sprains. Will reduce swelling. A strong stimulant that should not be taken internally.

Chamomile: Soothing and calming for anxiety. For insomnia used in a late bath. Will relax muscles as well as being anti-inflammatory.

Cinnamon: Indicated in exhaustion, especially following infections such as 'flu. Will help digestion and stimulate the heart. It is a strong antiseptic and makes a good inhalation.

Clary Sage: A good relaxing oil with euphoric effects on sensitive people! May help with insomnia.

Clove: Helps lift mental and physical debility. As an antiseptic it may be used as an inhalation or on the skin. Renowned for treating tooth infections and pain.

Cypress: Good for 'flu and coughs as an inhalation. Will clear the sinuses. It makes a good massage oil for use around varicose veins. Will help in menstrual problems.

Eucalyptus: A strong anti-microbial oil that has many uses as an inhalation and direct skin application. An insect repellent.

Sweet Fennel: A good carminative that eases wind, hiccoughs, indigestion and colic. Has been used as a massage oil for cellulitis.

Frankincense: A spicy oil that often eases anxiety. Makes a good inhalation for respiratory problems.

Ginger: An effective stimulating rubefacient for rheumatic aches and pains. A good general tonic. Used in the bath it will help ward off infections and colds.

Hyssop: A mild sedative and general nerve tonic. Helps regulate blood pressure, whether high or low.

Jasmine: A wonderful aroma that is anti-depressant and supposedly a sensual stimulant. It eases pain in the whole of the female reproductive system.

Lavender: If you only get one oil, let it be Lavender! It relaxes and eases aches and pains. It has a whole range of positive physical actions but is especially useful for migraines and headaches.

Lemon: A good remedy for sore throats as gargle with 2 per cent oil to warm water. An antiseptic that can be used on insect bites and stings. Is used straight on warts and verrucas.

Lemongrass: An invigorating oil that cleanses oily skin.

Marigold: An excellent vulnerary (healing) oil. Will reduce inflammation, help chilblains and chapped or cracked skin. Excellent for bruises and burns.

Marjoram: Useful for anxiety, grief and insomnia as well as easing muscular, menstrual and rheumatic pains. May help in migraine. A very warming remedy.

Myrrh: A strong healer with antiseptic properties. It is anti-catarrhal and as an inhalation will help in most respiratory conditions.

Orange Flower Absolute: A beautiful strong aroma that is quite effective for anxiety and its associated symptoms such as palpitations. It will ease depression as well. Good for shock and fear.

Patchouli: A stimulant to the nerves that lifts anxiety and depression. Has a reputation as an aphrodisiac.

Peppermint: A good remedy for all digestive problems and nausea. Used in orthodox medicine for irritable bowel syndrome. May help ease migraine. An insect repellent.

Pine: Primarily an antiseptic oil, but helps clear the mind and of benefit in mental fatigue.

Rose: Very soothing for the nerves and an anti-depressant. It can calm anger and alleviate hangovers.

Rosemary: An invigorating oil which may stimulate a weak memory and general dullness. Helpful for headaches.

Sandalwood: A stilling and refreshing oil that eases anxiety and nervous tension.

Thyme: A powerful antiseptic that is also good for all kinds of debility.

Verbena: An excellent nerve tonic that eases and strengthens at the same time. For all anxiety problems, especially palpitations and dizziness. An insect repellent.

Ylang-Ylang: A sweet exotic scent that is supposedly aphrodisiac. It stimulates the senses and brings about a sense of well-being. It is good for anxiety, tension and anger.

How to Use Essential Oils

As already pointed out, essential oils should not be used internally, but that leaves a whole range of ways to reap the benefit of these wonderful oils.

MASSAGE OILS: These aromatic oils blend well with any bland massage oil. This gives the opportunity to experiment with what is most appropriate for you. An example would be 10–12 drops of essential oil to 20 ml of almond oil, or 60 drops to 100 ml of almond oil.

BATH OILS: Add 5–10 drops of oil to a full bath. This way you absorb through the skin but also by inhaling.

PERFUMES: Any of the pleasant fragrances may be used as perfumes, alone or blended.

VAPOURIZATION: Place a few drops on a heat source, such as a radiator or a small bowl of hot water. All the oils evaporate easily.

TOILET WATER: Take 3 drops of essential oil and add to 100 ml of distilled water. Keep the mixture in a dark air-tight bottle. This will keep fresh for a few weeks.

5
_ THE CHEMISTRY OF PLANTS _

All the way through this book, reference has been made to the constituents of our herbal remedies. To a pharmacist these are the 'active ingredients' of the plant, the chemicals that have a marked, definable physiological and therefore possibly medical activity upon the body.

These active ingredients are not of immediate interest to a medical herbalist, because the focus is on using whole plants for whole people. Knowing chemical components and the actions in isolation from the rest of the plant, does not tell us much of use about the activity of the plant itself. Examples of this have been given throughout the book. It is worth reviewing what has been said about the cardiac glycosides in *Lily of the Valley* as opposed to those in *Foxglove*; look also at the actions of *Meadowsweet* even though it contains salicylates and the potassium-rich balance of the diuretic *Dandelion Leaf.*

None of this denies the value of studying such plant's constituents, as long as it takes its place within a holistic context of therapeutics. The pharmacists' search for the 'magic bullet' had produced potent and effective drugs but caused much havoc in the process. The 'magic bullet' is a chemical, often of plant origin, that can be put into the body and directed at a specific site to do a specific biochemical job. This may be anti-inflammation as in steroids, the destruction of micro-organisms with antibiotics or even the easing of mental and emotional tensions with tranquillizers. All are effective and even life-saving drugs.

However, by the very nature of the 'bullet', it has to smash through to get to its desired place of activity. So we get side-effects – an almost unavoidable result of treating human illness as biochemical and pathological problems without perceiving broader contextual patterns. The list of drugs that could be named here is unfortunately long indeed. We need only mention thalidomide and the point is made. Human beings are not bags of organs with biochemicals sloshing around! The uniqueness of each person and their divine gift of self-healing can be acknowledged and worked with in medicine. This is one of the gifts of using whole plants for whole people rather than active ingredients taken out of their botanical context.

Plant Constituents

When plant constituents are considered in the herbal context it usually refers to the groups that are described below. Of course, plant chemistry includes the miracle of photosynthesis, plant respiration, structure, growth, development and reproduction. Much of the chemical basis of life is common to both plants and animals, an example being acetyl choline which is a neurotransmitter in animals and a growth hormone in plants. Other examples abound. The chemical Gamma Amino Butyric Acid (GABA), an important chemical in the human nervous system, has recently been found in *Mistletoe*. This provides a chemical basis for this herb's use in epilepsy and raised blood pressure.

A brief overview of the main medicinally active plant constituents is included here. For some herbalists such information is the vital basis of their work while for others it is almost irrelevant. It is a sign of the applicability of plant medicine that it can be used successfully in such different contexts. From a holistic perspective the whole of the plant must be respected as an integrated biologically evolved unit that is beyond the analytical comprehension of science. It will only be when science steps beyond the analytical, reductionist limits it has placed on itself that a deeper understanding of plant chemical synergy will emerge.

The brief details given here assume a certain degree of chemical knowledge and are included to give those with such a background a chemical perspective on our healing remedies.

Physiologically active plant constituents are usually classified by their chemical structure rather than specific actions. This convention will be followed here.

Acids

Weak acids, usually in the form of salts or esters, are found throughout the plant kingdom. The ripening process in fruit is the transformation of fruit acids to fruit sugars. They are chemically differentiated upon how many carboxyl (acid) groups are present in the molecule. The simplest kind are straight chained molecules with one carboxyl group called the monobasic acids. An example is an ester of Valeric acid from *Valerian*, used as sedatives in orthodox medicine. Formic acid, found in *Nettles*, causes the sting but can also be used in a stimulating ointment. The acids with a large number of carbon atoms (over twelve) are the basis of the poly-unsaturated and saturated fats that play such an important role in nutrition.

The polybasic acids contain more than one acid grouping and are a large group. Perhaps the best known is oxalic acid, found in *Rhubarb* and *Sheeps Sorrel*. Because of its property of causing calcium to come out of solution it can cause kidney stones.

Aromatic acids are common. In their simplest form, benzoic acid, they consist of a benzene ring and a corboxyl group. The whole family is large and medically important. They are important in the activity of *Gum Benzoic,* and the balsams of *Tolu* and *Peru*. These make good inhalants for upper respiratory catarrh and infections, bronchial problems and externally for infections and irritations.

Alcohols

An alcohol in chemical terms is a molecule that contains what is called a hydroxyl group or groups. It is a vast class that includes many oils and waxes as well as the more recognizable substances such as the ethanol in whisky! Some of the groups described below are, strictly speaking, alcohols, but their properties are due more to the shape of the rest of the molecule. The most interesting group are those found in the volatile oils, described below.

Carbohydrates

These are a basic part of nutrition, either as the carbohydrate in grain and potatoes, or as the roughage of plant material. The whole range of sugars, monosaccharides and polysaccharides, will not be considered here, but have a valuable role to play in a healthy diet. The pectins, complex polysaccharides, can be healing in gut problems such as diarrhoea and externally for ulcers and deep wounds.

The gums and mucilages are medically useful types of carbohydrate, both for their actions and in pharmaceutical preparations such as ointments and lozenges. The action they have on different systems of the body is described in the section on demulcents on p. 54 and their practical use in Chapter 8.

Phenols and Phenolic Glycosides

These are molecules where a benzene ring is combined with an alcohol (hydroxyl) group. However, they differ from the straight chained alcohols in being weakly acidic. The basic example is the well known antiseptic phenol. Most of this class share phenol's antiseptic activity as well as being anthelmintic and caustic. To enable bodily absorption, in nature they are usually combined with a sugar to make a glycoside.

A common and important example is salicylic acid, which is found free or as methyl salicylate in many plants. Examples that are widely used herbally are *Black Willow, Poplar, Black Haw, Wintergreen* and *Meadowsweet*. This is the basis of aspirin and a whole class of non-steroidal anti-inflammatory drugs. The chemical has a whole range of properties which, it must be stressed, are not necessarily those of the plants it is found in. Perhaps the best example of this is the stomach irritation caused by salicylates, which can even lead to stomach haemorrhage. In plants such as

Meadowsweet, however, the whole remedy can actually stop bleeding in the stomach. Thus the actions of a whole plant *cannot* always be predicted from a knowledge of the ingredients.

Other actions of this group of chemicals include a fever-reducing action as well as a general anti-inflammatory effect. This is now know to be due to an anti-prostaglandin and bradykinin action which would appear to explain also the use of salicylates as anti-blood-clotting agents. In addition they increase the volume and concentration of bile. Externally they are rubefacient. Thus it is a generally useful chemical that proves quite safe when used in its natural plant context.

Of the many examples found in the plant kingdom we can mention eugenol from *Cloves* that helps in toothache. Thymol from *Thyme* and other aromatic remedies, is a useful antiseptic and anti-fungal oil.

Tannins

These widely found chemicals are described in more therapeutic detail in the section on astringents. Plants that act as astringents beause of their tannin content are described in that chapter. A diverse range of tannins are found that are classified by structural differences that do not concern us here.

Coumarins and their Glycosides

The coumarins are not well studied but are best known for their use in perfumery because of their 'newly mown hay' aroma. An excellent example of this is *Sweet Woodruff*. Recent research shows that they have a role to play therapeutically as anti-clotting agents. Coumarins are the basis of the anti-coagulant drug warfarin. Coumarin itself also has anti-bacterial actions and is the basis of the use of *Mouse-eared Hawkweed*. Other examples are umbelliferone found widely in the Umbelliferae family; aesculetin in *Horse Chestnut*; herniarin in *Rupturewort* and *Lavender*.

Anthraquinones and their Glycosides

These plant constituents have been long known to chemistry as the basis of the purgative and dyestuff properties of some plants. Anthraquinone or its close chemical relatives are usually found in plants as a glycoside, that is combined with a sugar. Plants containing such chemicals include *Senna, Yellow Dock, Turkey Rhubarb* and *Purging Buckthorn*.

The direct action of the anthraquinones on the gut may cause griping pains and these plants are often used in conjunction with carminatives to relieve such pain. It is for this reason they should never be used in constipation due to spastic colon. They would cause much pain and discomfort.

Flavones and Flavonoid Glycosides

A widely found group of phenolic compounds that get their name from the Latin word 'flavus' for their usual colour yellow. A list of plants containing this group would be enormous. It has been estimated that about 50 per cent of flowering plants contain flavonoids in their leaves.

This diverse chemical family has much of therapeutic value to offer humanity. They include anti-spasmodics, diuretics, heart and circulatory stimulants. Perhaps the best known flavonoids are what used to be called vitamin P, the bioflavonoids. It has been found that in nature vitamin C is never found without the bioflavonoids. By themselves they decrease capillary permeability and fragility while also reducing elevated blood pressure. Examples such as rutin from *Buckwheat*, can be used to strengthen capillaries and reduce tendencies to easy bruising. Bear in mind that yet again we have a situation where a chemical used in isolation will only give of its best when used

as nature provides it – in combination and with the synergy of the whole plant.

Volatile Oils

A universally recognized gift of plants to humanity is their aroma. In some spiritual traditions stages of inner attainment are characterized by the perfume that pervades the consciousness – wonderful things indeed. These plant aromas are given them by the volatile oils present. Not only do they provide sensory upliftment, but valuable medicines.

Any discussion of volatile oils should be many pages long. They are complex and fascinating in the extreme. It would be impossible to give them the treatment they deserve here. This is but a taste of the wealth of healing power inherent in the oils. Their therapeutic use is considered in Chapter 4 on aromatherapy and throughout the sections on body systems in Chapter 6.

Chemically they tend to be mixtures of oxygenated hydrocarbons and their polymers, all or multiples thereof, and alcohols. The monoterpenes have been well studied because they are used extensively in perfumery as are other volatile oil components such as pinene, geraniol, borneol, cineol, limonene and thujone. The list is very extensive.

A volatile oil from a specific plant will be a blend of a whole range of such component plants. Nature shows our perfumiers how to do their job!

Without getting into specifics it is possible to identify general areas of volatile oil activity. They can be strongly antiseptic, anti-fungal and insect repellent. Some can have the effect of increasing white blood cell formation and so increase resistance to infection. They act on the whole of the nervous system, being anti-spasmodic and relaxing. Externally some oils are warming, anti-inflammatory and may reduce itching, while others can be strongly rubefacient.

Saponins

This is an important class of plant chemicals for the pharmaceutical industry as it includes the natural precursors of sex-hormones, steroids and heart drugs. The name comes from the Latin 'sapo' meaning soap because of the property of plants containing them to froth up when in water solutions. In fact, *Soap Wort* is called Saponaria botanically.

They are extremely complex chemical structures that differ from each other in where on the basic framework of carbon atoms smaller groups are attached. They have been divided by the pharmacologists into steroidal and tri-terpenoid saponins depending on structural differences. To explore the saponins adequately would mean delving into organic chemistry far more than a book like this justifies. Briefly we can mention the steroidal saponins in *Wild Yam, Yucca, Beth Root, Fenugreek* and *Foxglove.* In many of these plants the saponins appear to fulfil the role of precursors of female sex hormones. The implications of this is discussed in the section on the reproductive system in Chapter 6. The new interest in the adaptogenic plants such as *Ginseng* focuses partly on the steroidal glycosides present.

A good example of tri-terpenoid saponins are glycyrrhizic acid and glycrrhizin found in *Liquorice.* These have a strengthening effect upon the adrenal gland as they mimic the activity of adrenocorticotrophic hormone (ACTH). This is implicated in many stress problems. Other valuable tri-terpenoid saponins are found in the lung remedies *Primrose, Senega* and *Blood Root. Horsechestnut leaves* also contain such constituents as do *Figwort, Golden Rod* and *Chickweed.*

Cardioactive Glycosides

These are specific steroidal saponins that have a marked action on the heart. Their mode of activity and use are discussed in the section on the circulatory system in Chapter 6.

They are far more widely found in nature than the usually recognized heart herbs *Foxglove* and *Lily of the Valley.* In addition we can mention *Mediterranean Squill, Figwort* and *Strophanthus.*

Cyanogenic Glycosides

This is a group of potentially lethal glycosides because on hydrolysis they yield prussic acid. They are the basic native poisons. However, some of the plants that contain milder examples are important medically, such as *Wild Cherry Bark, Almond, Elder* and *Red Clover.*

'Bitter Principles'

These are a vital part of herbal practice and are discussed therapeutically in the section on bitters on p. 44. Chemically they are a diverse group of chemicals that includes monoterpenes called iridoids, sesquiterpenes and a whole range of others that have a bitter taste.

In addition to the broad general actions of bitters described in the relevant chapter, certain bitters have quite distinct properties that can be related to their 'bitter principles'. Some are relaxing nervines, such as *Valerian* and *Hops. White Horehound* has pulmonary and expectorant actions while two good anti-inflammatories are *Bogbean* and *Devil's Claw.* The role of the 'bitter principles' here goes beyond the range of this book, but there can be no doubt that these chemicals play a vital role in Nature's healing work.

Alkaloids

This is an old term for vegetable alkali that covers a wide range of potent plant constituents. Fundamentally they are nitrogen-containing molecules that have a marked effect upon animal and human physiology. They are wonders of plant activity having little role in the life of the plant but profound effects on humanity and other animals. They can be interpreted as biochemical evolution and integration at work – a very real example of the links that bind all of nature.

These amazing chemicals have given humanity a range of natural products that include major painkillers, poisons and perhaps most potentially important the whole range of consciousness-expanding plant material.

The classification and differentiation of chemicals as diverse as nicotine, strychnine, caffeine and mescaline is beyond this book, but well worth exploring further.

6
BODY SYSTEMS

THE DIGESTIVE SYSTEM

Its Function and Role in Health and Wholeness

The health, integrity and proper functioning of the whole digestive system is fundamental to all life processes. Not only are we what we eat, but we are also what we are able to assimilate. If the digestive system is not breaking down and absorbing food properly, then the body will not be able to reap the rewards of a healthy diet. This makes a healthy gut almost a pre-requisite of a healthy life.

Herbal remedies are uniquely appropriate for healing and toning the digestive system, not just because they have a specific applicability, but as we appear to have evolved as plant eaters, they obviously work directly on the lining of the gut itself. As we shall see, this brings the unique qualities of the remedy directly to the place where it is needed.

However, the key to a healthy digestive system is healthy living in general and not simply taking the right herbs. This means a good diet, right lifestyle and ease in general.

This can be difficult to achieve, but then that is what health and wholeness is about!

In this book we are not concentrating on details of diet, relaxation techniques or counselling, but on how to use herbs. If the whole spectrum was considered in an integrated way we would end up with an encyclopaedia. Diet is vital and specific diets will be considered where necessary, but a good balanced wholefood diet is the foundation upon which all else is built.

What is a Good Diet?

Without creating a rigid dogma about 'natural foods' it is known that unrefined foods without man-made 'improvements' (colourings, stabilizers, pesticides and growth hormones) make up a good diet. There are countless dietary regimes which fall into this vague definition, and different people benefit from different foods. No one school of thought has the only truth so if you are looking for a set of guidelines on healthy diet, do just that and look! Read books, compare conflicting claims, talk to people and form your own conclusions. Nowadays most health food stores and bookshops have a selection of recipe books and books on nutrition.

Yet it can be said that in our culture and in this last quarter of the twentieth century, one will not go far wrong with approximately 30 per cent of raw vegetables in the diet, 20 per cent lightly cooked or steamed vegetables, 30 per cent complex carbohydrates (unrefined cereals or starchy vegetables like potatoes) and 20 per cent protein. The small amount of fats which are essential to health are well represented in many of these groups. Protein such as dairy, seafood or game contain saturated fats, while raw avocado is a good source of unsaturated fats. If cold-pressed vegetable oil is used over all those raw salads of different vegetables, that will also provide them. Protein need not be animal in origin. Some people thrive on a Vegan diet.

The exact form your own healthy diet will take is up to you. Equally important is your consciousness, for without your own caring attention, will you have the patience to scrutinize labels and eschew inappropriate items posing as food?

General Suggestions

The way we eat affects the digestion of food. Eating should be a time of ease and peace. Here are some suggestions.

1. Small meals should be taken at regular intervals, every 2 or 3 hours if possible.
2. Eat your meals slowly and chew your food carefully.
3. Avoid rush and hurry before and after meals. Try to arrange a short rest before and after eating.
4. Sufficient sleep at night is important; aim at 8 hours.
5. Remember that anxiety and worry can upset digestion.
6. Avoid large and heavy meals, fried food

and anything that disagrees with you.
7. Never smoke or drink before meals.
8. Drink only sparingly during meals but take plenty of fluids _between_ meals.

Herbs and the Digestive System

Herbal medicine offers not only potent and valuable remedies to put right digestive 'disease', but also tonics and normalizers that can help prevent problems developing. The question of how they can do this job of healing and strengthening is often unanswerable, either because no research has been done or because they work in a way that is more subtle than our scientists' method can perceive. In the hands of a skilled medical herbalist, there is little that cannot be achieved in digestive illness. Here we can talk only in generalities, as each person is unique. For example, each stomach ulcer will have a different set of factors to take into account.

Here we shall consider the actions that are most commonly called for and then look at how the herbs can be used for easing general patterns of digestive dis-ease and some specific illnesses.

Actions

Rather than thinking in terms of specific herbs or combinations for certain conditions, it is more fruitful in general to consider appropriate herbal actions. Of course there are specific herbs that may be right for specific people, but as a way to gain experience and insight, working with actions provides a solid foundation.

Some authorities speak of the action termed a 'stomachic'. This is a description that covers all herbal remedies that will aid and support the stomach and digestive process. It is so broad that you can consider most of the following plants as stomachic.

Demulcents

We have defined a demulcent as a plant rich in mucilage that soothes and protects inflamed and irritated tissue. With the way that many people abuse their stomachs with bad food, alcohol and swallowed tobacco tars, it may be obvious why this action can be so broadly helpful.

The soothing action of plants such as _Comfrey root, Marshmallow root_ and _Slippery Elm_ can help with conditions along the whole length of the gut. They can be freely used with little fear of side effects. The chapter on demulcents explains their mode of action.

Bitters

Bitters are of paramount importance in the toning of the digestive system. Please refer to the section on bitters in Chapter 3 where their mode of action on the digestive tract is explored in some depth. They provide the herbalist with remedies that tone and normalize the digestive process and so can help in the whole gamut of health problems by improving nutritional absorption. These remedies help the body to get the most out of the food eaten by stimulating the secretion of digestive enzymes from all the organs involved.

Of special importance for this system are _Wormwood, Gentian, Golden Seal_ and _Rue._ Milder Bitters that may be of value here include _Yarrow_ and _Centaury._ In addition to the herbs described in the chapter on bitters, _Golden Seal_ and _Centaury_ are discussed under 'Tonics', while _Yarrow_ is under 'Diaphoretics'.

Astringents

Because of the tannins contained in these plants, they cause the surfaces of tissues to be contracted while secretions or discharges are reduced. This makes astringents of great value in conditions of the gut that include diarrhoeal states in their symp-tom picture. Similarly with inflammatory conditions or even where there is bleeding, astringents can be most helpful. How they work is described in Chapter 3 where _Agrimony, Oak_ and _Cranesbill_ are especially mentioned. Amongst the astringents that can also be most helpful in the gut we can mention: _Bayberry, Bistort, Meadowsweet, Pilewort, Tormentil, Witch Hazel_ and _Yarrow._

Of course all the remedies that are astringent may be used for digestive problems but this range is especially good. In addition to those mentioned in the chapter on astringents and below. _Bayberry_ is discussed under stimulants, _Yarrow_ under diaphoretics and _Witch Hazel_ in the section on the skin.

MEADOWSWEET   _Filipendula ulmaria_
Part used: Aerial parts.
Collection: The fully opened flowers and leaves are picked at the time of flowering, which is between June and August. They should be dried gently at a temperature not exceeding 40°C.
Constituents: Essential oil with salicylic acid compounds called spiraeine and gaultherin; salicylic acid; tannin; citric acid.
Actions: Anti-rheumatic, anti-inflammatory, stomachic, antacid, antemetic, astringent.
Indications: Meadowsweet is one of the best digestive remedies available and as such may be used in most conditions if they are approached holistically. It acts to protect and soothe the mucous membranes of the digestive tract, reducing excess acidity and easing nausea. It is used in the treatment of heartburn, hyperactivity, gastritis and peptic ulceration. Its gentle astringency is useful in treating diarrhoea in children. The presence of aspirin-like chemicals explains Meadowsweet's action in reducing fever and relieving the pain of rheumatism in muscles and joints.

Preparation and dosage: Infusion: pour a cup of boiling water onto 1–2 teaspoonsful of the dried herb and leave to infuse for 10–15 minutes. This should be drunk three times a day or as needed.

Tincture: take 1–4 ml of the tincture three times a day.

PILEWORT (Lesser Celandine)
Ranunculus ficaria
Part used: The root.
Collection: The root should be unearthed during May and June.
Constituents: Anemonin, proto-anemonin, tannin.
Actions: Astringent.
Indications: As one would expect from the name, Pilewort is almost a specific for the treatment of haemorrhoids (or piles). For this condition it can be taken internally or made into a very effective ointment. It may also be safely used wherever an astringent is wanted.
Combinations: Pilewort combines well with *Plantain, Witch Hazel, Marigold* or *Agrimony* for the internal treatment of piles.
Preparation and dosage: Infusion: pour a cup of boiling water onto 1–2 teaspoonsful of the dried herb and leave to infuse for 10 minutes. This should be drunk three times a day.

Ointment: The ointment is best made in vaseline as described in Chapter 8.

Tincture: take 2–4 ml of the tincture three times a day.

Carminatives

These aromatic, pleasant herbs are usually rich in volatile oils and through the stimulation of the gut walls by these oils, there is an easing of the natural movement of the bowels and relaxation of over-activity and tension.

These are amongst the most familiar herbs as they are often those used in cooking in alcoholic drinks. In the section on this action in Chapter 3 we have explored *Fennel, Ginger* and *Caraway,* while *Aniseed* is described under 'aromatics', *Peppermint* under 'anti-cattarrhal', *Chamomile* as an 'anti-inflammatory', *Cayenne* as a 'Diaphoretic', *Lavender* and *Vervain* as 'Nervines' and *Balm* as an 'Antemetic'. These plants are often the source of the oils used in aromatherapy.

Carminatives can be safely used for the relief of colic and wind, but of course these symptoms must be seen as pointers to some cause. It may be physical, dietetic or tension, amongst many others. So with the wide range of remedies with this action we can choose those with any other actions called for in that unique individual's problems. An example is *Sweet Flag* which is not only carminative but also useful in treating excess stomach acid.

SWEET FLAG
Acorus calamus
Part used: Dried rhizome.
Collection: The rhizome should be harvested between September and October. A fork may be needed to extract it from muddy soil. Free the rhizome from leaves and root and clean it thoroughly. Halve it along its length and dry it in the shade.
Constituents: Mucilage, up to 3 per cent volatile oil, bitter principles, glycoside, tannin.
Actions: Carminative, demulcent, antispasmodic.
Indications: Sweet Flag combines demulcent effects of the mucilage with the carminative effect of the volatile oil and the stimulating effect of the bitters. It is thus an excellent tonic for the whole gastro-intestinal tract. It may be used in dyspepsia of all kinds, in gastritis and gastric ulcers. It will stimulate a flagging appetite and help to ease exhaustion and weakness when there is a digestive involvement. It may be considered a specific in colic due to flatulence.
Combinations: In flatulent colic it com-

bines well with *Ginger* and *Wild Yam*. In gastric conditions, it is best combined with *Meadowsweet* and *Marshmallow*.

Preparation and dosage: Infusion: pour a cup of boiling water onto 2 teaspoonsful of the dried herb and leave to infuse for 10–15 minutes. Drink a cup half an hour before meals.

Tincture: take 2–4 ml of the tincture three times a day.

Anti-spasmodics

These are remedies that ease the muscular spasms that lead to the colic pains that are commonly associated with digestive upsets. Simply using such remedies will rarely 'cure' anything; however the relief of pain is often thankfully received!

Cramp Bark and *Black Haw* have been described in the section on 'anti-spasmodics' in Chapter 3. Relaxant nervines such as *Valerian* and *Hops* may act in this way. A specific for the colon is *Wild Yam* described under 'anti-inflammatory'. The carminatives can relieve colic pain, especially *Chamomile* and *Peppermint*. *Hops* make a good relaxing carminative, although not in the form of beer: (see 'hypnotics' in Chapter 3).

Aperients and Laxatives

These remedies that relieve constipation are of much less value than is commonly thought. It is always best to ease such problems by dietary change, exercise or relaxation than by using external triggers. In the short run, of course they are most effective but if not used with discretion they will become more of a crutch than a help, with the body becoming dependent on them for normal motions to occur.

When longer term use is indicated then it is best to either use the bulk laxatives or the liver remedies that help the body to produce and release bile.

Hepatics and Cholagogues

These liver remedies often act as a core of many different herbal treatments for quite diverse illnesses. This reflects the approach of holistic treatment of aiding the body's own innate healing process. Herbalism can aid in cleansing and 'detoxifying' in ways that orthodox medicine cannot. Liver and pancreatic problems are discussed below, but the so-called liver herbs have a wide application. Many of them are also digestive bitters, but others work specifically on this most vital of organs.

As already described under 'hepatics', we can include *Dandelion Root, Boldo* and *Milk Thistle*. *Vervain* is described under 'nervine tonic' while the cholagogues *Balmony, Fringetree* and *Golden Seal* herbs find wide applicability.

Nervines

As there is often a close connection between our state of mind/feelings and the digestive process, nervines may often help in any holistic treatment. The expression having 'butterflies in the stomach' aptly shows the connection. Many nervines are also carminative or anti-spasmodic. In this broad context there is little point trying to be specific about nervine herbs other than those mentioned under other actions above.

Other Actions

While the actions and herbs mentioned are often those that are most indicated for the digestive system, by the very nature of the way the body is such an integrated miraculous whole, any other action may be right in any specific case. This may sound very vague but perhaps we have been conditioned by scientific rationality to expect specifics where there aren't any . . .

Anti-microbials can often be of value as may diuretics. While there is much specific advice given in herbals, from individual herbs to prescriptions, the wisdom of nature and plants is still beyond us all. Let us approach ourselves and our plant brethren with humility and discrimination. When it comes down to it, who knows other than God.

Using Remedies for the Digestive System

The health and integrity of the whole digestive tract is basic to all health and well being. With herbal remedies we have the possibility of safely treating most illnesses that might arise, but of much deeper significance is the preventative possibilities that open up.

Specific conditions will be discussed below, but it is more important to see how herbs can work with diet and general attitudes to ensure a well-integrated process of digestion and assimilation. In this way we can be well on the way to being whole and at ease with life.

As has already been pointed out, a well-balanced natural diet, rich in green vegetables and the right amount of fibre is vital to health. Inappropriate food may well block any attempt either to be well or regain health. Much digestive upset is due either to straight indigestion or to a more insidious food allergy. It is beyond the range of this book to explore this field adequately, but many excellent publications are now available.

In addition to correct diet (which may vary from person to person), one's state of mind and intensity of emotion have a direct impact on the digestive system. Relaxation and an easy approach to eating, taking time and enjoying what is being eaten, can often do as much as taking herbal teas!

Digestive symptoms need not be a sign of some pathological disease, but rather that of a functional under- or over-activity. Such functional problems can be corrected simply by using the wisdom of the herbs to normalize and return the gut to the harmonic miracle of integration it is.

It is not always possible to find the most appropriate herb for a person with wind or indigestion simply by looking it up in a book, but with a combination of skilled choice, intuition and the herbs themselves the problem can usually be cleared.

There are certain symptoms that are associated with a whole range of specific diseases that as symptoms can be cleared with herbs. We are blessed with remedies that work. This is a two-edged sword as the body is showing the symptoms to guide us to the cause. Suppression of symptomatic pain or diarrhoea can be dangerous. Skilled diagnosis is essential at all times.

Let's look briefly at these common symptoms:

Constipation: This will often be relieved by increasing the amount of fibre in the diet. This is best when in the form of natural vegetable or grain fibre rather than fibre supplements. Given that the diet is appropriate, the first herbal stage would be to use aperients and hepatics to aid the natural processes via the liver. Herbs to consider here would be *Dandelion, Yellow Dock* or *Rhubarb Root.* Of course, there are many more that could be used as gentle agents. *Butternut* can be a slightly stronger agent that is safe to use.

The next step for short-term use would be the stronger laxatives that work by stimulating the walls of the gut through chemical components. The best known of these is *Senna.* While being effective they can cause a form of colonic dependency if used for too long. This is to be avoided as the tone of the bowel is lost and there is then the need to retrain the bowel with bulk laxatives such as *Psyllium Seeds* and *Flax.* This is a long and involved process that should be supervised by a skilled medical herbalist.

A combination of herbs with supportive actions can tone the bowel to aid its natural functioning. Some herbalists have called such mixtures 'Lower Bowel Tonics'. They can take many forms but here is one example that can be mixed and taken as an infusion before going to bed:

Dandelion Root	2 parts
Yellow Dock	2 parts
Senna	1 part
Liquorice	1 part
Ginger	1 part

By studying the actions of these herbs you will see why they combine so well and augment positive properties and balance unwanted ones such as griping.

Diarrhoea: Mild or short term looseness of the bowels is often the body's way of clearing potentially dangerous material in the gut. If it is more long standing, then skilled diagnosis is essential. A herb that is especially relevant in mild diarrhoea and is safe for children is _Meadowsweet._ Other astringent remedies can then be tried in increasing strength such as: _Cranesbill, Agrimony, Bayberry, Bistort, Oak Bark._ These are but suggestions.

It is a good idea to become familiar with the herbs in your area and get to know which is the best astringent. For example, in parts of West Wales, in addition to the British herbs just mentioned, one of the commonest wild flowers is _Tormentil,_ an excellent and safe astringent that could be used in diarrhoea. In East Anglia or Australia it would be entirely different. Don't be dependent on herb suppliers!

Pain: Any severe abdominal pain is a warning sign to get to a skilled diagnostician, whether orthodox or herbal, as soon as possible. The colic-type pain of indigestion can often be cleared with herbs, but check that it is indigestion and not something else. Removal of symptoms can often mask problems that could be cured if found early enough. Herbs to think of here would be the carminatives, anti-spasmodics or possibly nervines.

Diseases of the Gastro-intestinal System

Take a look at any good medical textbook and you will see that a vast range of syndromes and specific diseases can be identified in the gut, from the mouth to anus. This book is not designed to be a training manual for herbal doctors. It is a guide to how to use plant remedies and ways to explore further their wealth of opportunity.

In this chapter we shall look at some conditions in depth to give an insight to the broader approach, while for other named diseases there will just be a brief outline. This does not belittle the importance of each condition, but is simply an acknowledgement of the limitations of this book.

The Mouth

The hygiene and wellbeing of the mouth is basic to the health of the rest of the system – if there are infections, the toxins and bacteria will be swallowed continually. The stomach acid is partially for the killing of such swallowed organisms, but if the teeth and gums are regularly attended to by a good dentist, then much that could go wrong is avoided. Wrong diet or lack of vitamin C will directly affect the mouth.

Infections of the gums such as gingivitis and the much more serious pyrrohoea can be treated herbally by a combination of internal and external medication. A wash or direct application of anti-microbials such as _Echinacea_ and _Myrrh_ are of great help, especially if combined with an astringent. _Krameria_ has an excellent reputation for this purpose, but is difficult to obtain. Any other may be used though. The common weed *Silverweed* can be very useful here. Internally the emphasis is on alternatives and anti-microbials that help the lymphatic system and the liver as well as their primary job of helping defend against infection. Herbs that are most useful include *Echinacea, Cleavers, Poke Root* and *Myrrh*. Of course these suggestions have to be seen in the context of that person's unique needs.

Mouth ulcers are a common problem with causes that range from ill-fitting dentures, through stomach problems to stress. The cause must be identified but the symptom of mouth ulcers can effectively be treated with high dosage vitamin B complex and C combined with a regular mouthwash of *Red Sage*. An internal treatment to cleanse the body will not go amiss..

RED SAGE   *Salvia officinalis*
Part used: Leaves.
Collection: The leaves should be gathered shortly before or just at the beginning of flowering in dry sunny weather in May or June. Dry in the shade or not above 34°C.
Constituents: Volatile oil including 30 per cent thujone, 5 per cent cineole, linalol, borneol, camphor, salvene and pinene; a bitter; tannins; triterpenoids; flavonoids; oestrogenic substances; resin.
Actions: Carminatives, spasmolytic, antiseptic, astringent, anti-hidrotic.
Indications: Red Sage is the classic remedy for inflammation of the mouth, throat and tonsils, its volatile oils soothing the mucous membranes. It may be used internally and as a mouthwash for inflamed and bleeding gums, inflamed tongue or generalized mouth inflammation It is an excellent remedy in mouth ulcers. As a gargle it will aid in the treatment of laryngitis, pharyngitis, tonsilitis and quinsy. It is a valuable carminative used in dyspepsia. It reduces sweating when taken internally and may be used to reduce the production of breast milk. As a compress it promotes the healing

of wounds. Red Sage stimulates the muscles of the uterus and so should be avoided during pregnancy.
CAUTION: Avoid during pregnancy.
Combinations: As a gargle for throat conditions it combines well with *Tormentil* and *Balm of Gilead*. In dyspepsia it can be combined with *Meadowsweet* and *Chamomile*.
Preparation and dosage: Infusion: pour a cup of boiling water onto 1–2 teaspoonsful of the leaves and let infuse for 10 minutes. This should be drunk three times a day.
Mouthwash: put 2 teaspoonsful of the leaves in half a litre of water, bring to the boil and let stand, covered, for 15 minutes. Gargle deeply with the hot tea for 5–10 minutes several times a day.
Tincture: take 2–4 ml of the tincture three times a day.

Peptic Ulcer

A peptic ulcer is a breach or defect in the lining of the upper part of the gut. Ulcers can occur in the first part of the small intestine (duodenal ulcers), in the stomach (gastric ulcers) or in the gullet (oesophageal ulcers). By far the commonest symptom of all these ulcers is pain followed by heartburn. The condition may not be as advanced enough to cause ulceration but may lead to inflammation which will lead to some of the symptoms. Herbally these can be approached in the same way.

Many people with a gastric ulcer find that food will aggravate their pain, while those with a duodenal ulcer often find their pain is relieved by eating and brought on by hunger. In both cases the pain is almost always eased by milk or antacids. However it is not unusual for someone to have 'typical' symptoms without there being an ulcer present.

The origin of peptic ulcers is suprisingly complex and somewhat puzzling, and appears to be different for each type of The strong acid in the stomach plays a leading role. The stomach normally produces a strong acid to aid digestion but protects itself by secreting a coating of mucous.

Food neutralizes stomach acid and it is during periods of stressful work on an empty stomach that the acid begins to damage the lining of the stomach. This will start ulcer formation. Alcohol, and particularly spirits drunk on an empty stomach, will further damage the stomach lining. Smoking affects the stomach in at least two ways, by increasing acid formation and interfering with the secretion of mucus, and by tiny amountgs of swallowed tar and nicotine directly irritating the lining. Smoking contributes to ulcer formation and slows down their healing.

A number of drugs will aggravate or even cause stomach ulceration. The commonest problem relates to aspirin and the anti-inflammatory drugs used in arthritis. As a general guideline, anyone suffering from indigestion or other stomach problems should avoid anything which contains aspirin or any drug which contains the word 'salicyl...' in the name of its components. It's worth pointing out that originally this group of chemicals was extracted from the bark of Willow. The Latin genus name is *Salix* and hence the chemical was called salicylic acid. *Willow bark*, however, does not cause the problems just mentioned.

Psychological factors may influence the workings of the stomach either directly through the vagus nerve (the stomach nerve) or by hormones and other biochemical factors. The effects of mood on gastric acid secretion are clear. People with duodenal ulcers tend to respond to the sight and smell of food with greater acid secretion than do others. There is no doubt that stress, anxiety, and depression are all pivotal in these digestive conditions.

Treatment

Psychological factors may not be para-mount in the causation of ulceration, but there can be no doubt that due care and attention to them will speed up healing and reduce the likelihood of relapse. Bed rest helps not only because it leads to a reduction of gastric acid secretion, but also in the way in which it allows the person to get away from a stressful environment. Successful healing must take into account stress, anxiety and depression as well as purely physical factors. Psychotherapy may have a lot to offer in helping the person review and re-evaluate their lifestyle and life purpose. At the very least the use of relaxation techniques to bring ease into one's life will soften the impact of the problem greatly.

Diet

The basis of dietary advice for peptic ulcers is the need to avoid anything that will act as an irritant. These may be chemical or physical.

Chemical irritants will include acid foods such as vinegar and pickles, any form of alcohol, cigarette smoking, fried and roast food, fizzy drinks, any rich sauces and sweet things. All of these will increase the impact of the stomach acid on the lining and so aggravate the ulcer.

Physical irritants will include too much roughage and extremes of temperature. Even though the virtues of a high fibre diet are unquestionable, if there is a peptic ulcer present it might act as sandpaper. Where an active ulcer is present it is best to be on a low or medium fibre diet. Forget about the F plan! Any drink or food that is too hot or too cold will also irritate and cause pain.

Herbs

The basis of treatment is initially calming down irritation and then promoting the healing of any damaged tissue with demulcent and vulnerary remedies. As we have seen, a wealth of such herbs is available, each of which acts in a slightly different way. The following are examples:

Marshmallow root: a demulcent rich in mucilage which coats the ulcer and calms down any inflammation present.

Comfrey root: another soothing demulcent and vulnerary remedy rich in mucilage, but also containing the chemical allantoin which stimulates the healing of wounds. This is the basis of its reputation as the paramount wound herb.

Meadowsweet: a natural antacid that acts to reduce the impact of excess acid formation in the stomach.

Slippery Elm: one of the best soothing remedies that is still freely available in chemist shops.

Other remedies that may prove useful are *Sweet Flag, Liquorice Root, Irish Moss* and *Iceland Moss.*

A particularly useful remedy because of its renowned tonic and healing action on mucous linings is *Golden Seal.*

Astringent remedies can often speed up the process of healing in these conditions, with *Comfrey, Cranesbill* and *Agrimony* coming to mind.

As already pointed out, anxiety and tension have a direct impact on the stomach and digestion in general. The nervine herbs have a lot to offer, and especially those from the *Peppermint* family (the Labiates) that also contain aromatic oils that settle the digestive system.

Lemon Balm: a wonderfully gentle relaxing herb that is quite safe to use regularly. It will also relieve wind and some sorts of indigestion.

Chamomile: a gentle relaxing nervine that will ease tension and at the same time act as an anti-inflammatory herb. A remedy that is applicable for all nervous problems of digestion.

Valerian: a stronger relaxing nervine that

because of its strong aromatic (though unpleasant) oil, also helps settle wind and indigestion.

Other relaxing herbs that can help are *Skullcap, St John's Wort, Pasque Flower, Hops* and *Passion Flower.*

From all of this it is possible to work out a prescription that will aid the person on many levels at once. Work out for yourself why this following mixture can be helpful. While giving an example here, it is purely theoretical and I guess that each person must be approached as a unique individual with unique needs.

Comfrey Root	2 parts
Marshmallow	2 parts
Golden Seal	1 part
Valerian	1 part

Mix together and make a decoction; drink three times a day or when needed.

Irritable Bowel Syndrome

This is a very common complaint that is also callen spastic colon or nervous bowel. It is characterized by colicy pain, which usually occurs in the lower abdomen, a tendency to alternate between diarrhoea and constipation, distension of the abdomen, wind and sometimes heartburn. It may come and go over a very long period of time and is often aggravated by stress and tension.

There are conflicting theories about the causes of this problem, but it appears to have a lot to do with a lack of fibre, or roughage, in the diet. This means that by the time the remnants of food reach the colon (large intestine), after the gut has absorbed the nutrients out, there is not enough bulk to enable it to be moved towards the back passage. Instead of small muscular contractions required to squeeze a large bulk down the colon, it has to squeeze very tightly to propel a small bulk. This leads to muscular spasms and so causes pain. The lack of bulk produces either diarrhoea or small hard stools.

With the muscular spasms going on, any stress causing tension and anxiety will amplify the spasms and aggravate the pain. In fact stress may just be the extra factor needed to cross the pain and discomfort threshold in the first place.

Treatment

From what has been said it is clear that herbs to help stress and reduce muscular spasms, in addition to a change in diet and a more relaxed approach to life, are the basis of treatment. Relaxation, yoga and meditation have a lot to offer here. A re-evaluation of the person's relationships, work and life purpose will often provide insights that if acted upon will remove the health problem.

Diet

Sometimes the simple addition of more roughage to the diet will alleviate the problem, but it is possible to aggravate it if too much bran, or its equivalent, are used too quickly. The increase in fibre is best achieved through eating plenty of green vegetables, salads, fruit and wholemeal bread. It may be appropriate to add bran to breakfast cereal or eat it as bran biscuits. While being a dry, tasteless and boring food it can be made palatable by mixing it with other food. Three tablespoons daily is enough.

Herbs

Nature provides us with remedies that relax the gut as well as soothing the digestive process, in addition to the herbal relaxing nervines for the nervous system itself: _Chamomile, Hops, Wild Yam, Fennel, Peppermint._

The more specifically relaxing remedies should also be considered. These include _Valerian, Skullcap_ and many discussed elsewhere in the book.

This can be a difficult problem to beat, but herbal medication is one of the best techniques for it.

Colitis

The colon is the site for a whole range of difficult health problems. These include colitis, ulcerative colitis and many others such as the less common problem called Crohn's disease. The symptoms may include attacks of constipation or diarrhoea which contains blood and mucous, associated with pain. Attacks are often precipitated or made worse by stress.

Treatment

Treatment in these colitis conditions should not be undertaken by unskilled people. Herbal remedies have much to offer in the easing of gut problems. If these are used in the context of working with any anxiety and other psychological patterns then there is much hope in this distressing and intransigent problem.

The core of a herbal approach would be based on astringents, demulcents, antispasmodics, carminatives and antimicrobials. While such cases necessitate a skilled medical herbalist, think about which herbs from these gorups may be useful and why. An antimicrobial that is especially valuable in such problems is garlic which is described in the section on the respiratory system on p.128.

Piles

It is difficult ending this brief review of digestive system disorders without referring to the healing properties of the herb _Pilewort_ in the treatment of Piles, as an ointment and as an internal remedy. Internally it works well if used with _Horse Chestnut_ and externally if mixed with _Witch Hazel._

Liver and Pancreas

These most vital organs of the body are part of the digestive system as a whole. Liver disease and pancreatic disorders call for skilled herbal attention, but there is some advice that can be given here.

The milder hepatics, cholagogues and bitters can be used in many diverse conditions for helping and supporting the action of the liver. It is worth becoming familiar with the uses and actions of *Dandelion Root, Vervain, Balmony,* and *Milk Thistle.*

The value of *Milk Thistle* in healing liver damage is becoming increasingly recognized. For gallbladder problems, assuming that correct diagnosis has been obtained, the following are of great value in aiding that much abused organ: *Balmony, Fringetree Bark, Dandelion Root.*

THE CARDIO-VASCULAR SYTEM

The plant kingdom has much to offer in the prevention and treatment of the ills that effect the circulatory system. As has been said repeatedly, there are limitations to self-help and this diagnosis and correct usage of the plants enables much to be done, but needs skilled herbalists. But there is still much that can be done in the way of self-help and this we shall explore here.

The heart and circulatory system can, on one level, be viewed as a straightforward mechanistic set-up. Blood is pumped around and it does its job. On other levels we have a profound symbol of human life and the vital force that pumps through our veins. In all cultures the heart is a symbol of feelings, of love, of the ineffable – not of hydraulic pumps!

In treating these problems holistically we have to include a perception of subtler aspects of the person's life and nature. This goes beyond the herbal remedies that are indicated and into a wider sphere. Herbal remedies not only provide a valid therapeutic tool but also link us with the planet that is our source and foundation. In a way, our taking herbs as medicine is linking in with the planetary circulatory system.

In this chapter we shall briefly review what is known of herbal action on the heart, which actions can help in this system and look at certain specific problems.

How do the Remedies Work?

Much research has gone into the mode of action of potent herbal heart remedies. This power shows in the still pre-eminent place that *Foxglove* plays in orthodox treatment of heart failure. There is a range of plants that contain active ingredients called cardiac glycosides.

A glycoside is a chemical made of two parts, an active 'aglycone' which is often a steriodal base, combined with a sugar. This combination makes a biologically absorbable entity that will get the active bit into the body with ease. This structure was not designed by a Nobel Laureate but is a produce of nature – evolutionary integration at work!

The cardiac glycosides are those in which the aglycone acts on the heart. There are many other glycosides that do not concern us here. The group is characterized by a wide range of chemical structures; subtle differences in shape or position of various chemical radicles have a profound effect on the action of the heart. Thus some of the cardiac glycosides are poisonous and were discovered by western science through their use as arrow poisons in various parts of the world. Others are relatively safe because their structures control the rates at which they are absorbed and used up by the body. In fact, the sugar part can be as critical to availability of the aglycone to the heart as the specific activity of the aglycone itself.

How they act on the heart is a miracle of efficiency. Through an effect on potassium and sodium levels intracellularly, there is an increase of the action of calcium on muscles causing muscle contraction. The biochemistry of this is complex. The result of all of this is a twofold action on the heart itself. First there is a so-called 'inotropic' action of increasing the power of contraction, and secondly a 'chronotropic' action of slowing and normalizing excessive heart rate.

This has a total effect of increasing the efficiency of the heart beat so that cardiac output per unit of oxygen consumed is much improved. It is this effect which may be life saving in conditions such as congestive heart failure. Nature does indeed know what we need. This effect was not duplicated by drugs for many years.

A whole range of plants has cardiac glycosides naturally present but only a handful are used therapeutically. Of these the medical profession favours *Foxglove* while medical herbalists prefer *Lily of the Valley*. The reasons for this are worth exploring. Due to the sort of structural differences referred to above, the glycosides in *Lily of the Valley* have less potential for cumulative poisoning, as must be guarded against using *Foxglove*. This is partly due to the main component of the cardiac glycoside fraction of *Lily of the Valley* being more water soluble and therefore excreted more readily. Also, a lower dose of the plant has a proportionally greater activity than *Foxglove* because other less active components, such as convallatoxol, are metabolized into the active convallatoxin as it is needed. So we have an extended effect from each dose. This guards

against potential dangers. More can be said about this but it would become exceedingly technical. The research has been done and borne out in herbal practice. *Lily of the Valley* has equal status in the Official Pharmacopoeias of Russia, Hungary and Poland.

Other herbal remedies act on the circulatory system but without containing cardiac glycosides. Usually the claims made by herbal practitioners have not been examined by researchers and so we have little scientific understanding of how they work. This does not mean they don't do it! One important exception is the cardiotonic *Hawthorn Berries*, which has been well researched.

Due to flavonoids and other constituents it has the effect of gently dilating the arteries of the heart and others in the body. The importance of this in angina and arteriosclerosis is clear. In a complex way it has the paradoxical effect of stimulating coronary circulation while easing the intensity of heart overactivity. It has properties that lower raised blood pressure yet increase low blood pressure. It normalizes rather than moving in any specific direction. Published research in the *British Medical Journal* shows that it helps lower blood pressure due to arteriosclerosis and kidney disease while also supporting the heart in cases of heart disease. Here is a herb that has been described as 'heart food'.

Actions for the Circulatory System

The remedies that have most direct effect on the heart itself are the cardiac tonics. While their mode of action has been reviewed above, please refer to the section on them in Chapter 3. From the list here please refresh your memories as to their specific actions where they are individually described: *Lilly of the Valley, Hawthorn Berries, Broom, Motherwort, Bugleweed, Figwort*.

The last two may be a bit of a surprise. *Bugleweed* has its main use in the treatment of the thyroid gland while *Figwort* is thought of as a 'skin' remedy. However, both have an action on the heart that must be taken into account.

Diuretics are often vital in the treatment of this system as water retention is a common accompanying symptom. *Lily of the Valley* can act as a diuretic in cases of heart failure as it enables the heart to beat with more strength, so more blood passes through the kidney and thence more water is removed. Of the more general diuretics we can mention *Dandelion Leaf, Broom,* and *Yarrow.*

The value of *Dandelion* here lies in its high potassium content as well as the diuresis it produces.

Circulatory stimulants can have a large role to play. This group of remedies are also called peripheral vasodilators as they cause the aterioles and capillaries to dilate. This is what happens when someone blushes. The effect is to improve the heat and oxygen getting to the outer surfaces of the body and so help in bad circulation, cramp and even high blood pressure. Review *Cayenne, Ginger, Prickly Ash, Mustard, Rosemary* and *Horseradish.*

Nervines and anti-spasmodics are often useful.

Conditions of the Circulatory System

There is no way that the whole range of heart and circulatory problems can be adequately discussed in a book of this sort. As has been said, heart problems need skilled attention, and what is said here does not replace that. But it must be said that in the hands of a skilled medical herbalist problems such as angina pectoris, heart failure and arteriosclerosis are treatable.

We shall consider heart disease, blood pressure problems, anaemia, poor circulation and varicose veins.

Heart Disease

Here we shall talk in general terms rather than about specific syndromes. The advice given covers many heart problems.

The blood which supplies oxygen and food to the heart moves through the coronary arteries which encircle the heart. If these arteries become narrowed, the blood supply is restricted and may become insufficient. The narrowing usually is due to the deposition on the walls of the blood vessels of a fatty substance called atheroma. If the blood supply is inadequate when an extra load is put on it, for example, during exercise or in cold weather, the person may have an angina attack. That is a gripping pain across the chest and sometimes into the neck and jaw or down one or both arms. When the exercise is stopped and the extra demand reduced, the pain will pass in a couple of minutes.

Anxiety, fear and stress may bring on such attacks as there is an increase in adrenaline and noradrenaline release at such times. These hormones increase the work of the heart, making it beat faster. The pain experienced is itself so that the person will become afraid of having an attack, the heightened anxiety making one more likely.

A heart attack occurs when the blood supply to the heart muscle is abruptly stopped. It is often due to clotting in a coronary blood vessel. As we shall see, stress can contribute to this. The details are not entirely clear but stress factors increase the stickiness of the blood and make it more likely to clot.

The origins of these common problems are complex and confusing. Some of the factors involved are well known and can lead to clear guidelines for possible prevention, but simplistic statements about saturated fats or jogging can be misleading. The search for factors that contribute to the scourge of heart disease has highlighted diet, socio-economic conditions, psychological and behavioural characteristics and life events.

Food

Whole forests have been turned into pulp to provide paper for the articles about cholesterol, poly-unsaturated fats and heart disease. Anyone trying to read them all or even follow the broad arguments, will get very stressed from the disagreements!

It is clear that heart disease has definite links with too much fat in the diet, raised blood cholesterol, raised blood pressure, smoking, obesity, short stature and underactivity. The precise role each of these factors plays is unclear but general guidelines about a possible preventative diet appear.

Something that is certain is the involvement of fats. While the so-called saturated fats may be worst, it seems that it is an over-preponderance of all fat in the total diet that is to blame.

In this book we shall not explore specific diets in much depth, but these ideas are basic to heart problems.

● Animal fats and cholesterol-rich foods should be kept to a minimum. These include red meat, dairy products and eggs.
● An absolute minimum of salt. Ideally don't add any salt to food, either in cooking or on the table.
● DON'T SMOKE!
● Excessive alcohol should be avoided.
● Generally avoid becoming overweight.
● Avoid refined food, white sugar and white bread, and artificial additives of any kind.

Personality

An association between a particular type of personality and heart disease has been suggested. There is a difference in the risk of developing heart disease between two types of behaviour; these are called type A and type B.

Type A behaviour is characterized by a chronic sense of time-urgency, aggressiveness which may be repressed, and striving for achievement. Type A people will often drive themselves on to meet deadlines, many of which will be self-imposed. There are feelings of being under pressure of time and responsibility, often doing two or three things at once. They are likely to react with hostility to anything that seems to get in their way and are temperamentally incapable of letting up. They are liable to think of themselves as indispensable. All of which adds up to a state of constant stress!

Type B behaviour is the opposite of these characteristics. They are less preoccupied with achievement, less rushed and generally more easygoing, not allowing their lives to be governed by a sense of deadlines. They are less prone to anger and do not feel constantly impatient, rushed and under pressure. They are also better at separating work from play and know how to relax.

Studies done over an 8½ year period with a group of type A and type B people showed that there was a 31 per cent increased risk of developing heart disease in type As.

There is much debate on the methods for assessing type A and B behaviour. The important insight is the association of types of behaviour with disease development. However, there are *not* two types of people! Everyone is an individual, and while people can always be fitted into artificial categories, these categories do not identify them.

Treatment

The treatment of heart disease must be undertaken by a skilled practitioner. To do the best that is possible it is essential, however, that the sufferer of the condition be involved in its treatment. This might sound like a truism, but unfortunately we have become isolated from our own healing process by the very expertise of the doctors and even the herbalists.

This is especially so when the emotional and mental aspects are considered and from a holistic perspective it is obvious that the psychological aspects of treatment and recuperation must be taken into account. It comes as no surprise that a great reduction in the chance of any repeat occurrence of the attack or the development of complications follows the management of psychological and social problems.

Ways of dealing with tension and anxiety must be found that will suit the person involved. There are many different ways of relaxing and not all of them suit everyone. Treatment should be based on a broad reappraisal of lifestyle and life goals, not simply in medical approaches to the illness. Diet, exercise, relaxation, meditation, etc. are all potentially appropriate.

Herbs

Herbal remedies have a lot to offer in the treatment, prevention and alleviation of heart problems. It must be stressed, however, that any herbal treatment of the heart must be undertaken under the supervision of a well-trained medical herbalist, especially if the heart is already being treated with drugs.

There are a number of remedies that have a direct action on the heart itself. These include the following: _Broom, Hawthorn Berries, Lily of the Valley, Lime Blossom_ and _Mistletoe._ These have all been discussed elsewhere except _Broom._

BROOM TOPS   _Sarothamnus scoparius_
Part used: Flowering tops.
Collection: May be gathered throughout

spring, summer and autumn. The tops may be dried in the sun or by heat.
Constituents: Alkaloids including spartein and cystisine; flavonoid glycosides; tannin; bitter principle; volatile oil.
Actions: Cardioactive diuretic, hypertensive, peripheral vasoconstrictor, astringent.
Indications: Broom is a valuable remedy where there is a weak heart and low blood pressure. Since it is also a diuretic and produces peripheral constriction of the blood vessel while increasing the efficiency of each stroke of the heart, it can be used where water retention occurs due to heart weakness. Broom is used in cases of overprofuse menstruation.
Combinations: Broom can be combined with _Lily of the Valley_ and _Hawthorn Berries_ when treating the heart.
CAUTION: Do not use Broom in pregnancy or hypertension.
Preparation and dosage: Infusion: pour a cup of boiling water onto 1 teaspoonful of the dried herb and let infuse for 10–15 minutes. This should be drunk three times a day.
Tincture: take 1–2 ml of the tincture three times a day.

You will notice that I have not included the well-known heart herb _Foxglove._ In modern medical herbalism this is considered too poisonous as described above and is only used under certain circumstances. It should never be used in the home.

Lime Blossom is especially helpful when used with the main Cardio-tonics such as _Hawthorn Berries,_ for reasons described below under 'Blood Pressure'.

A whole range of herbs can be used to aid and support the heart through generally helping the body by their actions elsewhere. Diuretics are valuable to help any build-up of water in the body. _Dandelion Leaves_ are especially indicated as they are so rich in potassium, a mineral that is essential to people under treatment for heart problems.

There is much that can be done with herbs to help the anxiety and tension that accompanies and contributes to heart problems. The nervine tonics and relaxants can all play a role in such cases, but one which has particular relevance where the heart is affected by stress and anxiety is *Motherwort*. This can be specific for nervous palpitations. Other remedies in this large group that may prove useful include the following: *Balm, St John's Wort* and *Skullcap*. Remember, however, that different remedies may suit some people more than others. They are safe, so try them out.

Blood Pressure

Blood pressure is the pressure created by the heart pumping the blood around the body. As the heart contracts in its beat, the blood pressure in the arteries increases quite abruptly and as the heart relaxes again, the blood pressure drops to about two-thirds of its peak value.

There are always two figures for blood pressure because it is measured at its highest (the systolic) and lowest (the diastolic) points. Peaks of high blood pressure are usually reached several times during the day, but are transient in most people. However, in people with raised blood pressure, these abnormal levels are maintained. There are health risks involved if either the systolic or diastolic pressures are constantly raised.

Periods of stress in people's lives are often associated with a rise in blood pressure. With most people the blood pressure will return to normal if the stress is removed, but with some people this is not the case. If the blood pressure rise has been severe and prolonged, changes can take place in the arteries which result in raised blood pres-

sure being maintained even after the stress has been reduced or removed.

High blood pressure is associated with many other effects. When the pressure is up the heart must pump harder and so is under more strain. This may lead to the oxygen supply to the heart becoming insufficient, which will result in an angina attack. Hardening and narrowing of the arteries becomes much more likely. This may in turn produce heart attacks and strokes as the high pressure can burst blood vessels, resulting in brain haemorrhage. In extreme cases this may lead to the kidneys becoming affected to the point of kidney failure. From all of this it is clear why high blood pressure is a major health risk, liable to cut down life expectancy considerably.

Blood pressure may become high without any symptoms at all. It is often discovered during routine medical checkups. It may be heralded by headaches, dizziness, palpitations or unexplained fatigue.

Treatment

To treat raised blood pressure effectively there needs to be a reappraisal of lifestyle, diet, degree of relaxation and medicines used.

Life style: It is important in the reduction of high blood pressure for the person to learn how to recognize and control stress in their lives. A re-evaluation of lifestyle and life goals may be called for, and is often far more effective than any medical treatment, whether herbal or chemical. Relaxation exercises and possibly meditation have a lot to offer.

Diet: There is commonly a dietary connection in the elevation of blood pressure. The broad approach described for heart problems should be the basis for a diet to combat or prevent high blood pressure. There are some quite specific additional suggestions. Salt should be avoided completely in the food of anyone with blood pressure problems. It should not be used in cooking or added to food on the table. Milk, butter and cheese may contribute to the problem and it is worth cutting them out of the diet completely for at least one month to see if there is a change in the condition. This change will not only show in the blood pressure reading, but as an improvement in the general state of well being. Oily foods and fats should be avoided.

Herbs

As high blood pressure can be caused by a whole range of factors, from stress and anxiety to kidney failure, there are many herbs that can be used with benefit. There are a number of remedies that have a quite specific role in the normalizing of blood pressure. There are two which always come to mind: *Hawthorn Berries* and *Lime Blossom*.

Hawthorn is discussed above and in the section on 'Cardiac tonics', here we shall review *Lime Blossom*.

LIME BLOSSOM   *Tilia europea*
Part used: Dried flowers.
Collection: The flowers should be gathered immediately after flowering in the mid-summer. They should be collected on a dry day and dried carefully in the shade.
Constituents: Essential oil containing farnesol; mucilage; flavonoids; hesperidin; coumarin fraxoside; vanillin.
Actions: Nervine, anti-spasmodic, diaphoretic, diuretic, mild astringent.
Indications: *Lime Blossom* is well known as a relaxing remedy for use in nervous tension. It has a reputation as a prophylactic against the development of arteriosclerosis and hypertension. It is considered to be a specific in the treatment of raised blood pressure associated with arteriosclerosis and nervous tension. Its relaxing action combined with a general effect upon the circulatory system give *Lime Blossom* a role

in the treatment of some forms of migraine. The diaphoresis combined with the relaxation explain its value in feverish colds and 'flu.
Combinations: In raised blood pressure it may be used with *Hawthorn* and *Mistletoe,* with *Hops* or other relaxing nervines in nervous tension and with *Elder Flower* in the common cold.
Preparation and dosage: Infusion: pour a cup of boiling water onto 1 teaspoonful of the blossoms and leave to infuse for 10 minutes. This should be drunk three times a day. For a diaphoretic effect in fever, use 2–3 teaspoonsful.
Tincture: take 1–2 ml of the tincture three times a day.

A herb that has a long tradition of use in high blood pressure is *Mistletoe.* Its use has come under scrutiny recently because of potential dangers. These dangers have been exaggerated and a generation of experience cannot be gainsaid.

MISTLETOE   *Viscum alba*
Part used: Dried leafy twigs.
Collection: The young leafy twigs should be collected in the spring.
CAUTION: The berries are poisonous.
Constituents: Viscotoxin (a cardio-active polypeptide); triterpenoid saponins; cholins; histamine; 'anti-tumour' proteins.
Actions: Nervine, hypotensive, cardiac depressant, possibly anti-tumour.
Indications: It is a relaxing nervine that has a wide range of uses. It acts directly on the vagus nerve to reduce heart rate while strengthening the wall of the peripheral capillaries. Because of this it will lower high blood pressure and ease the effects of arteriosclerosis. It can help in a nervous quickening of the heartbeat and will ease headaches due to high blood pressure.
Combinations: For high blood pressure it may be used with *Hawthorn Berries, Lime Blossom* and *Yarrow.*

120

Preparation and dosage: Infusion: pour a cup of boiling water onto ½-2 teaspoonsful of the dried herb and leave to infuse for 10-15 minutes. This should be drunk three times a day. The tincture may be used at a dose of 1-2 ml three times a day.

There may be associated water retention or the suspicion of such, in which case gentle herbal diuretics have a role to play. Whenever medicines are used to help the body get rid of water it is always necessary to ensure that there is a supplement of potassium. If this is not seen to, there may be a potentially dangerous depletion in this vital mineral. With herbal remedies we can take care of this by using nature's best natural diuretic, *Dandelion leaf.* This will get rid of excess water build-up but there will be a net increase in potassium in the body. Another diuretic that is particularly useful for the circulatory system is *Yarrow.*

A wealth of herbs to relax both psychological as well as physical tension are available to us. It is worth emphasizing again that the relaxants described here will not replace the development of a more relaxed, less stressed approach to life. The key is being at ease. This is but a partial list of the possible herbs that could be used: *Cramp Bark, Motherwort, Wood Betony, Valerian* and *Skullcap.*

Having said all of this it is possible to suggest the outlines of a combination of herbs that is effective in reducing raised blood pressure. If you have followed the discussion so far and reviewed the herbs mentioned you will see the value of a combination like this. However, each person is different and it is unique individuals that have hypertension, so the mixture must be moulded to their needs.

Hawthorn Berries	2 parts
Lime Blossom	2 parts
Yarrow	2 parts
Mistletoe	1 part
Wood Betony	1 part

Of the nervines that could have been used here, *Wood Betony* was chosen as it will ease headaches due to raised blood pressure. *Cramp Bark* can be of great service here as well. *Garlic* eaten daily, preferably raw, has a deserved reputation as a remedy for lowering blood pressure.

CAUTION: Do not use *Broom* in high blood pressure as it may raise it even more.

Having pointed out that possible herbal danger I must stress that the herbs mentioned in this section are safe and will not produce a rebound low blood pressure. They will normalize to an optimum for the person concerned.

Low Blood Pressure

This problem does not carry with it the long-term dangers that hypertension does; however, it is distressing and worth sorting out. Of course any underlying cause must be sought. If there is no clear-cut reason found it can be related to debility and exhaustion.

Herbally we can strengthen a debilitated body while toning the circulatory system. This will usually return the blood pressure to normal levels. *Broom* is especially indicated here; part of its action is due to a constriction of peripheral blood vessels. This has the effect of gently raising the blood pressure because of a slightly reduced volume in the whole system. Any treatment should include the cardiovascular tonic *Hawthorn.* Nervine tonics and bitters can often have a role to play. This is one time that stimulants such as *Kola* can be most useful. Herbs to consider are: *Broom, Hawthorn Berries, Oats, Kola, Gentian* and *Wormwood.*

Anaemia

Anaemia is a complex subject that we cannot adequately cover here. But, simply, because of the reduction in iron in the blood-stream there is a reduced ability to carry oxygen. However, the reasons for this are diverse indeed and can range from blood loss to blood chemistry to infection to genetic problems. So again I must stress the importance of accurate diagnosis. Anaemia is a symptom, not a disease. The cause must be sought and that treated. Having said that, herbs and diet can aid in the supply of iron and help the body metabolize it healthily.

Iron supplements are notorious in producing constipation. There are vegetables that are rich in this mineral and include: *Parsley, Nettles, Apricots* and *Pumpkin Seeds.*

Another natural source is a good full-bodied red wine such as Beaujolais. However, there are obvious problems with using this as an iron supplement!

For non-vegetarians meat and fish will provide a certain amount of iron, especially liver. However, if the cause of the anaemia is rooted in absorption problems in the gut then a simple supplement will be of no use whatsoever.

Herbally the use of bitter remedies will aid the digestive process and stimulate the body's natural processes. Herbs to consider include: *Gentian, Condurango* and *Wormwood.*

Bad Circulation

This can be a real problem for some people in cold weather, where the blood going to the body's extremities does not warm them enough. It can be painful and lead to cramping. The stimulants and vaso-dilators will help in conjunction with vessels' tonics, but causes must be sought. Consider: *Cayenne, Ginger, Prickly Ash* and *Hawthorn.*

Where chilblains have developed, an application of *Cayenne* powder or an ointment of that herb will locally increase circulation and so improve the condition. Don't do this if there are any cuts or cracks – It is simply too painful!

Varicose Veins

These are often a complication of circulatory problems and can have their root causes in the lower abdomen where pressure from the child in the womb, a prolapse or hip misplacement, can lead to a restricted flow of blood into or out of the legs. Assuming that such causes have been looked for, and they often aren't, exercise is of great help to get the thigh muscles pumping and the blood returning into the trunk. The feet should be raised whenever sitting as this gets gravity working in the right direction for you.

Herbs can help by toning the walls of the vessels and getting the strength back. We can mention *Hawthorn Berries, Horsechestnut* and *Buckwheat.*

Diuretics will help remove the water build-up that often accompanies this problem, but remember this is symptomatic relief only. Use *Yarrow* and *Dandelion Leaf.*

The stimulants mentioned in the previous section can help as can gentle aperients and laxatives as it is essential that constipation be avoided. All the above herbs are described elsewhere except for *Horsechestnut*, which follows.

HORSECHESTNUT
Aesculus hippocastanum
Part used: The fruit, that is the Horsechestnut itself.
Collection: The ripe chestnuts should be gathered as they fall from the trees in September and October.
Constituents: Saponins, tannin, flavones, starch, fatty oil, the glycosides aesculin and fraxin.
Actions: Astringent, circulatory tonic.
Indications: The unique actions of Horse-

chestnut are on the vessels of the circulatory system. It seems to increase the strength and tone of the veins in particular. It may be used internally to aid the body in the treatment of problems such as phlebitis, inflammation in the veins, varicosity and haemorrhoids. Externally it may be used as a lotion for the same conditions as well as for leg ulcers.

Preparation and dosage: Infusion: pour a cup of boiling water onto 1-2 teaspoonsful of the dried fruit and leave to infuse for 10-15 minutes. This should be drunk three times a day or used as a lotion.

Tincture: take 1-4 ml of the tincture three times a day.

If there is surface irritation, a sensation of burning or discomfort, a lotion of distilled _Witch Hazel_ and _Hawthorn Berries_ will usually help.

Varicose ulcers are a common and very difficult problem. Their treatment is not simply one of external applications around the ulcers to promote healing, but internally to get things moving again in the face of circulatory stasis in the lower limbs. This is difficult to do and should be done in conjunction with a qualified medical herbalist.

THE RESPIRATORY SYSTEM

Its Function and Role in Health and Wholeness

The clear and open flow of breath in our bodies is one of the keys not only to health but to a deep experience of wholeness. There is a technique of meditation that focuses attention on the free flow of the tides in and out of the chest, and at the 'right' moment poses the question – 'who is the breather?'.

The ebb and flow of life, prana or breath provides us with a direct experience of the vitality and dynamism of our world. All that lives breathes, and we partake of this planetry lung whenever we inhale and give to it with each exhalation. Our oneness with the whole in action!

But what do we do with this miracle. We smoke, have cars, oil-fired power stations, acid rain, and all manner of air-borne pollutants. A very sorry state for the planetary lung, but even more for our own!

The best preventative measure against lung disease is clean air, which of course means cleaning it up and changing our social lifestyle. The implications of all of this are wide, but if you have asthma, don't just take medical steps – join Friends of the Earth!

The health and vitality of the lungs is not only important for the body to obtain its oxygen, but the lungs are also a pathway of excretion. Even if _Garlic_ is rubbed into the soles of the feet, the absorbed oil will be smelt on the breath within twelve hours! If someone has a chest disease then there will be extra pressure on the other organs of elimination. If this is taken into account herbally by supporting the kidneys etc., the lungs have some of their excretory load removed and can recover faster. Similarly, promoting respiratory health may be appropriate in digestive or skin problems. How this is done we shall see below.

The lungs are prone to infections, allergies, pollution, dietary overload as well as the more inherent auto-immune and genetic problems. A vast field which we shall only review here. As has been stressed throughout the book, competent diagnosis is essential and for more complex problems herbal advice should be sought from a qualified medical herbalist.

Herbs and the Respiratory System

Not only does herbal medicine offer valuable remedies to put right respiratory 'disease', but also tonics and normalizers that can help prevent problems developing. The question of how they do this job of healing and strengthening is often unanswerable, either because no research has been done or that they work in a way that is subtler than our methods can perceive. In the hands of a skilled medical herbalist, there is little that cannot be achieved in respiratory illness. Here we can only talk in generalities as each person is unique and each person with asthma will have a different set of factors to take into account.

Here we shall consider the actions that are most commonly called for and then see how the herbs can be used for easing general patterns of respiratory dis-ease and some specific illnesses. There will be much overlap here with the section on 'Ear, Nose and Throat'.

Actions

Rather than thinking in terms of specific herbs or combinations for certain conditions, it is more fruitful in general to consider appropriate herbal actions. Of course, there are specific herbs that may be right for specific people, but as a way to gain experience and insight, working with actions provides a solid foundation.

Expectorants

This action has been discussed in general in its own section in Chapter 3 but here we shall explore it in a more differential way. The classic definition of expectorant is a remedy that stimulates the removal of phlegm from the lungs. This is the result, but it can be achieved in a number of ways. The extremes are a stimulation of the lungs

and that expels the phlegm through coughing, or an easing of tissue tension allowing a loosening of the phlegm and letting the body's own reflexes remove it. This may be by coughing or movement to the back of the throat for swallowing. This differentiation can often be difficult to make with all herbs as many of the excellent remedies we have can, paradoxically, work in both ways when the need arises.

A good example of a stimulating expectorant is *Ipecacuanha*, which is described in the section on 'Emetics' in Chapter 3. It is a common finding with these strong remedies that if they are used at too strong a dose they will cause vomiting, as the mechanism in the body is not too dissimilar.

Most of the remedies that act as useful expectorants do act in between the two extremes. Good examples are *Coltsfoot, White Horehound, Mullein, Aniseed, Hyssop, Angelica, Sweet Violet, Elecampane* and *Bloodroot.*

There are more that will be described later. Of those just mentioned all have been looked at other than *Angelica* and *Hyssop,* which follow.

ANGELICA   *Angelica archangelica*
Part used: Roots and leaves are used medicinally, the stems and seeds are used in confectionery.
Collection: The root is collected in the autumn of its first year. If it is very thick it can be cut longitudinally to speed its drying. The leaves should be collected in June.
Constituents: Essential oils including phellandrene and pinene, angelica acid, coumarin compounds, bitter principle, tannin.
Actions: Carminative, anti-spasmodic, expectorant, diuretic, diaphoretic.
Indications: This herb is a useful expectorant for coughs, bronchitis and pleurisy, especially when they are accompanied by fever, colds or influenza. The leaf can be

used as a compress in inflammations of the chest. Its content of carminative essential oil explains its use in easing intestinal colic and flatulence. As a digestive agent it stimulates appetite and may be used in anorexia nervosa. It has been shown to help ease rheumatic inflammations. In cystitis it acts as a urinary antiseptic.

Combinations: For bronchial problems it combines well with _Coltsfoot_ and _White Horehound_; for indigestion, flatulence and loss of appetite with _chamomile._

Preparation and dosage: Decoction: put a teaspoonful of the cut root in a cup of water, bring it to the boil and simmer for two minutes. Take it off the heat and let it stand for 15 minutes. Take one cup three times a day.
Tincture: take 2–5 ml of the tincture three times a day.

HYSSOP   _Hyssopus officinalis_
Part used: Dried aerial parts.
Collection: The flowering tops of Hyssop should be collected in August and dried in the sun.
Constituents: Up to 1 per cent volatile oil; flavonoid glycosides; diosmin; tannin.
Actions: Anti-spasmodic, expectorant, diaphoretic, sedative, carminative.
Indications: Hyssop has an interesting range of uses which are largely attributable to the anti-spasmodic action of the volatile oil. It is used in coughs, bronchitis and chronic catarrh. Its diaphoretic properties explain its use in the common cold. As a nervine it may be used in anxiety states, hysteria and petit mal (a form of epilepsy).
Combinations: It may be combined with _White Horehound_ and _Coltsfoot_ in the treatment of coughs and bronchitis. For the common cold it may be mixed with _Boneset, Elder Flower_ and _Peppermint._
Preparation and dosage: Infusion: pour a cup of boiling water onto 1–2 teaspoonsful of the dried herb and leave to infuse for

10–15 minutes. This should be drunk three times a day.
Tincture: take 1–4 ml of the tincture three times a day.

SWEET VIOLET   _Viola odorata_
Part used: Leaves and flowers.
Collection: The leaves and flowers are gathered in the spring, in March and April. Dry with care.
Constituents: Saponins, menthyl salicylate, alkaloids, flavonoids, essential oil.
Actions: Expectorant, alterative, anti-inflammatory, diuretic, anti-neoplastic.
Indications: Sweet Violet has a long history of use as a cough remedy and especially for the treatment of bronchitis. It may also be used to aid in the treatment of upper respiratory catarrh. With the combination of actions present, it has a use in skin conditions such as eczema and in a long-term approach to rheumatism. It may be used for urinary infections. Sweet Violet has a reputation as an anti-cancer herb; it definitely has a role in a holistic approach to the treatment of cancer.
Preparation and dosage: Infusion: pour a cup of boiling water onto 1 teaspoonful of the herb and let infuse for 10–15 minutes. This should be drunk three times a day.
Tincture: take 1–2 ml of the tincture three times a day.

The more overtly relaxing remedies for the chest are very useful in conditions such as asthma and some forms of bronchitis. Apart for sedative nervines that act in this way, such as _Cowslip_ and _Wild Lettuce_, we can mention the following: _Lobelia, Wild Cherry Bark, Grindelia, Pill-bearing Spurge._

Let's look at those herbs not discussed elsewhere.

GRINDELIA   _Grindelia camporum_
Part used: Dried aerial parts.
Collection: The aerial parts are collected

before the flower buds open. They are dried as soon as possible in the sun.

Constituents: Saponins, volatile oil, bitter alkaloids, resin, tannins.

Actions: Anti-spasmodic, expectorant, hypotensive.

Indications: Grindelia relaxes the smooth muscles of the chest and heart muscles. This helps to explain its use in the treatment of asthmatic and bronchial conditions, especially where these are associated with a rapid heart beat and nervous response. It may be used in asthma, bronchitis, whooping cough and upper respiratory catarrh. Because of the relaxing effect on the heart and pulse rate, there may be a reduction in blood pressure. Externally the lotion is used in the dematitis caused by poison ivy.

Combinations: In the treatment of asthmatic conditions it may be used with *Lobelia* and *Pill-bearing Spurge*.

Preparation and dosage: Infusion: pour a cup of boiling water onto 1 teaspoonful of the dried herb and leave to infuse for 10–15 minutes. This should be drunk three times a day.

Tincture: take 1–2 ml of the tincture three times a day.

PILL-BEARING SPURGE
Euphorbia pilulifera

Part used: Aerial parts.

Collection: Gather aerial parts while it is in flower.

Constituents: Glycoside, alkaloids, sterols, tannins, phorbic acid.

Actions: Anti-asthmatic, expectorant, anti-spasmodic.

Indications: Pill-bearing Spurge has a relaxing effect upon the smooth muscles of the lungs and acts with great benefit in conditions such as asthma and bronchitis. It will also relieve spasms in the larynx, helping nervous coughs. It will help to relieve upper respiratory catarrh. This herb has a specific action of destroying the organisms that cause amoebic infections in the intestines.

Combinations: For the treatment of asthmatic conditions it will combine well with *Grindelia* and *Lobelia.*

Preparation and dosage: Infusion: pour a cup of boiling water onto ½–1 teaspoonful of the dried leaves and let infuse for 10–15 minutes. This should be drunk three times a day.

Tincture: take 1–2 ml of the tincture three times a day.

WILD CHERRY BARK   *Prunus serotina*

Part used: Dried bark.

Collection: The bark is gathered from young plants in the autumn. The outer bark is stripped off and the inner bark is carefully dried in the shade to avoid losing the oils. It must be stored in an airtight container and protected from sunlight.

Constituents: Cyanogenic glycosides including prunasin; volatile oil; coumarins; gallotannins; resin.

Actions: Anti-tussive, expectorant, astringent, sedative, mild digestive bitter.

Indications: This remedy has a specific sedative action on the body's cough reflex and is mainly used in irritating coughs. This gives it a role in bronchitis, whooping cough and asthma when used with other pectoral remedies. Just suppressing a cough is *never* a good thing to do. A cold infusion of the bark may help as a wash for inflamed eyes.

Preparation and dosage: Infusion: pour a cup of boiling water onto 1 teaspoonful of the dried bark and leave in a covered pot for 10–15 minutes. This should be drunk three times a day, or when needed.

Tincture: take 1–2 ml three times a day.

COWSLIP   *Primula veris*

Part used: The yellow petals and the root.

Collection: The flower corollae should be

gathered without the green calyx, between March and May. Dry quickly in the shade. The roots should be unearthed either before Cowslip flowers or in the autumn. Over-collecting has led to this plant becoming increasingly rare. Only pick if present in abundance and then pick only limited amounts.

Constituents: Up to 10 per cent saponins; glycosides; essential oil; flavonoids.

Actions: Sedative, anti-spasmodic, expectorant.

Indications: Cowslip is an excellent, generally applicable relaxing, sedative remedy. It will ease reactions to stress and tension, relaxing nervous excitement and facilitating restful sleep. It may be used with safety in bronchitis, colds, chills and coughs. Try it in nervous headaches and insomnia.

Combinations: For stress-related problems it may be used with any of the relaxing nervines such as _Lime Blossom_ or _Skullcap_. For coughs it may be used with _Coltsfoot_ and _Aniseed_.

Preparations and dosage: Infusion for petals: pour a cup of boiling water onto 2 teaspoonsful of the petals and let infuse for 10–15 minutes. This should be drunk three times a day.

Decoction for root: put 1 teaspoonful of the root in a cup of water, bring to the boil and simmer for 5 minutes. Take a cup three times a day.

Tincture: take 2–4 ml of the tincture three times a day.

Pectoral

Any herb that strengthens and tones the tissue of the lungs can be called a pectoral. Most of the herbs just mentioned under 'Expectorants' can be classed in this way. To remind you, these following remedies are herbs that while being pectorals also have a range of expectorant or relaxing actions: _Elecampane, Mullein, Lobelia_ and _Coltsfoot_.

Demulcents

As was pointed out in the section on 'Demulcents' in Chapter 3, we cannot claim that the soothing action of mucilage has a direct effect upon the irritated lining of the lungs. On the other hand there can be no practical doubt that chest demulcents exist and have a wonderful effect where there is much irritation and soreness. Amongst herbs that may have this action we can mention: _Elcampane, Comfrey Root, Mullein, Coltsfoot, Golden Rod, Marshmallow Root, Liquorice, Lungwort_ and _Plantain_.

These are all discussed under other headings, except for _Lungwort,_ which I shall leave for you to make your own notes about.

Anti-spasmodics

These remedies can help where there is much spasmodic coughing. This can lead to sleepless nights, pain and general discomfort. I must repeat, however, that coughing as such should not simply be stopped; either the body is trying to clear material or there is inflammation or obstruction. The anti-spasmodics are most useful in asthmatic-type problems.

Anti-microbials

With the respiratory system such a common site for infection, the value of the anti-microbials should be obvious. However, if the environment of the lungs is just not healthy because of smoking, pollution or chronic illness then such remedies may not be enough to clear the infection. As we shall see, the aim is to aid the body's own defence system rather than replace it. In addition to the basic anti-microbials there are _Echinacea, Wild Indigo_ and _Myrrh_.

We can add two other remedies, _Garlic_ and _Thyme_, that while having wide applications are of special service in the chest.

GARLIC *Allium sativum*
Part used: Bulb.
Collection: The bulb with its numerous cloves should be unearthed when the leaves begin to wither in September. They should be stored in a cool dry place.
Constituents: Volatile oil, mucilage, gluco-kinins, germanium.
Actions: Antiseptic, anti-viral, dia-phoretic, cholagogue, hypotensive, anti-spasmodic.
Indications: Garlic is among the few herbs that have a universal usage and recognition. Its daily usage aids and supports the body in ways that no other herb does. It is one of the most effective anti-microbial plants avail-able, acting on bacteria, viruses and alimen-tary parasites. The volatile oil is an effective agent and as it is largely excreted via the lungs, it is used in infections of this system such as chronic bronchitis, respiratory catarrh, recurrent colds and influenza. It may be helpful in the treatment of whoop-ing cough and as part of a broader approach to bronchitic asthma. In general it may be used as a preventative for most infectious conditions, digestive as well as respiratory. For the digestive tract it has been found that Garlic will support the development of the natural bacterial flora while killing patho-genic organisms. In addition to these amazing properties it will reduce blood pressure when taken over a period of time as well as reducing blood cholesterol levels. Garlic should be thought of as a basic food that will augment the body's health and protect it in general. It has been used exter-nally for the treatment of ringworm and threadworm.
Combinations: For microbial infections it will combine well with *Echinacea*.
Preparation and dosage: A clove should be eaten three times a day. If the smell becomes a problem, use Garlic oil capsules. Take three a day as a prophylactic or three times a day when an infection occurs.

THYME *Thymus vulgaris*
Part used: Leaves and flowering tops.
Collection: The flowering branches should be collected between June and August on a dry sunny day. The leaves are then stripped off the dried branches.
Constituents: More than 1 per cent volatile oil rich in thymol, carvacrol, cymol, linalol and borneol; bitter principle; tannin; flavo-noids; triterpenoids.
Actions: Carminative, anti-microbial, anti-spasmodic, expectorant, astringent, mildly anthelmintic.
Indications: The oil in this popular herb is strongly antiseptic and when used in the context of the plant it has a wide range of uses. As an extracted oil it can prove too strong for internal use. It makes the plant a good carminative for indigestion but also digestive system infections. It will benefit both lower and upper respiratory infections such as laryngitis, tonsilitis, and bronchitis. It is a safe basis for a holistic approach to bronchitis, whooping cough and asthma. Externally it can be used as an antiseptic wash for cuts, sores and infected wounds.
Preparation and dosage: Infusion: pour a cup of boiling water onto 2 teaspoonsful of the dried herb and let it infuse in a covered pot for 10 minutes. This should be drunk three times a day. Use a small handful of fresh leaves.
Tincture: take 2–4 ml of the tincture three times a day.

Anti-catarrhals
If there is much build up of cattarh and phlegm, these remedies should come to mind. Of course many of them have already been mentioned, but it is worth remember-ing that the following remedies are specifi-cally anti-catarrhal while also helping the lungs: *Golden Rod, Golden Seal, Elder Flowers, Hyssop.*

Nervines

It is always worth considering the potential value of nervines in chest problems such as asthma, and irritable coughs. However, with the right herbal and dietary approach these nervine remedies are less indicated than is thought. They are of inestimable value when stress, tension or debility are part of the person's life experience.

Diet

With congestion being such a common accompaniment to respiratory problems, it is always worth giving attention to diet. Of course, it should go without saying that for everyone and especially those with chest problems. . . DO NOT SMOKE!

As the phlegm that builds up is mucous in nature a diet that is low in mucus or the materials that are metabolized into mucus is worth considering. The basis of any good diet is plenty of fresh green vegetables and fruit with the right balance of protein/fibre/carbohydrate and fats. This is discussed in the section on the digestive system in Chapter 3. In addition to all the advice there, consider the following for a low mucus diet: Avoid or keep to a minimum:

- Dairy products, including goat's milk and yoghurt,
- Eggs,
- Grains, especially the mucus-rich ones such as wheat and oats,
- Sugar,
- Potatoes and other starchy root vegetables like swedes and turnips.

Common Problems of the Lungs

The lungs are prone to much major illness in these times of pollution and abuse. While we shall look at remedies to help in a range of respiratory problems, it in no way replaces skilled diagnosis. Lung cancer is one of the major causes of death in the western world, a condition that is largely avoidable. Its successful treatment needs early diagnosis and must be in the hands of a well-qualified practitioner.

Self-help with herbal medication will go a long way to keep a person healthy and remove illness, but there are exceptions. We shall consider only the basic and common problems here. Herbs will help in the whole range of problems from cancer, auto-immune conditions such as sarcoidosis, infections such as T.B. and industrial disease such as pneumoconiosis. This will need qualified herbal support and not just self-help.

We can divide respiratory problems into those that are characterized by a cough and those by breathing difficulties. This gross simplification has value when it comes to self-help and dealing with simple ailments in the home. It is not a strict divide as any chest condition can in some phase of its development manifest any symptom, but it's a place to start.

Coughs

A cough is the body's way of attempting to clear phlegm or other material from the lungs. As such it should not be automatically suppressed. It is an essential process for internal health. The cough may be due to infection, straight congestion because of phlegm, some foreign matter in the lungs or more serious medical problems.

IF ANY COUGH DOES NOT CLEAR WITH HERBAL REMEDIES, CONSULT A DOCTOR.

What can we do? The list of herbs that help with coughs is almost endless. One of the best standby remedies is *Coltsfoot,* whose latin name, *Tussilago,* actually comes from the word for cough! To this we can add the stronger and rather bitter herb *White Horehound,* as well as *Mullein* and *Aniseed.*

In fact, most of the remedies described at

the beginning of this chapter will help. A cough mixture need not be syrupy; this is often to mask a bitter component. *Liquorice* will add a flavour that masks unpleasantness.

A good mixture for a productive cough might be:

Coltsfoot
White Horehound
Liquorice.

These should be mixed in equal parts and infused.

This is but an isolated suggestion. Get to know the herbs so that you have a better base to make selections from. If a demulcent is needed for a cough, then consider *Comfrey* for example. If there is much irritation with it and there is perhaps a nervous involvement, then *Motherwort* may be useful.

There is a well-known and effective mixture for coughs recommended in Potters herbal which consists only of flowers:

Marshmallow Flowers
Mallow Flowers
Coltsfoot Flowers
Sweet Violet Flowers
Mullein Flowers
Red Poppy Flowers.

These are mixed in equal parts and infused.

It may be appropriate to add anti-microbials to the medication, the best here being *Garlic, Echinacea, Thyme* and *Eucalyptus*. If the cough is part of an infection such as bronchitis or even pneumonia, herbs have much to offer, but skilled advice and nursing care are needed as well. In addition to anti-microbials and expectorant pectorals, consider using lymphatic remedies to aid the body in its cleansing process. If there is fever, then diaphoretic remedies will also have a place in the treatment. Please consult the section on infections on p. 182.

Apart from taking the herbs internally there is benefit in inhalations from steam baths – old fashioned, but effective! A few drops of the oil of *Eucalyptus* and *Thyme* in a bowl of steaming water is all that is needed. When covering your head with a towel to keep the oils in, remember to keep your eyes closed, they can sting. A whole body bath can be made from the dried plants by taking equal amounts of both herbs to make up to 4-5 tablespoonsful. Pour a litre of boiling water over the mixture and let it stand for thirty minutes. Strain and then add to the bath.

The coughs of more chronic congestive disease such as emphysema and bronchiectasis can be helped with herbs such as *Elecampane, Comfrey* and *Blood Root*, combined with others as appropriate.

Shortness of Breath

This common experience can be caused by a wide range of problems including food allergy, heart failure, kidney problems, anxiety, asthma, exertion etc. This shows how important correct diagnosis is here. There is no point in looking for a food allergy if it is the beginnings of heart problems! We have discussed a range of herbs that ease spasms in the lungs and so often help in this group of conditions. Let's look at asthma in more depth to see what can be done herbally.

Asthma

In an attack of asthma, the tubes through which air is carried in and out of the lungs become narrowed. This has the effect of making it more and more difficult to get air in and out of the lungs. This leads to a shortness of breath, wheezing and a cough. The worse the breathlessness, the greater is the feeling of anxiety and even panic, which will tend to make the attack worse.

Cause

The problem is a reversible obstruction of the small airways of the lungs. Knowing this does not tell us the precise sequence of the physiological process. An all-encompassing cause for asthma has not been found, but a whole range of triggers are known. Attacks can be triggered in different people by allergies, chest infections, irritant gases, smoke, and psychological factors such as stress and anxiety.

Food allergies are a common predisposing factor. They do not always take the form of overt allergies since taking the food may not trigger an attack. They predispose. The worst culprits here are dairy products; that is cow's milk, butter and cheese. They are especially implicated in asthma in children who were either not breast-fed or weaned onto cow's milk in the first nine months of life. Other widely involved foods include white sugar, sweets and artificial additives of any kind. It is possible for any food to be involved in individual cases, and specialist help should be sought. There is much that herbal medicine has to offer in the alleviation of allergies but it is best to work with a medical herbalist, whose training includes nutrition and 'clinical ecology', as it is now called.

If a chest infection gets out of hand or a very prone person succumbs to such an infection, the congestion that develops will trigger attacks. The usual course is for people to get antibiotics from their doctor. There are problems with this, especially with young children who may be on repeated courses. Please consult the chapter on infections because with herbs we can strengthen the lungs and increase bodily resistance.

Any irritating gas or dust may trigger an attack. This could be smoke from a coal fire or even cold air. By far the commonest and worst such irritant is tobacco smoke. Unfortunately, this is not just from smoking cigarettes but from being around smokers. Any one with asthma should not feel reticent about asking smokers to stop in their presence.

Anxiety and stress do not cause asthma, but in most sufferers it can act as an initiating trigger or at least prolong an attack. Usually it will be a combination of factors that produce the attack.

Treatment

In addition to dietary advice and herbs, breathing exercises can be especially helpful in young people. Relaxation and stress-management are vital and are discussed in other parts of the book.

Herbs that are particularly useful include the following which have already been discussed. It is impossible to give a specific mixture for asthma as each person will have a different range of factors in play: _Lobelia, Grindelia, Pill-bearing Spurge, Sundew, Wild Cherry Bark, Mullein , Elecampane._

If there is much catarrhal build-up then consider: _White Horehound, Blood Root, Coltsfoot._

Herbs that ease nervous tension can be used freely as well as muscle relaxants. It is worth considering: _Cramp Bark, Motherwort, Skullcap, Valerian, Wild Lettuce._

All are described elsewhere except _Sundew_, which follows.

SUNDEW   _Drosera rotundifolia_
Part used: Entire plant.
Collection: The whole of the plant is gathered during the flowering period in July or August.
Constituents: Naphthaquinones including plumbagin; flavonoids; tannins; citric and malic acid.
Actions: Anti-spasmodic, demulcent, expectorant.

Indications: Sundew may be used with great benefit in bronchitis and whooping cough. The presence of plumbagin helps to explain this as it has been shown to be active against streptococcus, staphylococcus and pneumococcus bacteria. Sundew will also help with infections in other parts of the respiratory tract. Its relaxing effect upon involuntary muscles helps in the relief of asthma. In addition to the pulmonary conditions it has a long history in the treatment of stomach ulcers.

Combinations: In the treatment of asthma Sundew may be used with *Grindelia* and *Pill-bearing Spurge.*

Preparation and dosage: Infusion: pour a cup of boiling water onto 1 teaspoonful of the dried herb and leave to infuse for 10–15 minutes. This should be drunk three times a day.

Tincture: take 1–2 ml of the tincture three times a day.

EAR, NOSE AND THROAT

The upper respiratory system, the ears and eyes are usually considered as one integrated system. This is only part of the story as, in fact, the whole body is an integrated system that can only be adequately treated if the whole is approached coherently. Much that is said in the sections on the 'Respiratory system', 'Fevers and infections' and the 'Digestive system' are totally relevant here.

As the focus for much sensory perception and personality expression, this system has to be seen as far more than the tissue that makes it up. It is quite straightforward to concentrate upon the medical syndromes that commonly are found and herbal approaches to the treatment, but there are often much deeper psycho/spiritual roots to such problems. This fascinating insight into the nature of disease expression is one that cannot be dealt with fully here.

However, a simple and rather surface example of this deep-rooted integration is the proneness of this system to infections. It is commonly said that we 'catch' a cold. This is not so. For the virus, or any infection, to become active the body's resistance must have been lowered. If this was not the nature of openness to infection humanity would have a constantly running nose! The nature of resistance is discussed in the section on 'Infections' on p. 183.

Herbs for the Ear, Nose and Throat

As with all bodily systems there are remedies that are quite specific for this system, and we shall consider them in the context of their actions. It must be pointed out again that for resistance and healing power to be at their peak, each person will need what *they* uniquely need, and as such it may be something entirely other than the remedies suggested here that do the trick.

Anti-catarrhals

These remedies provide a firm foundation for any treatment within this system. The remedies that help remove catarrh by initially producing a more watery secretion can be most effective in the early stages of treating sinusitis etc. We can mention the following amongst a long potential list: *Elder Flowers, Golden Rod, Hyssop, Peppermint, Red Sage, Vervain.*

All of these are described elsewhere except the useful garden plant *Red Sage.*

RED SAGE   _Salvia officinalis_
Part used: Leaves.
Collection: The leaves should be gathered shortly before or just at the beginning of flowering in dry sunny weather in May or June. Dry in the shade or not above 34°C.
Constituents: Volatile oil including 30 per cent thujone, 5 per cent cineole, linalol, borneol, camphor, salvene and pinene; a bitter; tannins; triterpenoids; flavonoids; oestrogenic substances; resin.
Actions: Carminative, spasmolytic, anti-septic, astringent, anti-hidrotic.
Indications: Red Sage is the classic remedy for inflammations of the mouth, throat and tonsils, its volatile oils soothing the mucous membranes. It may be used internally and as a mouthwash for inflamed and bleeding gums, inflamed tongue or generalized mouth inflammation. It is an excellent remedy in mouth ulcers. As a gargle it will aid in the treatment of laryngitis, pharyngitis, tonsilitis and quinsy. It is a valuable carminative used in dyspepsia. It reduces sweating when taken internally and may be used to reduce the production of breast milk. As a compress it promotes the healing of wounds. Red Sage stimulates the muscles of the uterus and .so should be avoided during preganancy.
CAUTION: Avoid during pregnancy.
Combinations: As a gargle for throat conditions it combines well with _Tormentil_ and _Balm of Gilead._ In dyspepsia it can be combined with _Meadowsweet_ and _Chamomile._
Preparation and dosage: Infusion: pour a cup of boiling water onto 1–2 teaspoonsful of the leaves and let infuse for 10 minutes. This should be drunk three times a day.
Mouthwash: put 2 teaspoonsful of the leaves in half a litre (one pint) of water, bring to the boil and let stand, covered, for 15 minutes. Gargle deeply with the hot tea for 5–10 minutes several times a day.
Tincture: take 2–4 ml of the tincture three times a day.

In addition there is a remedy that has a tonic action on the mucous membranes and will tend to dry up the secretions, though this is not the best thing to do initially. This herb is _Golden Seal._

Anti-microbials

All of these remedies can play a role in the preservation of resistance in the face of infective organisms or help throw off such an infection should it arise. See sections on _Garlic, Echinacea_ and _Wild Indigo._

Of these _Wild Indigo_ is also anti-catarrhal, while _Garlic_ is especially appropriate. The anti-septic oils can all be useful for inhalants etc. Consider this partial list and refer to the section on aromatherapy: _Peppermint oil, Eucalyptus oil, Thyme oil, Balsam of Tolu, Balsam of Peru, Marjoram oil._

Lymphatics

All the herbs mentioned in the chapter on the lymphatic system can play a useful role in helping the glands of the throat and neck do their allotted task. Refer to that section and consider especially: _Cleaver, Poke Root_ and _Echinacea._

Alteratives/Tonics

For anyone with an ongoing experience of catarrhal or sinus problems, herbs that aid elimination and general tonic activities in the body can be of great help. It is a mistake to limit the range of remedies to the groups mentioned above. In broader healing terms actions such as alterative, tonic, diuretic, hepatic or even laxative can play an important role on the path back to health and wholeness.

Diet

For some people, the general balance of diet can play a fundamental part in the causation and proneness to catarrhal problems. Without exploring it in too much detail we can identify two broad areas of concern. I would repeat here my general avoidance of extreme or fad diets. Having said that, however, in a bad case of sinus catarrh extreme measures may well help.

To prevent the body needing to remove excess catarrah from the body, the simplest thing to do is to reduce the intake of foods that are metabolized into catarrh. Thus we can talk of a 'low mucous diet'. In most people this goes a long way to eliminating the experienced problems. However, it does not always work. Sorry! In such cases herbs used as well increase the success rate greatly.

The basis of the diet is avoidance of high carbohydrate foods such as wheat flour products (bread and cakes etc.); root vegetables such as potatoes; sugar-containing foods or the use of sugar itself. In addition all cow's milk products, butter and cheese must be avoided.

This diet can be initiated with a 2–3 day fast followed by the introduction of fruit and fruit juices leading to a regular diet rich in vegetables and fruit.

The Ear

Here we immediately come to major limitations of herbal medicine. There is very little that our remedies can do for neurological deafness, and while catarrhal problems of the ear are discussed below, the very structure of the ear poses problems for herbs to get to the place they are needed. Having acknowledged the limits let us explore what herbs have to offer.

Infections

The general guidelines for the herbal treatment of infections described elsewhere holds good for the ear as well. Infections of the middle ear can be extremely painful and may lead to damage of the inner ear. It is one of the cases where it may be appropriate to

use herbal remedies in the context of medically prescribed antibiotic treatment.

The anti-microbials and anti-catarrhals act as the basis of treatment. They are especially helpful with children who have been exposed to repeated courses of antibiotics which give only short-term relief followed by another attack. The use of herbs will not immediately solve the problem, but will enable the child's body to regain its innate powers of healing over a period of time.

For earache, a number of herbs will relieve the pain. Two points must be borne in mind. Such pain relief is not a treatment of the underlying infection, and never introduce anything into the ear if there is a suspicion of a perforated ear drum. A traditional Welsh remedy is the expressed juice of *Pennywort,* a common herb found on old walls and rocks. A drop or two of this juice at body temperature, introduced into the ear canal and stoppered with cotton wool will usually ease the pain and stop the screaming. Another remedy is to use warm oil of *Mullein.* However, this is difficult to obtain and takes time to make. See the instructions for making *St John's Wort* oil in the appropriate section.

Chronic Catarrh Problems

These can take a number of forms which often get treated by the surgical insertion of grommets to ensure drainage of the middle ear and so clear the build-up.

It is possible to help such conditions with a combination of strict adherence to the dietary advice given above plus the continued use of remedies such as: *Golden Rod, Wild Indigo* and *Golden Seal.*

This is an intransigent problem, however, and can take many months to control adequately.

Balance and Tinnitus

These problems of the inner ear are usually

due to nerve damage, or to a lesser degree to catarrhal build-up. This is one of those cases where in theory herbs should not be able to help, but certain remedies can help and in some people even control conditions such as Menier's disease. For such problems skilled advice is needed. The herbal basis is: *Black Cohosh* and *Golden Seal.*

The Nose

Many of the problems that affect the nose can be explained by pollution, whether from unclean air or self-inflicted cigarette smoking. The first step for problems of the nose is to stop smoking and ensure as clean an environment as possible. The sinuses are common sites for catarrhal build up so the advice on diet earlier in this chapter is especially relevant.

It is worth repeating that we don't 'catch' a cold, it will thrive on the right kind of 'soil'. So while we shall talk about relevant remedies for such problems, the first step should always be an attempt to improve bodily resistance to infection. This can be found in the appropriate section.

Colds and the Flu

The common cold is not a bane but a friend, a chance for the body to cleanse and, given the chance, to rest. Remedies most appropriate are anti-catarrhals, anti-microbials and diaphoretics. Of the many household remedies that can work we can mention: *Elder Flower, Peppermint, Yarrow* and *Ginger.*

This is a partial list because many different herbs will help different individuals to reach their own balance point. Influenza is a different matter. It can be a potentially dangerous and at best a debilitating infection. If the 'flu does set in even though you have followed the advice about maintaining resistance, there is a herb that will help you

deal with the miseries – *Boneset.*

This can be used with other diaphoretics if needed.

Sinusistis

A common and sometimes chronic problem that is quite amenable to herbal treatment. The basis must be the dietary advice given above combined with anti-catarrhals, anti-microbials and aromatic decongestant oils. Herbs to choose from are all of those mentioned above.

Hayfever

This catchall phrase for allergic reactions in the whole system can prove very open to herbal remedies. It is best to start any treatment about a month before one's personal hayfever season starts. The general advice given in the section on allergies should be followed. Herbs that may be useful include: *Ephedra, Golden Rod, Golden Seal* and *Eyebright.*

The Throat

As one of the main sites of personal expression, the throat can be a focus for much psychologically related health trauma, as well as the obvious sore throats and infections. This might sound rather extreme, but repeated problems with the throat might have a causal basis in problems around expressing oneself. If crying, expressing anger or speech problems occur, it is feasible that the local stresses on the throat might lower resistance and tone, opening the door to ill health.

Sore Throats

As was said for the nose and sinuses, it can be a site of first entry for infectious organisms and so sore throats can be unpleasantly common. If they do occur, of course, the first step is to strengthen health in general with dietary and vitamin support described in the section on infections. Herbs to consider would include antimicrobials, astringents and anything else specifically indicated such as remedies for coughs or catarrh. Herbs to consider internally include: *Echinacea, Myrrh, Golden Seal* and *Garlic*.

Many different remedies have reputations as gargles, especially the antiseptic labiates and oil-rich plants such as *Thyme* and *Eucalyptus*. Of particular importance are *Red Sage* and *Balm of Gilead*.

Of these *Red Sage* is by far the most pleasant!

Tonsilitis and Adenoids

These common childhood complaints are the expression of the body defending itself and so working well, rather than a sign of disease and malfunction. They are their epitome of where herbal support is preferable to antibiotic suppression. This does not deny the value of using such drugs in extreme situations, but they should ideally not be first choice. The following antimicrobials and lymphatic alteratives are the most appropriate, although different people respond better to different remedies, as usual: *Cleavers, Echinacea, Myrrh, Wild Indigo, Garlic*.

General dietary aid and support should be given as described in the section on Infections and Fevers.

The Eye

There is little that can be done with herbal remedies to alleviate problems that can arise within the eye itself or relating to eyesight. It is of interest to note that *Marijuanha* appears to be of value in the treatment of glaucoma. Research in America suggests that it may lower the intra-eye pressure. For obvious reasons this has not been taken very far yet.

When eye problems are related to the cir-

cultory system, as in high blood pressure, a trained and qualified herbalist may be able to help through a holistic approach to the body.

Stress and tension can lead to symptoms of eye strain and pain. If this is a component in the individual's case then the advice given in the chapter on the nervous system is relevant.

For weak or strained eyes, a number of herbs can make easing compresses. In its simplest form a compress is a piece of cloth soaked in a tea of the herb concerned. It is best to lie down otherwise the compress falls off! Good herbs include: *Eyebright, Marigold Petals, Elder Flowers* and *Cucumber*.

The simplest way of doing this is to put thin fresh slices of cool cucumber on the eyes and replace when they have become warm or too dry.

Let's consider *Eyebright*.

EYEBRIGHT   *Euphrasia officinalis*
Part used: Dried aerial parts.
Collection: Gather the whole plant while in bloom in late summer or autumn and dry it in an airy place.
Constituents: Glycosides including aucubin, tannins, resin, volatile oil.
Actions: Anti-catarrhal, astringent, anti-inflammatory.
Indications: Eyebright is an excellent remedy for the problems of mucous membranes. The combination of anti-inflammatory and astringent properties make it relevant in many conditions. Used internally it is a powerful anti-catarrhal and thus may be used in nasal catarrh, sinusitis and other congestive states. It is best known for its use in conditions of the eye, where it is helpful in acute or chronic inflammations, stinging and weeping eyes as well as oversensitivity to light. Used as a compress and taken internally it is used in conjunctivitis and blepharitis.

Combinations: In catarrhal conditions it combines well with _Golden Rod, Elder Flower_ or _Golden Seal._ In allergic conditions, where the eyes are affected, it may be combined with _Ephedra._ As an eye lotion it mixes with _Golden Seal_ and distilled _Witch Hazel._

Preparation and dosage: Infusion: pour a cup of boiling water onto 1 teaspoonful of the dried herb and leave to infuse for 5-10 minutes. This should be drunk three times a day.

Compress: place a teaspoonful of the dried herb in half a litre of water and boil for 10 minutes, let cool slightly. Moisten a compress (cotton wool, gauze or muslin) in the lukewarm liquid, wring out slightly and place over the eyes. Leave the compress in place for 15 minutes. Repeat several times a day.

Tincture: take 1-4 ml of the tincture three times a day.

Infections of the eyelids or coating of the eye can often be successfully cleared with herbs. However, if they do not work within a few days, please seek medical advice. The herbs should be made into the appropriate teas and put into an eyebath and this used three to four times a day. Drops of tincture can be used diluted with distilled water. The strength here is variable and advice should be sought from a qualified practitioner. The safe herbs to consider include: _Marigold Petals, Golden Seal, Eyebright_ and _Elder Berries._

THE LYMPHATIC SYSTEM

Strictly speaking, this is a part of the circulatory system as one of its functions is to return cellular fluids back into the bloodstream. It is collected from all over the body and re-introduced into the blood system in the major veins. It also has an important job to play in the body's defence systems as it is a site where the immune system brings into play much of its anti-infectious might.

Much of this anti-microbial activity goes on in the lymphatic glands which are found all over the body. There are major collections of them below the jaw and at the side of the neck, in the axillae of the arms, the groin and in the breasts. The tonsils and adenoids are also lymphatic tissue. When these glands get swollen it is a sign that they are doing their job, that of protecting the body as a whole against infection. Herbal medicines will aid this process and greatly reduce the need for antibiotics.

The health and integrity of the lymphatic system appears to be fundamental to the general cleansing process that is continually going on. It is no wonder then that in the holistic approaches to health and prevention of disease as well as its treatment, so much emphasis is placed on helping the lymphatic system. Supporting this system is basic in most anti-cancer treatments as well as cleansing programmes for a whole range of health problems.

Here we shall consider herbal agents for the system as well as dietary factors. How to treat infections in general and specifics such as tonsilitis and adenitis will be discussed in another section.

Herbs for the Lymphatic System

Certain actions are especially indicated. The anti-microbials and alteratives can all play a role in helping to maintain the healthy functioning of the lymphatic system. Diuretics and hepatics may be indicated if the body needs especially cleansing. Diaphoretics will help if infection is actively present.

Herbs that can be thought of as being ~ific here that, as you will see, can fit into more than one of the categories mentioned are: *Cleavers, Marigold, Poke Root, Echinacea, Golden Seal, Wild Indigo, Blue Flag* and *Garlic.*

All are discussed elsewhere except *Cleavers.*

CLEAVERS   *Galium aparine*
Common name: Goosegrass.
Part used: Dried aerial parts and the fresh expressed juice.
Collection: The plant should be gathered before flowering and dried in the shade.
Constituents: Glycoside asperuloside, gallotannic acid, citric acid.
Actions: Diuretic, alterative, anti-inflammatory, tonic, astringent, anti-neoplastic.
Indications: Cleavers is perhaps the best tonic to the lymphatic system available. As a lymphatic tonic with alterative and diuretic actions it may be used in a wide range of problems where the lymphatic system is involved. Thus it would be used in swollen glands anywhere in the body and especially in tonsilitis and in adenoid trouble. It is widely used in skin conditions, especially in the dry varieties such as psoriasis. It will be useful in the treatment of cystitis and other urinary conditions where there is pain and may be combined with demulcents for this. There is a long tradition for the use of Cleavers in the treatment of ulcers and tumours, which may be the result of the lymphatic drainage. Cleavers make an excellent vegetable.
Combinations: For the lymphatic system it will work well with *Poke Root, Echinacea* and *Marigold.* For skin conditions it is best combined with *Yellow Dock* and *Burdock.*
Preparation and dosage: Infusion: pour a cup of boiling water onto 2–3 teaspoonful of the dried herb and leave to infuse for 10–15 minutes. This should be drunk three times a day.

POKE ROOT   *Phytolacca americana*
Part used: Root.
Collection: The root should be unearthed in the late autumn or spring. Clean it and split lengthwise before drying.
Constituents: Tripterpenoid saponins, alkaloid, resins, phytolacic acid, tannin, formic acid.
Actions: Anti-rheumatic, stimulant, anti-catarrhal, purgative, emetic.
Indications: Poke Root has a wide range of uses and is a valuable addition to many holistic treatments. It may be seen primarily as a remedy for use in infections of the upper respiratory tract, removing catarrh and aiding the cleansing of the lymphatic glands. It may be used for catarrh, tonsilitis, laryngitis, swollen glands, mumps etc. It will be found of value in lymphatic problems elsewhere in the body and especially for mastitis, where it can be used internally and as a poultice. Poke Root also has a use in rheumatism, especially where it is long standing. Care must be taken with this herb as in large dosage it is powerfully emetic and purgative. Externally as a lotion or ointment it may be used to rid the skin of scabies and other pests.
CAUTION: In large doses Poke Root is a powerful emetic and purgative.
Combinations: For lymphatic problems it may be used with *Cleavers* or *Blue Flag.*
Preparation and dosage: Decoction: only small amounts of this herb should be used. Put ¼–½ teaspoonful of the root in a cup of water, bring to the boil and simmer gently for 10–15 minutes. This should be drunk three times a day.
Tincture: take ½–1 ml of the tincture three times a day.

Diet and Lymphatic System

Much has been written about cleansing

diets for the lymphatic system, and cleansing diets in general. The different diets often recommend quite divergent things.

It is not possible to outline the basis of a cleansing diet that removes the possible weight of inappropriate foods while replacing them with foods that will actively aid and support the work of the lymphatic system.

There should be an initial day of fast followed by two days of fluid only. This should be fresh fruit or vegetable juice. The diet should then be based on fruit and a high preponderance of raw vegetables. If meat is desired it should be fish or poultry only.

Certain foods should be avoided to give the body a rest! These include: red meats, fatty and fried foods, dairy products, vinegar and pickles of all kinds, alcohol, sugar and sugar-rich products. Artificial additives of all kinds should be avoided. DO NOT SMOKE.

THE URINARY SYSTEM

Its Function and Role in Health and Wholeness

The urinary system plays a crucial role in the inner hygiene of the body. Through the miracle of design and physico/chemical functioning of the kidney tissue, excess water is taken from the blood along with unwanted chemicals that are the result of the cellular respiratory processes. In our times of pollution and crazy diets, the kidney is also one of the main sites of removal of toxic or potentially toxic chemicals in the blood-stream.

It does not simply remove water, however; it is part of a complex body-wide process of maintaining a steady, regular internal environment, or homoeostasis. So sometimes it will remove very little salt or water, while at other times apparently too much is flowing. The control involves the brain, hormones, and receptors all over the body. It is such a wonderful organ that we could write a vast scientific textbook about its form, function and integration, or just as easily write a poetic epic. As a medical herbalist I shall do neither!

Proper activity in the kidneys is vital to health – if the movement of salts, proteins or other complex chemicals across the selective membranes of the kidney nephrons goes awry a whole range of health problems can arise. These can vary from mild water retention associated with premenstrual tension to major kidney failure and protein loss. Herbal treatment of the whole system can be directed in two broad directions, which (as in all things) overlap. Either specific diseases can be treated, or a supportive and tonic role can be played by aiding natural kidney activity.

In a book of this kind, far more emphasis will be placed on the latter. This is partially because of the need for skilled diagnosis in the first case. More importantly by strengthening over-pressured kidneys the general work of body cleansing and thus general systemic health can be greatly helped. This brings us back to the preventative role herbal remedies can play.

Herbs and the Urinary System

Herbal medicine offers not only potent and valuable remedies to put right urinary 'disease', but also tonics and normalizers that can help prevent problems developing. The question of how they can do this job of healing and strengthening is often unanswerable, either because no research has been done or that they work in a way that is subtler than our scientists' methods can perceive. In the hands of a skilled medical herbalist, there is little that cannot be achieved in digestive illness. Here we can talk only in generalities as each person is unique and each bladder infection may have a different set of factors to take into account.

Here we shall consider actions that are most commonly called for and then look at how the herbs can be used for easing common urinary system problems.

Actions

Rather than thinking in terms of specific herbs or combinations for certain conditions, it is more fruitful in general to consider appropriate herbal actions. Of course, there are specific herbs that may be right for specific people, but as a way to gain experience and insight, working with actions provides a solid foundation.

Diuretics

The different kinds of diuretic and their modes of action (where understood) are described in Chapter 3. Please refer to it now to refresh your memory about this range of remedies. As pointed out there, many herbs that have an action on the urinary system as a whole are described as diuretic in traditional herbal texts. This is not the correct usage as a diuretic is an agent that increases the flow of urine from the body.

An example of the way in which Nature appears to know our needs before we do is shown by that excellent diuretic _Dandelion Leaf_. Apart from being perhaps the strongest diuretic we have herbally, it is also an excellent source of potassium. When diuretics are taken it may lead to a loss of potassium from the blood-stream. This will be dangerous, and especially so for people with heart problems that lead to water retention. By using _Dandelion Leaf_ there will not only be the desired water loss but also a net increase in potassium, so avoiding the potential problems.

Some of the commonest foods eaten have diuretic effects. For example with _Parsley_ we have a salad vegetable that cleanses the body as well as feeding it.

PARSLEY   _Petroselinum crispum_
Part used: The tap root, leaves and seeds.
Collection: The root is collected in the autumn from two-year-old plants. The leaves can be used any time during the growing season.
Constituents: Essential oil including apiol and myristicin, vitamin C, glycoside apiin, starch.
Actions: Diuretic, expectorant, emmenagogue, carminative, supposed aphrodisiac.
Indications: The fresh herb, so widely used in cookery, is one of our richest sources of vitamin C. Medicinally, Parsley has three main areas of usage. First, it is an effective diuretic, helping the body to get rid of excess water and so may be used wherever such an effect is desired. Remember, however, that the cause of the problem must be sought and treated – don't just treat symptoms. The second area of use is an emmenagogue stimulating the menstrual process. It is advisable not to use parsley in medicinal dosage during preganancy as there may be excessive stimulation of the womb. The third use is as a carminative, easing flatulence and the colic pains that may accompany it.
CAUTION: Do not use during pregnancy in medicinal dosage.
Preparation and dosage: Infusion: pour a cup of boiling water onto 1–2 teaspoonsful of the leaves or root and let infuse for 5–10 minutes in a closed container. This should

be drunk three times a day.
Tincture: take 2–4 ml of the tincture three times a day.

Demulcents

There is a range of demulcent herbs that work specifically on the urinary tract and can be most helpful where irritation has occurred, either through infection, stones or calculus or chemical damage. These urinary demulcents include: _Corn silk, Couchgrass_ and _Marshmallow Leaf._

Anti-microbial

This system can be particularly prone to infection, either because of organisms entering from outside the body, or because of infection developing as a complication or repercussion of problems elsewhere in the body. This highlights the cleansing role of the kidney but also explains how some very difficult infections can develop in that organ.

There are certain herbs that have a specific anti-microbial action on this system. This is sometimes because of oils from the plant that are excreted via the kidney. A good example of this would be _Juniper._ Others work for a whole range of reasons. Their use should always be in conjunction with systemic anti-microbials to augment their activity and strength. Of most importance are: _Bearberry, Yarrow, Couchgrass_ and _Buchu._

To these we can add the more widely applicable remedies such as _Echinacea, Wild Indigo_ and _Garlic._

Astringents

Astringency can be a useful adjunct to herbal treatments in the urinary system as they help to tone tissue and heal the minor cuts and abrasions that are occurring all the time. You will remember that this action will reduce bleeding from wounds, and

there are herbs with the power to do this in the urinary tract. However, if there is ever blood in the urine it is a sign of great medical importance and the person involved must seek skilled help. Having said that, herbal urinary astringents have a great supportive role in broader treatments.

Many herbs can play this role, but perhaps the most important specifics are: _Horsetail, Couchgrass, Yarrow_ and _Periwinkle._

Below we shall consider the one we have not already covered elsewhere – _Horsetail._

HORSETAIL   _Equisetum arvense_
Part used: Dried aerial stems.
Collection: Collect in early summer. Cut the plant just above the ground, hang in bundles and dry in an airy place.
Constituents: Silicic acid (a source of silicon); saponin; flavone glycosides; organic acids; nicotine; palustrine.
Actions: Astringent, diuretic, vulnerary.
Indications: Horsetail is an astringent for the whole genito-urinary system, reducing haemorrhage and healing wounds thanks to its high silica content. While it acts as a mild diuretic, its toning and astringent actions make it invaluable in the treatment of incontinence and bed-wetting in children. It is considered a specific in cases of inflammation or benign enlargement of the prostate gland. Externally it is a vulnerary (healing wounds). In some cases it has been found to ease the pain of rheumatism and stimulate the healing of chilblains.
Combinations: Horsetail is often combined with _Hydrangea_ in the treatment of prostate troubles.
Preparation and dosage: Infusion: pour a cup of boiling water onto 2 teaspoonsful of the dried plant and let infuse for 15–20 minutes. This should be drunk three times a day.
Bath: a useful bath can be made to help in rheumatic pain and chilblains. Allow 100

grams of the herb to steep in hot water for an hour. Add this to the bath.
Tincture: take 2–4 ml of the tincture three times a day.

You will see from this example as throughout herbal medicine, plants have a wide range of use and not just those in which the herb is described.

Anti-lithics

From a study of this action in previous sections you will know that there is a whole range of remedies with a reputation for helping the body rid itself of renal stones or gravel. How to use them will be described below, but in addition to *Hydrangea, Parsely Root* and *Pellitory of the Wall* described in the anti-lithic section there are two more to consider. *Stone Root* we shall describe here, but to help you in your exploration of herbalism, make your own notes on the herb *Gravel Root.*

STONE ROOT   *Collinsonia canadensis*
Part used: Root and rhizome.
Collection: Roots and rhizome are unearthed in the autumn.
Constituents: Saponins, resin, tannin, organic acid, alkaloid.
Actions: Anti-lithic, diuretic, diaphoretic.
Indications: As its name suggests, Stone Root finds it main use in the treatment and prevention of stone and gravel in the urinary system. It can be used as a prophyl-axis but is also excellent when the body is in need of help in passing stones or gravel. It can also act as a strong diuretic in some people.
Combinations: For urinary stone and gravel, it may be combined with *Parsley Piert, Gravel Root, Pellitory of the Wall* or *Hydrangea.*
Preparation and dosage: Decoction: put 1–3 teaspoonsful of the dried root in a cup of water, bring to the boil and simmer for 10–15 minutes. This should be drunk three times a day.
Tincture: take 2–4 ml of the tincture three times a day.

Anti-spasmodics/Nervines

Muscle spasm, either due to colic from a stone or muscle tension from other causes, can be very painful. In extreme pain the legal herbs have little to offer, but it is worth noting that orthodox medicine uses drugs from plant sources to relieve such extreme pain.

Nervines to relax the general state of tension, or anti-spasmodics to relax the smooth muscle in the area, may be helpful. Perhaps the most applicable of the range available to us are: *Cramp Bark, Black Haw* and *Valerian.*

Tonics/Alteratives

Many of the tonic and alterative remedies have a diuretic action to some degree. This is understandable as they all work to improve general health and this will often involve a cleansing of some sort. Perhaps the best remedies in this vast range for urinary problems are: *Cleavers* and *Buchu.*

Ways Remedies can be Used

The treatment of many of the problems that arise in the urinary system can prove quite straightforward for a herbalist. However, it must be stressed that some forms of kidney disease are potentially life-threatening and must not be treated without skilled supervision. It is because of this that kidney disease will not be discussed here. Herbs may be of value in the treatment of the gamut of such problems but only in the hands of a skilled practitioner.

Recent research has shown that *Golden Rod* will reduce the loss of protein from a damaged kidney. This is surprising as it is usually thought of as an anti-catarrhal remedy. Other herbs have similarly valuable specific and unique uses. However, if there is protein in the urine then something is not at all right in the kidney and calls for immediate diagnosis.

A number of plants act to help heal a damaged kidney, whatever the cause. These herbs can be used long term to strengthen and support the organ without fear of side-effects or dependancy. Perhaps the best all-round such remedy is *Buchu*. This is described in the section on 'Diuretics' in Chapter 3.

In general it is not advisable to use strong diuretics over too long a period of time as this will either mask an underlying condition, or prove a strain on the kidneys in time. With the diuretics used by herbalists there is no problem in the short or medium term. *Juniper Berries,* which are a strong diuretic, should not be used for anyone with a history or kidney infection or damage. This is because the oil is too irritating to the kidney. Water retention, or to give it its medical name, oedema, can be due to a whole range of problems from heart failure to pre-menstrual tension. The simple use of herbal diuretics is not an adequate approach as again this is a sign that the body is showing that all is not well. However, once the cause has been identified there are remedies that can be safely used. Perhaps the best is *Dandelion Leaf,* preferably fresh, made into a tea and drunk three times a day. The leaves can also be used in salads.

Infections

As has already been pointed out, the bladder and other parts of this system are rather prone to infection. While pathologically we can differentiate between different sites or variety of infection, herbally the approach is often very similar. The commonest of such infections is *Cystitis,* an infection of the bladder. It can often be cleared by drinking large amounts of *Yarrow* tea each day, especially if the herb is picked wild.

To treat a more persistent case consider using a mixture of herbs that acts as an anti-microbial, demulcent or even astringent. By such an approach not only will the infection be cleared but the burning and general irritation will soon go. A good diet is essential with a minimum of acid foods. An example of such a mixture would be: *Bearberry, Couchgrass, Yarrow* or *Corn Silk,* in equal parts.

This should be drunk as an infusion three or four times a day. We shall describe *Corn Silk* here. The others are discussed elsewhere.

CORN SILK   *Zea mays*
Part used: Stigmas from the female flowers of maize. Fine soft threads 10–20 cm long.
Collection: The stigmas should be collected just before pollination occurs, the timing of which depends upon climate. It is best used fresh as some of the activity is lost with time.
Constituents: Saponins, a volatile alkaloid, sterols, tannin.
Actions: Diuretic, demulcent, tonic.
Indications: As a soothing diuretic, Corn Silk is helpful in any irritation of the urinary system. It is used for renal problems in children and as a urinary demulcent combined with other herbs in the treatment of cystitis, urethritis, prostatitis and the like.
Preparation and dosage: Infusion: pour a cup of boiling water onto 2 teaspoonsful of the fresh or dried herb and leave to infuse for 10–15 minutes. This should be drunk three times a day.
Tincture: take 3–6 ml of the tincture three times a day.

Kidney Stones and Gravel

Herbal remedies have a lot to offer here with

a combination of anti-lithics and demulcents. There is a common assumption that herbal remedies exist that 'dissolve' stones. It is only rarely that this is the case. What they will do is enable the tissue of the urinary tract to pass the material with less pain and trauma than would otherwise be the case. Whatever happens it will probably be a painful and unpleasant process, however. It is important to be on a low acid diet and to drink at least 3 litres of fluid a day.

Review the anti-lithics and get to know their other actions to give a basis on which to select for an individual. The irritation that almost always accompanies such problems suggests that demulcents would be useful. This sort of irritation can create the environment in which an infection can establish itself so anti-microbials may be necessary at some stage. A good mixture for daily use could be one based on the following remedies: *Stone Root, Hydrangea, Corn Silk.* This is only a basic suggestion. Remember that each herb has a range of actions and must be suited to the individual's unique needs.

If there is associated pain, herbs such as *Cramp Bark* or *Valerian* may help. However, the pain can be too severe for such remedies to do much. In severe cases get medical attention immediately.

THE REPRODUCTIVE SYSTEM

Here we have life at work, the vital force renewing itself, perpetuating and creating afresh. No wonder that nature is so prolific in herbal remedies that support and aid the whole system. To treat the system, however, we need to see it in a broader context.

In Western societies, all kinds of emotional and mental disorders are commoner in women than men. This bald fact opens up vast areas of psychological, sociological, physiological and political exploration, most of which is inappropriate to enter now. The main suggested reasons for the difference are genetic, and the social pressures on women and differences in patterns of upbringing and cultural expectations. However, it would seem to say something is wrong with a society that causes such suffering in half its population.

While we shall focus on the medical 'syndromes' common to women it must be remembered that the atmosphere of mental illness that pervades our society can be easily seen as a result of the patriarchy that runs it. The alienation and depersonalization of the high rise, militarism, multi-national corporate oppression, the nuclear threat and inequality of world resources leading to massive misery could all be seen as aspects of male mental disorders. This could all get too political but to view health holistically means that such perspectives cannot be avoided.

Perhaps there should be some attention given to male menopause and the male version of pre-menstrual tension. While that may sound like a joke I am afraid there is something to it!

Herbs for the Reproductive System

Nature is rich in herbs and actions that help the whole process of reproduction. This is only to be expected from a holistic perspective as this is such a fundamental and profound aspect of life. There are a number of actions quite unique to the female reproductive system. Here we shall discuss them and the general actions applicable.

Tonics

These remedies have the unique property

of toning and strengthening the whole of the system, helping it to function and providing a basis for dealing with specific disorders. Each of the uterine tonics has associated actions which provide a broad herbal matrix within which selection of the appropriate remedy can be done. They can be used where no overt 'disease' is present but a constitutional strengthening is indicated. They are healers in a truly holistic sense. Nature at work again! – *Black Cohosh, Blue Cohosh, Chasteberry, False Unicorn Root, Life Root, Motherwort, Raspberry, Squaw Vine.*

Five of these herbs come to us from the American Indians. Perhaps it is no coincidence that a culture so in tune with Mother Earth has given us herbs to help our Mothers.

All are discussed elsewhere except *Blue Cohosh, False Unicorn Root, Life Root* and *Squaw Vine.*

BLUE COHOSH *Caulophyllum thalictroides*
Part used: Rhizome and root.
Collection: The roots and rhizome are collected in the autumn, as at the end of the growing season they are richest in natural chemicals.
Constituents: Steroidal saponins, alkaloids.
Actions: Uterine tonic, emmenagogue, anti-spasmodic, anti-rheumatic.
Indications: Blue Cohosh is a plant that comes to us from the North American Indians, which shows in its other names of *Squaw Root* and *Papoose Root.* It is an excellent uterine tonic that may be used in any situation where there is a weakness or loss of tone. It may be used at any time during pregnancy if there is a threat of miscarriage. Similarly, because of its anti-spasmodic action, it will ease false labour pains. However, when labour does ensue, the use of Blue Cohosh just before birth will help ensure an easy delivery. In all these cases it is a safe herb to use. As an emmenagogue it can be used to bring on a delayed or suppressed menstruation while ensuring that the pain that sometimes accompanies it is relieved. Blue Cohosh may be used in cases where an anti-spasmodic is needed such as in colic, asthma or nervous coughs. It has a reputation for easing rheumatic pain.
Combinations: To strengthen the uterus it may be used well with *False Unicorn Root, Motherwort* and *Yarrow.*
Preparation and dosage: Decoction: put 1 teaspoonful of the dried root in a cup of water, bring to the boil and simmer for 10 minutes. This should be drunk three times a day.
Tincture: take 1–2 ml of the tincture three times a day.

FALSE UNICORN ROOT
Chamaelirium luteum
Part used: Dried rhizome and root.
Collection: The underground parts are unearthed in the autumn.
Constituents: Steroidal saponins which include chamaelirin.
Actions: Uterine tonic, diuretic, anthelmintic, emetic.
Indications: This herb, which also comes to us via the North American Indians, is one of the best tonics and strengtheners of the reproductive system that we have. Though primarily used for the female system, it can be equally beneficial for men. It is known to contain precursors of the oestrogens (female hormones). However, it acts in a way to normalize function. The body may use this herb to balance and tone and thus it will aid in apparently opposite situations. While being of help in all uterine problems, it is specifically useful in delayed or absent menstruation. Where ovarian pain occurs, *False Unicorn Root* may be safely used. It is also indicated to prevent threatened miscarriage and ease vomiting associated with

pregnancy. However, large doses will cause nausea and vomiting.

Preparation and dosage: Decoction: put 1–2 teaspoonsful of the root in a cup of water, bring to the boil and simmer gently for 10–15 minutes. This should be drunk three times a day. For threatened miscarriage it may be drunk copiously.

Tincture: take 2–4 ml of the tincture three times a day.

LIFE ROOT   *Senecio aureus*
Part used: Dried aerial parts.
Collection: It is collected just before the small flowers open in the summer.
Constituents: Alkaloids including senecifoline and senecine, tannins.
Actions: Uterine tonic, diuretic, expectorant, emmenagogue.
Indications: This is a safe uterine tonic that can be used wherever toning is called for. It will normalize menstrual disturbances of all kinds, especially where delayed or suppressed. It can be used as a douche in vaginal infections or discharges.
Combinations: It goes well in menopausal problems with *St John's Wort, Pasque Flower* and *Chasteberry.*
Preparation and dosage: An infusion is made with 1–3 teaspoonsful of the dried herb to a cup of boiling water. Leave to infuse for 10–15 minutes and drink three times a day.
Tincture: take 1–4 ml of the tincture three times a day.

SQUAW VINE   *Mitchella repens*
Part used: Dried aerial parts.
Constituents: Saponins, mucilage.
Actions: Uterine tonic, emmenagogue, diuretic, astringent, tonic.
Indications: Another wonderful remedy from North America, especially useful for preparing the womb for childbirth. It should be taken for some weeks before birth to ensure a safe experience. It may

relieve painful periods. It has been used to treat colitis.
Combinations: For childbirth it may be used with *Raspberry,* and for painful periods with *Cramp Bark* or *Pasque Flower.*
Preparation and dosage: An infusion is made with 1 teaspoonful to a cup of boiling water, leave to steep for 10–15 minutes and drink three times a day.
Tincture: take 1–2 ml of the tincture three times a day.

Emmanagogues

In herbal literature this is a greatly overused word. It has been used to describe remedies that are generally beneficial to the female reproductive system. However, strictly speaking, the emmenagogues stimulate and promote a normal menstrual flow. Most of the uterine tonics can act as emmenagogues through their tonic and normalizing activity. These are quite powerful herbs that have a specific stimulating action on the womb. This is not necessarily all that healing and they can be very irritating and potentially dangerous in too high a dose. Because of this the powerful emmenagogues must not be used in pregnancy. A list of these is given below. The most useful ones might be: *Blue Cohosh, False Unicorn Root, Life Root, Pennyroyal, Rue, Southernwood, Squaw Vine, Yarrow.*

All are described elsewhere except *Pennyroyal* and *Southernwood.*

PENNYROYAL   *Mentha pulegium*
Part used: Aerial parts.
Collection: Just before flowering in July.
Constituents: Volatile oil, tannin, flavone glycosides.
Actions: Carminative, emmenagogue, diaphoretic, stimulant.
Indications: Its main use is as a stimulating emmenagogue to promote the menstrual process and to strengthen uterine contractions. It should be avoided in pregnancy for

this reason. Because of the aromatic oil it can be used to ease flatulence and colic. It has a reputation for easing anxiety and tension. The oil of *Pennyroyal* should not be used internally without professional guidance.

CAUTION: Avoid during pregnancy.

Preparation and dosage: An infusion is made using 1–2 teaspoonsful of the dried leaves to a cup of water. Leave to steep for 10–15 minutes and drink three times a day.

SOUTHERNWOOD *Artemisia arbortanum*
Part used: Aerial parts.
Collection: In late summer with flowering tops, although it rarely flowers in Britain. Dry with care.
Constituents: Volatile oil.
Actions: Bitter, emmenagogue, anthelmintic, antiseptic.
Indications: A good all-round bitter tonic that has valuable properties in aiding menstrual flow and in stronger doses actually bringing on a delayed period. It can help in clearing threadworm in children.
Combinations: For period problems it is best used with a uterine tonic such as *False Unicorn Root.*
Preparation and dosage: An infusion is made with 1–2 teaspoonsful to a cup of boiling water. Leave to steep for 10 minutes and drink three times a day.
Tincture: take 1–4 ml of the tincture three times a day.

Hormonal Normalizers

A number of herbs contain the chemical precursors of the sex hormones. These remedies can act to provide the body with building blocks that allow it to normalize a hormonal imbalance. This will not always happen as it depends on what the basis of the imbalance is, but in most cases they can work most effectively, as we shall see in the section on menopause. As they do not contain the hormones themselves, the herbs are safe to use with no fear of inducing hormonal imbalance. The uterine tonics can work in this way, but by far the most important remedy here is *Chasteberry*.

CHASTEBERRY *Vitex agnus-castus*
Part used: The fruit.
Collection: The very dark berries should be picked when ripe, which is between October and November. They may be dried in sun or shade.
Constituents: Iridoid glycosides which include aucbin and agnoside; flavonoids including casticin, isovitexin and orientin; essential oil.
Actions: Tonic for the reproductive organs.
Indications: Chasteberry has the effect of stimulating and normalizing pituitary gland functions, especially its progesterone function. It can produce apparently opposite effects though in truth it is simply normalizing. It has for instance a reputation as both an aphrodisiac and an anaphrodisiac! It will always enable what is appropriate to occur. The greatest use of Chasteberry lies in normalizing the activity of female sex hormones and it is thus indicated for dysmenorrhoea, pre-menstrual stress and other disorders related to hormone function. It is especially beneficial during menopausal changes. In a similar way it may be used to aid the body to regain a natural balance after the use of the birth control pill.
Preparation and dosage: Infusion: pour a cup of boiling water onto 1 teaspoonful of the ripe berries and leave to infuse for 10–15 minutes. This should be drunk three times a day.
Tincture: take 1–2 ml of the tincture three times a day.

Astringents

This action will help reduce excessive bleeding and increase the rate of healing of inflammations in the reproductive system. Most of the astringents described in the section on actions (Chapter 3) are valuable here, but especially so are *Beth Root, Cranesbill, Lady's Mantle* and *Periwinkle*.

Let us consider *Beth Root, Lady's Mantle* and *Periwinkle*.

BETH ROOT   *Trillium erectum*
Part used: Root or rhizome.
Collection: The underground parts are unearthed in late summer or autumn.
Constituents: Steroidal saponins, steroidal glycosides, tannins, fixed oil.
Actions: Uterine tonics, astringent, expectorant.
Indications: This is another plant with natural sex hormone precursors present, and so has the normalizing action described above. It is a good uterine tonic but is most often used as a uterine astringent for excessive blood loss during or between periods. It can help in blood loss associated with the menopause. It has been used as an ointment for ulcers and wounds.
Combinations: For excessive bleeding during periods it will combine well with *Cranesbill* or *Periwinkle*.
Preparation and dosage: A decoction is made with 1-2 teaspoonsful of the dried herb simmered in a cup of water for 10-15 minutes. This is drunk three times a day.

LADY'S MANTLE   *Alchemilla vulgaris*
Part used: The aerial parts.
Collection: The leaves and stems are collected in the summer.
Constituents: Tannin, bitter principle, traces of essential oil, salicylic acid.
Actions: Astringent, diuretic, anti-inflammatory, vulnerary.
Indications: The whole genus of *Alchemilla* has a long reputation in Europe for 'women's complaints'. It will ease both period pains and excessive bleeding. It will aid in the changes of the menopause. As a general astringent *Lady's Mantle* can be used internally in diarrhoea and externally for cuts and wounds.
Preparation and dosage: An infusion is made with 2 teaspoonsful to a cup of water. Steep for 10-15 minutes and drink three times a day.

PERIWINKLE   *Vinca major*
Part used: Aerial parts.
Collection: This herb is collected in the spring.
Constituents: Alkaloids, tannins.
Actions: Astringent, sedative.
Indications: Periwinkle is an excellent all-round astringent that may be used internally or externally. Its main use is in the treatment of excessive menstrual flow, either during the period itself or with blood loss between periods. It can be used in digestive problems such as colitis or diarrhoea where it will act to reduce the loss of fluid or blood while toning the membranes. It may also be used in cases of nose bleed, bleeding gums, mouth ulcers or sore throats. It has a reputation for aiding in the treatment of diabetes.
Combinations: It will combine well with *Cranesbill* and *Agrimony*. For menstrual problems it may be used with *Beth Root.*
Preparation and dosage: Infusion: pour a cup of boiling water onto 1 teaspoonful of the dried herb and let infuse for 10-15 minutes. This should be drunk three times a day.
Tincture: take 1-2 ml of the tincture three times a day.

Demulcents
These may often be useful to soothe inflamed and sore tissue. The urinary demulcents are especially helpful here. We can mention *Blue Cohosh, Corn Silk, Golden Seal* and *Marshmallow Leaf.*

Antiseptics
The urinary system is a common site for

infection to get a hold. The reasons why this should be are numerous; partially it is a result of anatomy but with the use of the IUD, antibiotic drugs etc. the natural defences break down. This is discussed more in the section on infections. Important herbs here include: *Bearberry, Echinacea, Garlic, Juniper, Wild Indigo* and *Yarrow.*

Alteratives and Lymphatic Tonics
These gentle cleansing and toning remedies will help the system both as a whole deal with a focus of illness in the reproductive system and speed the recovery from any specific illness. Try *Blue Flag, Burdock, Cleavers, Echinacea, Poke Root* and *Sarsaparilla.*

Nervines and Anti-spasmodics
Remedies to help the nervous system and ease stress and tension reactions will often help in problems of this system. The anti-spasmodic remedies will ease cramping of periods. Of the vast range of such herbs we can mention: *Black Haw, Cramp Bark, Pasque Flower, Skullcap, Lady's Slipper, Valerian* and *Vervain.*

Diuretics
Water retention is often associated with period problems, either because of direct water retention or congestion of the lower abdomen leading to a water build-up in the legs. Diuretics will help remove excess water, but the basic problem must be addressed. Appropriate remedies include: *Dandelion Leaf, Yarrow* and *Juniper Berries.*

Problems of the Reproductive System

In a book of this kind there is a limit to what can usefully be covered, so only certain topics will be examined. This does not mean that herbal medicine cannot help in the wide range of gynaecological conditions that arise, but that many of these problems call for a skilled practitioner. There are limits to self-help.

The Menstrual Cycle

The uterine tonics will usually normalize irregularities in the normal cycle. The right one to use must be worked out for each individual depending on the broader picture. A detailed study of these herbs will show how they each can be used in the context of the whole body or combined with other herbs. The context of the whole body or combined with other herbs. The suggestions given here for specific problems must be seen in this context.

Where there is delayed onset of menstruation, which can cause distress and a whole range of physical problems in adolescent girls, a combination of uterine tonics and emmenagogues will often initiate normal activity and so relieve the physiological tension that builds up. Possible remedies are: *Blue Cohosh, Chasteberry, Rue, Southernwood, False Unicorn Root.*

In adult females a similar range could be used but with more emphasis on the emmenagogues. Remember, however, that the commonest cause for lack of periods is pregnancy. So check this out first.

Excessive bleeding during periods, or menorrhagia, can be successfully controlled with herbs. It is important to ensure that such treatment is not masking an underlying reason for the blood loss. This will involve skilled diagnosis. Given that this is the case, a combination of astringents and uterine tonics will usually help. Of course, as already stressed, the treatment must be in the context of the needs of that individual woman. The herbs suggested may be used in combination with whatever is appropriate: *Cranesbill, Beth Root, Periwinkle.*

A similar approach will often help bleeding in between periods. This, however, is a sign that must be taken very seriously and medical advice be sought. Herbally it is worth considering *Chasteberry* as well as those just mentioned.

Painful periods, with cramping etc. can be relieved quite easily with herbs. There are two specifics that relax the muscles involved: *Black Haw* and *Cramp Bark.*

Other nervines will help, but at this point it is worth considering pre-menstrual tension, as it will often be associated with period cramps.

Pre-menstrual Tension

Herbal remedies are uniquely successful in easing the miseries of this very common problem.

It can be described as a condition of physical, behavioural and mood changes related to the menstrual cycle. The commonest symptoms include irritability, depression, breast tenderness and a 'bloated' sensation. Pre-existing disorders such as migraine or skin problems are likely to be exacerbated premenstrually. Life generally becomes more of a strain, the degree of pressure varying between women.

Little clarity has come from physiological research about the root causes of this problem. Localized water retention in various parts of the body has been implicated as a possible cause of the tension, as have hormonal changes. Cyclical changes in certain brain chemicals have been suggested in the same way. There is no doubt that marked body changes occur at all levels of study.

Such research ignores, to its loss, the involvement of mind and emotion in PMT, and menstruation in general. There is a suggestion that such problems are a response to the hormonal changes resulting from the women's experience of her mother's attitudes and approaches to periods. If these attitudes were not open and healthy then as a child the girl would develop resistance and psychological blockage around the whole subject. As she grew and matured this would surface as premenstrual tension. There are many other such theories, the point being that this problem has a range of causative factors feeding it. There is no one thing to blame.

Herbs that can be used to relieve the symptoms when they arise include the following nervines: *Skullcap, Valerian, Motherwort, Cramp Bark, Pasque Flower.*

The specific remedies chosen will depend on the ones that work best, obviously, but also on the degree of associated cramping or water retention etc. Herbs such as *Skullcap*, almost a specific here, are best used when the problem is active just before the menstruation starts.

Long-term treatment is best based on the use of *Chasteberry* in the context of a balanced herbal approach to the person's whole being. It works over a period of time to balance hormone levels without interfering with any of the body's necessary work.

Herbal diuretics are sold in chemist shops for the relief of PMT. The value of diuretics is debatable as the water retention may be secondary to the emotional tension rather than the other way round. Thus *Skullcap* may relieve the water retention while diuretics may not ease the tension. If diuretics are indicated, consider *Dandelion Leaf* and *Yarrow.*

Pregnancy and Childbirth

This most profound and magical of human experiences is blessed by nature with many herbs to aid and support both mind and body, mother and baby, throughout the whole time.

However, of much more importance than which herbs to use are the attitudes, experiences and energies that surround the mother and developing baby. The mother's experience of love and support, or lack of it, are an integral part of the development of the foetus. it is a time to put one's loving attention within to experience the unfolding of life. To be able to do this completely involves creating an environment and relationship that are whole and loving in themselves. This asks a lot of mother, father, relations, the world, but it is the least the baby deserves.

A whole and healthy diet, rich in fresh vegetables and fruit, is going to be a firm foundation for the child to build its body from, just as the quality of the mother's emotional and mental experience during pregnancy lay the foundations for the child's experience and perception of themselves and their world.

Herbs that can be used to ensure a strong mother, easy birth and healthy child are numerous. The first point is to ensure that the mother is well, and so herbs that are appropriate for her and her unique needs are central to any prescribing at this time. If digestive problems arise, then the advice given in the section applies. Similarly if blood pressure rises, the herbs that lower it can be safely used if the advice given in the section on 'Circulation' is followed.

Certain herbs have a reputation of helping to strengthen the womb. The two main ones here are _Squaw Vine_ and _Raspberry Leaves._

These can be taken throughout pregnancy to ensure as much uterine strength and health as possible. Here we will describe _Raspberry._

RASPBERRY   _Rubus idaeus_
Part used: Leaves and fruit.

Collection: The leaves may be collected throughout the growing season. Dry slowly in a well-ventilated area.

Constituents: Leaves: fruit sugar, volatile oil, pectin, citric acid, malic acid.

Actions: Astringent, tonic refrigerant, parturient.

Indications: Raspberry leaves have a long tradition of use in pregnancy to strengthen and tone the tissue of the womb, assisting contractions and checking any haemorrhage during labour. This action will occur if the herb is drunk regularly throughout pregnancy and as a drink during labour. As an astringent it may be used in a wide range of cases, including diarrhoea, leucorrhoea and other loose conditions. It is valuable in the easing of mouth problems such as mouth ulcers, bleeding gums and inflammations. As a gargle it will help sore throats.

Preparation and dosage: Infusion: pour a cup of boiling water onto 2 teaspoonsful of the dried herb and let infuse for 10–15 minutes. This may be drunk freely.

Tincture: take 2–4 ml of the tincture three times a day.

The alteratives and tonics can be helpful, especially ones such as _Nettles_ and _Cleavers._

If constipation develops, gentle laxatives may be used: _Yellow Dock, Dandelion Root._

Blood pressure problems may be normalized with anti-hypertensives such as _Hawthorn Berries, Lime Blossom, Yarrow_ and _Cramp Bark._

Morning sickness, which is due to hormonal changes in the early stages of pregnancy, can often be stopped with the following herbs taken regularly through the first few weeks: _Black Horehound, Peppermint, Chamomile._

The galactogogues can be astoundingly effective at increasing milk production. The best even gets it name from its use to increase milk yields in goats, that is _Goat's Rye._ Others include the aromatic herbs _Fennel, Fenugreek_ and _Aniseed._ To stop milk production use *Red Sage* liberally.

Menopause

The menopause is one of the biggest transistions a human being can go through. Much has been written, and much said about its multiple problems; however, it can be a time of release and freedom. The ties of a lifetime and roles with which society has bound women can be loosened.

The undoubted physical problems of the hormonal transformation can be eased and in some cases removed altogether. Whether the hormonal changes lead to the rather too common mental and emotional problems is unclear. However it is a time of major life events – children leaving home, parents dying, husband retiring etc.

There can be no doubt that this time period has profound implications for the woman involved, the major changes in personal role often being seen as her becoming 'useless'. Valuable counselling work can be done based on an exploration of the opportunities that open up in the 'Change of Life', as a new start where the woman can create what she wants and not simply what her children and husband need, if previously these defined her activities. It can be a release rather than a rejection, no matter what she is changing *from* and moving *to*.

Herbal medicine can help both with the hormonal and psychological problems. Herbs to consider include: *Chasteberry, Blue Cohosh, Life Root, False Unicorn Root, Golden Seal* and *Ladies Mantle*.

Of these, *Chasteberry* is the most important because of its action in balancing hormonal disruptions. It will gradually, but effectively, reduce hot flushes.

A whole range of the herbal relaxing and anti-depressant remedies may be indicated. The specifics will vary from woman to woman and so should ideally be prescribed by a good herbalist. Certain plants are worth emphasizing: *St John's Wort, Motherwort, Pasque Flower, Skullcap, Valerian.*

The Male Reproductive System

Certain remedies act as tonics for the male reproductive system. Apart from the general strengthening tonics we can mention *Saw Palmetto, Damiana* and *Ginseng*.

They work in different ways, the *Ginseng* being a more general hormonal and endocrine adaptogen. All three have traditional use as aphrodisiacs; however, this can probably be explained through their action as tonics. When health is renewed the natural strengths and urges will be more alive. Let us consider *Saw Palmetto*.

SAW PALMETTO BERRIES
Serenoa serrulata
Part used: Berries.
Collection: The berries of this impressive palm are gathered from September through until January.
Constituents: Volatile oil, steroids, dextrose, resins.
Actions: Diuretic, urinary antiseptic, endocrine agent.
Indications: Saw Palmetto is a herb that acts to tone and strengthen the male reproductive system. It may be used with safety where a boost to the male sex hormones is required. It is a specific in cases of enlarged prostate glands. It will be of value in all infections of the genito-urinary tract.
Combinations: For debility associated with the reproductive system it will combine well with *Damiana* and *Kola*. For the treatment of enlarged prostate glands it may be used with *Horsetail* and *Hydrangea*.
Preparation and dosage: Decoction: put ½–1 teaspoonful of the berries in a cup of water, bring to the boil and simmer gently

for 5 minutes. This should be drunk three times a day.

Tincture: take 1-2 ml of the tincture three times a day.

The Prostate Gland

A common problem that effects men in later life is an enlargement of the prostate gland. This will cause problems with passing water and can be painful. Accurate diagnosis is essential as it may be due to infection or even cancer. In cases where a simple, or benign, enlargement is occurring the following herbs can be helpful when used over a few months: *Horsetail, Saw Palmetto, Hydrangea.*

If infection is present then in addition consider: *Bearberry, Echinacea.*

THE NERVOUS SYSTEM

In no other system of the body is the connection between the physical and the psychological aspects of our humanity as apparent as in the nervous system. Clearly, the tissue of the nervous system is part of the physical make-up of the body and, just as clearly, all psychological processes take place in the nervous system. Therefore, if there is dis-ease on a psychological level, it will be reflected physiologically. One wonders why the physical side of being was ever regarded as separate from the psychological.

A holistic approach to herbal healing acknowledges this interconnectedness, and regards nervous tissue and its functions as a vital element in the treatment of the whole being.

Orthodox medicine tends to reduce psychological problems to the mere biochemical level, and assumes that 'appropriate' drugs will sort out or at least hide the problem sufficiently to allow 'normal' life to continue.

Interestingly enough, some techniques in the field of complementary medicine assume or imply the other extreme, namely that psychological factors are the cause of *any* disease and that treatment of the psyche is the *only* appropriate way of healing, and will take care of any physical problem.

By bringing these two reductionist views together, we come closer to a holistic approach. With herbal medicine we can treat the nervous system as part of the whole body. We can feed and strengthen it, helping the psyche. For our being to be truly healthy, we have to take care of our physical health through right diet and right lifestyle, but we are also responsible for a healthy emotional, mental and spiritual life. The emotional atmosphere we live in should be fulfilling, nurturing, and support emotional stability. Our thoughts should be creative and life-enhancing, open to the free flow of intuition and imagination, not conceptually rigid. And equally, we have to stay open to the free flow of the higher energies of our soul, without which health is impossible.

Any disease that manifests in the body must be seen in an emotional, mental and spiritual, as well as a physical, context. We must also remember that as part of the greater whole of humanity we are, in a deep and mysterious way, connected with humanity's diseases, and immersed in a sea of impulses and factors not directly under our control. Many 'neuroses' met in today's western society are quite possibly normal responses to an absurdly abnormal environment, *sane* reactions of the psyche and emotions to the *insanities* of a diseased society.

In this sense, there is a limit to the healing of an individual, when the disease is really a reflection of society's disease. To be a healer in the late twentieth century involves an awareness of the whole and a certain amount of political insight, if not activity. For us to be whole, our society must be whole. For our society to be whole, *we* must be whole. For our society to truly reflect our highest aspirations, *we* have to live, embody and reflect those aspirations.

Herbal medicine can be an ecological and spiritually integrated tool to aid the nervous system of humanity, so that humanity can help itself. It is an ideal counterpart on the physical level for therapeutic techniques on the psychological level, to help people to embrace their wholeness.

For a more detailed look at herbal medication and its dovetailing with relaxation, meditation etc. see *Successful Stress Control* by D.L. Hoffman (pub. Thorsons).

Herbs for the Nervous System

There are a number of ways in which herbs can benefit the nervous system in addition to the rather simplistic ones of stimulation and relaxation. As was described in Chapter 3 on 'Actions', herbs that benefit the nervous system are called nervines and are usually divided into *nervine tonics, nervine relaxants* and *nervine stimulants*. It may be superfluous to point this out again, but any successful treatment of illness with herbs will involve treating the whole body and not simply the symptoms. This holds as true for the complexities of the nervous system as for any other part of the body. Of course, the symptoms of anxiety, depression or nerve damage can be reduced greatly, but the whole system must be strengthened in the face of the storm! In addition to these nervines we have also discussed anti-spasmodics, adaptogens and sedatives.

Please review the sections on these actions and familiarize yourself with the herbs mentioned there.

In addition to ordinary herbal remedies it is worth considering Diet and Bach Flower remedies when dealing with this system.

Bach Flower Remedies

The Bach Flower Remedies represent an approach to herbalism that is an alchemical amalgam of the spiritual essence of the flower in co-operation with the emotional/mental need of the person.

They are not used directly for physical illness, but for the individual's worry, apprehension, hopelessness, fear, irritability, etc. The state of someone's psychic being has a major bearing on the causation, development and cure of any physical illness. The remedies appear to work with the life-force, allowing it to flow freely through or around the block and so speed healing and a return to wholeness.

Thirty-eight remedies were developed by the late Dr Edward Bach. The story of how he found them is wonderful indeed and worth reading about. The contact address for any information about the Remedies is:

Dr E. Bach Centre, Mount Vernon, Sotwell, Wallingford, Oxon, OX10 OPZ, England

He found thirty-eight flowers to cover the negative states of mind from which we so often suffer, catagorizing them under seven major headings with further subdivisions. These headings are apprehension, indecision, loneliness, insufficient interest in circumstances, over-sensitivity, despondancy and despair, over-care for others.

These flower remedies are ideal for self-use and again much more information and supplies are obtainable from the Centre. They are inherently benign in action and have no unpleasant reactions and can be used by anyone. The dose is simply a few drops of the special extracts in water.

I shall quote from a brief guide to remedies produced by the centre to give a taste of the uses of the remedies.

Agrimony: for those who suffer inner torture which they try to hide behind a facade of cheerfulness.

Aspen: for apprehension and forboding. Fears of unknown origin.

Beech: for those who are arrogant, critical and intolerant of others.

Centaury: weakness of will in those who let themselves be imposed upon and become subservient, who have difficulty in saying 'no'.

Cerato: those who doubt their own judgement and overly seek the advice of others. Often influenced and misguided.

Cherry Plum: for a fear of mental collapse, desperation or loss of control. Vicious rages.

Chestnut Bud: a refusal to learn by experience and continually repeating the same mistakes.

Chicory: over-possessive and demanding attention. Selfishness. For those who like others to conform to their standards. Will often make martyrs of themselves.

Clematis: indifferent, inattentive, dreamy and absent-minded. Mental escape from reality.

Crab Apple: a cleanser for those who feel unclean or ashamed of ailments. For self-disgust and the house-proud.

Elm: temporarily over-come by responsibility or inadequacy, although normally very capable.

Gentian: despondent, easily discouraged and dejected.

Gorse: extreme hopelessness.

Heather: for people who are obsessed with their own troubles and experiences. Poor listeners.

Holly: for those who are jealous, envious, revengeful and suspicious. For those who hate.

Honeysuckle: for those with nostalgia who constantly dwell in the past. Also home-sickness.

Hornbeam: procrastination, 'Monday morning' feeling.

Impatiens: impatience and irritability.

Larch: despondency due to lack of self-confidence. An expectation of failure so they fail to make an attempt. They feel inferior although have the ability.

Mimulus: fear of known things, shyness and timidity.

Mustard: deep gloom that descends for no known reason but which can lift just as suddenly. Melancholy.

Oak: determination. Struggles on in illness and against adversity despite setbacks. A plodder.

Olive: exhaustion-drained of energy –everything is an effort.

Pine: feelings of guilt. They blame themselves for mistakes of others and feel unworthy.

Red Chestnut: excessive fear and over-caring for others held dear.

Rock Rose: terror, extreme fear or panic.

Rock Water: for those who are hard on themselves, rigid-minded and self-denying.

Scleranthus: uncertainty, indecision and vacillation.

Star of Bethlehem: for all the effects of bad news or fright following an accident.

Sweet Chestnut: anguish of those who have reached the limits of endurance and absolute dejection.

Vervain: over-enthusiasm, over-effort and straining. Fanatical.

Vine: dominating, inflexible, ambitious and autocratic. Arrogance and pride.

Walnut: a protection remedy from powerful influences and helps adjustment to any transition or change, e.g. menopause or divorce.

Water Violet: proud, reserved, 'superior'.

White Chestnut: persistent unwanted

thoughts. Pre-occupation with a worry or event. Mental arguments.

Wild Oat: helps determine one's intended path in life.

Wild Rose: resignation, apathy. For drifters who accept their lot, making little effort for improvement.

Willow: resentment and bitterness with a 'poor me' attitude.

RESCUE REMEDY: a combination of *Cherry Plum, Clematis, Impatiens, Rock Rose, Star of Bethlehem.* An all-purpose emergency composite for causes of trauma, anguish, bereavement, and any stress.

Rescue Remedy is to treat the effect that a sufferer may experience through serious news, bereavement, terror, severe mental trauma, a feeling of desperation or a numbed, bemused state of mind. Every home should have a dropper bottle of it, and it is worth travelling with it. It is taken orally, at a dose of about four drops in water.

Diet

By now everyone has heard the expression 'you are what you eat'. Nowhere is this more true than in a person with neurological problems or under stress and suffering from subsequent tension.

Ideally the food we eat and the way that we eat it supplies us with all the nutrition we need and a time of relaxation in which to digest it. Most people are not ideal, however!

The normal diet of our society has been commented on so many times by everyone from dieticians to the government that I shall focus here on how to ensure that the nervous system is fed as well as the whole of body and mind. One point: avoid fad diets. They may be good for weight loss or whatever, but they are very bad for awareness and conciousness. Diet is discussed in more depth in the section on the digestive system.

In general a healthy diet would be one rich in fresh, raw green vegetables and fruit with a small amount of good meat if you can morally justify it to yourself. A major problem with meat in stress-related conditions is the feed stuff given to the animals, the chemicals that may have been used to stimulate growth. Much of current animal husbandry is straight out of a chemistry laboratory that we as the consumers know nothing about. The diet should contain a fair proportion of roughage, but not buckets of bran! Wholemeal bread and a proportion of raw vegetables is fine.

A key to any dietary approach to health has to be the avoidance of artificial additives in any form. This will include flavours, colours and preservatives — extremely difficult but vital.

A good supply of the vitamin B complex and vitamin C is essential. The C will come from fruit and most green vegetables while the B is found in wholegrains, eggs, some fish, molasses and brewer's yeast.

There is much that should be avoided to help reduce anxiety and tension in general. As a priority there must be no caffeine-containing food or drink as this adds to any agitation–this means no coffee, tea and chocolate. Too much red meat can act as a physical stimulant and so might be avoided.

Alcohol will be deleterious to the nervous system, amongst its other problems. Avoid it as well as tobacco.

The Nervous System and Illness

This system has a multifaceted pattern of illnesses that affect it. We can talk about the purely physical problems, such as Motor Neurone Disease or Parkinson's Disease or the purely psychological problems such as anxiety neuroses and depression. There are, of course, a whole range of overlapping 'syndromes'.

We shall not consider the major neurological problems that are so common today. Their adequate treatment involves the help of skilled practitioners or the healing arts, whether orthodox or complementary. Much can be done in problems such as, Parkinson's, Multiple Sclerosis, Motor Neurone Disease, etc., but it lies beyond the scope of this book.

Here we shall consider stress and anxiety, depression, insomnia, headaches and migraine, hyperactivity and pain.

Stress

A major contributing factor in all illness these days is the stress under which we live. There are many herbs that help the body deal with the extra pressures laid upon it in such times. Here we shall look at ways they can be used.

Daily Use of Herbal Remedies for Stress

If it is known that a period of stress and strain is about to descend and fill your life with its usual basket of 'goodies', it is worth recognizing this beforehand. There are certain herbs that will minimize the impact.

These herbs will help as gentle relaxing remedies for regular use. They can be used as teas, as cold drinks, as relaxing foot baths, infused in massage oil, or even as full baths. As oils, in aromatherapy, is a wonderful way of absorbing the herbal benefits. The remedies can make quite delicious wines, but it could be a very herbal way to become alcoholic so they should be used with discretion. The different ways of using the herbs are described in detail in Chapter 8.

It may be best to list the plants that can be used as safe daily easers of stress and calmers of anxiety. Choose the ones for yourself by their effect on *you*. Taste and general intuition may tell which would be the most suitable to use. All these suggested here are safe and are not tranquilizers. This is a partial list. The sections in Chapter 3 contain much more detailed information: *Oats, Chamomile, Limeblossom, Wood Betony, Balm, Lavender, Skullcap.*

In addition to herbal remedies it is important that your food is feeding you well and this especially applies to the nervous system. In addition to all the guidelines for good diet, this is a time when a vitamin supplement may be called for. A daily supplement of the B complex of vitamins, perhaps one combined with vitamin C, would be most beneficial.

Apart from healthy responses to stress – enjoying herbs and improving diet – try to see if the stress itself can be reduced. This is occasionally impossible but surprisingly often quite possible. Don't just put up with something or someone because they are there. You can change both you and your life. It helps to re-evaluate your choices. Are you doing what you really want to do? If not, what is it that you would like to do? Give yourself permission to ask some searching questions of yourself and about your lifestyle. Don't censor any of the answers that may come up!

After checking out your inner motivation you have the choice of what you do with it. If changing the apparent cause is too difficult or painful . . . well, you are free to not change also. With herbs, and possibly counselling combined with relaxation, it will be possible to ease the strain and live a less tense and anxious life. However, if you choose to change, then herbal medicine, if used wisely will aid you in the process of transformation.

So from all of this it is clear that the daily use of herbs to help with the stresses and strains of daily life have much to offer. Give them a try.

When Stress Continues For a Long Time

The borderline is blurred between this degree of stress impact and the daily levels we all seem to put up with. For a gentle soul with a not too strong constitution it will be sooner than for the stronger one who copes well. Neither of these extremes of personality is 'better' than the other, we just live in a world of human diversity. That is sometimes a joy and sometimes the cause of the strain itself!

The advice given above still holds here, but in addition there are two remedies that should become staples. Not both together, but the one that is most suitable for the person concerned.

The remedies are the adaptogens, *Ginseng* and *Siberian Ginseng*. As it happens there is no close botanical relationship, the similarity in names comes from commercial interests. Of these two perhaps *Siberian Ginseng* is of widest relevance, aiding and supporting the whole of the hormonal system that deals with the impact of stress.

Immediate Relief

There are times in most people's lives where things get too much and the pain of existence builds to a crescendo. At such times herbs can be only an aid, a part of a whole approach to the difficulties being faced. These difficulties can be so multifarious in our crazy and chaotic times that I shall simply talk about herbs that can be used. It may be appropriate to seek aid from the various caring professions, go on holiday or retreat, or even go to hospital.

Immediate herbal relief may be needed in a whole range of traumatic situations, from being involved in a car accident to some personal emotional crisis. In all cases the herbs will take the edge off the intensity but will rarely remove it. Pain, physical and emotional, appears to be part of the 'gift', of our being human. Pain, be it emotional or physical, is a message from ourself to ourself and as such it must be listened and responded to. To suppress the pain with painkillers or tranquilizers only pushes the trauma deeper–either deeper into our psyche or deeper into the body.

There are plants that will suppress this intensity but in our society they are considered dangerous and are restricted drugs, and as such will be ignored here.

We can mention herbs that safely ease the intensity: *Valerian, Passion Flower, Jamaican Dogwood, Wild Lettuce, Ladies Slipper.*

These are discussed in depth elsewhere in the book.

Anti-spasmodic drops: these are a combination of herbs, not all nervines, that ease shock and trauma. There are a number of proprietary makes available and it is easier to buy a bottle from a reputable herb supplier than try and concoct them yourself. The remedy can safely be used to ease the trauma of a shock. Take as directed on the label.

Rescue Remedy: this is discussed in much more detail in the section on Bach Flower Remedies, but it is one of the best treatments for shock available.

Anxiety and Tension

The remedies already described for stress management all have a role to play in dealing with what the medical profession call 'anxiety neurosis'. However, herbs by themselves will not always be enough. Counselling, relaxation techniques, meditation or a whole range of other physical or psychological approaches may be called for. Herbs will work well in conjunction with such approaches which are beyond the scope of this book to discuss in any valid form.

Aromatherapy has much to offer in conjunction with internal herbal medication.

Please consult the section on the use of aromatic oils.

Depression

We have all at some time or other experienced depression. It is a word that describes a whole range of feelings from a mild case of the 'blues' to an all-encompassing black cloud that can be unendurable for the person in it.

Herbal aid and support in depression can help in raising this cloud but the only truly effective way is to find the roots of it. If there is a clear-cut external reason that produces an 'understandable' depression, herbs can help in supporting the person through the time of trial. This would be the case in depression following bereavement or loss of some sort.

However, when the depression appears out of the depths of one's being with no apparent cause, treatment poses problems. The roots need to be found and helped. This will often necessitate skilled psychotherapy, for which herbal medication will support. In extreme depression there can be no doubt that drug therapy has much to offer that herbs do not. There can be a useful blending of therapies here with the herbs helping the broader body picture and drug therapy helping the psychological state.

Treatment of Depression

All that has been said above in the section on stress about diet, relaxation and a reappraisal of lifestyle and purpose holds true here. There is a range of herbal remedies that will raise a depressed state. However, we have to be careful about claiming specific anti-depressant action as different herbs will work in different ways with different people.

Actions that can have the desired effect include nervine tonics, adaptogens and bitters. It is possible to talk about thymoleptics meaning anti-depressants, but it is somewhat outmoded as a term. Of the herbs that have a reputation as useful direct anti-depressants we can mention *Damiana, Vervain, St John's Wort, Lavender, Lemon Balm* and *Skullcap.*

These have all been discussed excepted *Damiana.*

DAMIANA *Turnera aphrodisiaca*
Part used: Dried leaves and stems.
Collection: The leaves and stems are gathered at the time of flowering.
Constituents: Essential oil that includes pinene, cineol, cymol, arbutin, cymene, cadinene and copaenen; alkaloids, bitter; flavonoid; cyanogenic glycoside; tannins; resin.
Actions: Nerve tonic, anti-depressant, urinary antiseptic, laxative.
Indications: Damiana is an excellent strengthening remedy for the nervous system. It has an ancient reputation as an aphrodisiac. While this may or may not be true, it has a definite tonic action on the central nervous and the hormonal system. The pharmacology of the plant suggests that the alkaloids could have a testosterone-like action (testerone is a male hormone). As a useful anti-depressant, Damiana is considered to be a specific in cases of anxiety and depression where there is a sexual factor. It may be used to strengthen the male sexual system.
Combinations: As a nerve tonic it is often used with *Oats.* Depending on the situation it combines well with *Kola* or *Skullcap.*
Preparation and dosage: Infusion: pour a cup of boiling water onto 1 teaspoonful of the dried leaves and let infuse for 10–15 minutes. This should be drunk three times a day.

From the herbs mentioned you will see that most are nervine tonics, which is to be expected as they work to strengthen and feed the nervous system directly. Others in this group not mentioned here can be anti-depressive.

Aromatherapy can aid in a general experience of upliftment and self-worth. To avoid repetition please consult Chapter 4.

When depression is associated with debility or after illness such as the 'flu then in addition to nervine tonics it is worth considering bitters, adaptogens or even nervine stimulants. The adaptogens can help lift a depression if taken over a period of time. However some very sensitive people develop headaches with _Ginseng_ and so should avoid it. The stimulants should be used in moderation as caffeine takes more out of the nervous system than it apparently gives and can give rise to a debility after its effects have worn off.

Bitters often lift debilitated depression through their general tonic action on the body. Ones worth mentioning here are _Wormwood, Mugwort, Rue_ and _Gentian_. All are considered in the section on 'Bitters' except _Mugwort,_ which follows.

MUGWORT   _Artemisia vulgaris_
Part used: Leaves or root.
Collection: The leaves and flowering stalks should be gathered just at blossoming time, which is between July and September.
Constituents: Volatilve oil containing cineole and thujone; a bitter principle, tannin, resin, inulin.
Actions: Bitter tonic, stimulant, nervine tonic, emmenagogue.
Indications: Mugwort can be used wherever a digestive stimulant is needed. It will aid the digestion through the bitter stimulation of the juices while also providing a carminative oil. It has a mildly nervine action in aiding depression and easing tension, which appears to be due to the volatile oil, so it is essential that this is not lost in preparation. Mugwort may also

be used as an emmenagogue in the aiding of normal menstrual flow.
Preparation and dosage: Infusion: pour a cup of boiling water onto 1-2 teaspoonsful of the dried herb and leave to infuse for 10-15 minutes in a covered container. This should be drunk three times a day. Mugwort is used as a flavouring in a number of aperitive drinks, a pleasant way to take it! Tincture: take 1-4 ml of the tincture three times a day.

Psychosomatic Illness

Most illness is either caused or contributed to by psychological factors. In its more medically obvious forms it is called psychosomatic illness. We could as easily talk of somatopsychic illness as the body and mind are one whole integrated reality. It is a therapeutic mistake to create such divisions.

With herbal medicine there is the chance to work holistically by using remedies for the physical manifestation while aiding the mind and emotions through the right nervines. This is mentioned throughout this book but please consult _Successful Stress Control_ (pub. Thorsons).

Insomnia

Good sleep is fundamental to good health and lack of sleep will hurt either immediately or eventually. On a day-to-day basis, pain, stress and anxiety may all be disruptive to a good night's sleep, leaving you fatigued the next day. This fatigue will reduce the body's ability to cope with stress and discomfort, so that you are even more uncomfortable and probably more anxious. This makes it more likely that the following night's sleep will be spoiled. And so you enter into a vicious cycle of stress-anxiety-insomnia-fatigue-increased stress and pain.

The lack of enough sleep may be voluntary. It may seem that the body has got used to operating on a tired basis. However, this will tell in the long run via serious disease or disorder, increasing vulnerability to stress symptoms, and faster ageing.

Herbs to Help Sleep

Nature is rich in plant remedies that help soothe the way towards sleep. If the mind will not stop or the body is too agitated, herbs can be of much help.

The strong and potentially dangerous narcotic plants are, of course, illegal and will not be discussed here. All the plants mentioned are safe and non-addictive.

They can be used in a number of ways. The specific details are discussed in the section on preparations, but to aid sleep they are most effective as teas or used as additives in baths. This works best with relaxing plants that have a pleasant aroma. The combination of a relaxing nervine herb such as a few drops of *Lavender* oil added to the bath, followed by a cup of sleep-inducing *Valerian* tea is both pleasant and effective.

The actions to consider are the hypnotics, sedatives and nervine relaxants. All the relaxing remedies may be enough to help relax the body and mind enough for sleep to come. Herbs such as *Skullcap, Lavender* and *Motherwort*, while not for insomnia, may have the desired effect. Here I shall list the plants with a reputation for inducing sleep, all of which are described elsewhere: *Hops, Jamaican Dogwood, Lime Blossom, Passion Flower, Valerian, Wild Lettuce.*

With the wide range of plants that can help and the different ways to use them it would be a book in itself exploring all the ramifications of herbs for sleep. There are a few favourites that I have.

A mixture of equal parts of *Skullcap,* *Valerian* and *Passion Flower* makes an effective sleep potion. It can be made by mixing equal parts of the dried herb or the tinctures. If using the dried herb then an ounce of the herb mixture to a pint of boiling water should be left to infuse for 10 minutes. If the insomnia is a major problem then take a wineglassful of the tea after each meal and two before going to bed. It is difficult to be too specific about dosage as there is such variation between people.

In addition to herbal remedies there are some dietary things that can help. With some people a light snack an hour before going to bed may, especially if it is a *Lettuce* sandwich. This is because, as the cultivated cousin of the wild species, it may help.

The natural amino acid L-Tryptophan taken regularly for about a month will usually help the sleep process. It is a natural precursor to a sleep-inducing chemical found in the brain. Another supplement that can help is Dolomite tablets. In addition, remember the guidelines for diet and low stress. Don't take any caffeine drinks such as tea, coffee, hot chocolate or 'colas' from 5 p.m. onwards, as these will tend to keep awake those with a sleep problem.

Various relaxation techniques can help with this problem. For guidance in relaxation for sleep, please consult *Successful Stress Control* (pub. Thorsons).

Headaches

Headaches must be the commonest complaint to affect us today. Turn on the television at any time and you will see the most common type of head pain illustrated in advertisements for aspirin or its substitutes. Unfortunately, these drugs offer no lasting relief for chronic pain. If the roots of the headache are sought and dealt with, the headache will go and not return.

Broadly speaking, there are two types of headache, both of which may be aggravated or triggered by stress. There is the muscular tension sort and the vascular or migraine type.

Tension Headaches

Tension headaches are not only due to emotional or mental tension. Tight muscles can result from poor posture, from working in awkward positions, and from a too sudden strain. Stress, however, is the commonest catalyst for transforming painless muscle tension into a headache.

Even though we are all under the stresses of our competitive society, not everyone suffers from chronic headaches. Why do some people collapse under the same pressures that others seem to thrive on? Each person has a different stress threshold, which allows one person to cope easily with life's events, while another will suffer fits of anxiety in the face of a minor crisis. The anxious person is more prone to headaches.

Relaxation, massage and other ways of easing tension are as important as herbs for this sort of headache. A simple exercise can help to keep the neck and shoulders relaxed and poised. Sit back for a moment and do a few slow head rolls. Bring your chin down to your chest, slowly circle your head to the left, drop it back, bring it to the right and back to your chest. It is best to do five in one direction and then five in the other. These head rolls stretch the muscles that tend to get tense under pressure; this will help relieve any muscle spasms and so any consequent pain.

Herbs for Tension Headaches

The herbal advice given for the easing of tension will be generally useful for head-aches. However, some herbs can produce headaches in sensitive people. The relaxing herb *Valerian* can do this in some people. *Ginseng* may cause headaches if used over too long a period, or at too high a dose.

As such headaches may be caused by a whole range of factors, there is a similarly wide range of remedies that have reputations in the easing of head pain. It is best to study the associated virtues of the plants and choose those most appropriate in a broader picture. A partial list would include: *Balm, Cayenne, Chamomile, Elder Flower, Jamaican Dogwood, Lady's Slipper, Lavender, Marjoram, Peppermint, Rosemary, Rue, Skullcap, Thyme, Valerian, Wood Betony, Wormwood.*
All of these are discussed eleswhere except *Wood Betony*, which follows.

WOOD BETONY   *Stachys betonica*
Part used: Dried aerial parts.
Collection: The aerial parts should be collected just before the flowers bloom. They should be dried carefully in the sun.
Constituents: Alkaloids including betonicine, stachydrene and trigonelline.
Actions: Sedative, nervine tonic, bitter.
Indications: Wood Betony feeds and strengthens the central nervous system, combined with a gentle sedative action. It is used in nervous debility especially when associated with anxiety and tension. It will ease headaches and neuralgia when they are of nervous origin.
Combinations: For the treatment of nervous headache it combines well with *Skullcap* and *Lavender*.
Preparation and dosage: Infusion: pour a cup of boiling water onto 1–2 teaspoonful of the dried herb and leave to infuse for 10–15 minutes. This should be drunk three times a day.
Tincture: take 2–6 ml of the tincture three times a day.

Migraine

Most of the headaches that people describe as migraines are simply severe head pain. These can be bad enough, but migraine describes a specific type of headache due to the contraction and dilation of blood vessels in the membranes that cover the brain. It seems that first a blood vessel constricts, but then the blood flow forces it open again. This dilation irritates the walls of the vessel, causing them to become inflamed and painful. When the blood passes through it produces the characteristic symptoms and pain.

There appears to be a number of different causes. Its origins may, for example, lie in a spinal problem that could possibly be corrected by an osteopath or chiropractor. The most frequent triggers appear to be food, stress and hormonal changes.

When the migraine is triggered by stress, relaxation, meditation and gentle soothing exercise can do much to relieve such people of their pain. It is well worth taking a close look at environmental conditions such as working under flourescent lighting or watching a computer VDU all day. The physical environment and quality of emotional relationships all play a role in generating excess stress.

It is well established that foods containing tyramine, nitrite, monosodium glutamate or alcohol all have the property of triggering migraines in sensitive people. Many books have been written about the dietary approach to the alleviation of migraine, so here I shall just give the outlines of things to avoid.

- Dairy products: especially cheese, yogurt and sour cream,
- Chocolate and cocoa,
- Meat and fish: especially pickled herring, salted fish, sausages, liver,
- Some vegetables: broad beans, sauerkraut,
- Alcohol: especially beer, red wine, champagne and sherry.

The last main cause for migraine is hormonal changes in women. Migraines that come on at the time of a period or start during menopause, may seem intractable, but can be alleviated using the right herbal remedies. This should be done by a qualified medical herbalist, however, and is discussed elsewhere.

Herbs

There are many herbs that have reputations as being good for migraines. As has been pointed out, to find the right one(s) depends on being sure of the cause. Most of the remedies mentioned for headaches are of value with perhaps *Lavender* being a good all-round help. The Oil of Lavender may be rubbed into the temples or a couple of drops on a sugar cube could be taken. The flowers can be infused to make a tea.

The invaluable herb *Feverfew* must be mentioned here. While not quite the wonder remedy the media has led us to believe, the regular use of it either fresh, as a tablet or tea will often clear the migraines given a month or so of treatment. If you have migraine then plant Feverfew in your garden!

FEVERFEW   *Tanacetum parthenium*
Part used: Leaves.
Collection: The leaves may be picked throughout the spring and summer, although just before flowering is best.
Actions: Anti-inflammatory, vasodilatory, relaxant, digestive bitter, uterine stimulant.
Indications: Feverfew has regained its deserved reputation as a primary remedy in the treatment of migraine headaches, especially those that are relieved by applying warmth to the head. It may also help arthritis when it is in the painfully active inflammatory stage. Dizziness and tinnitus

163

may be eased, especially if used in conjunction with other remedies. Painful periods and sluggish menstrual flow will be relieved by Feverfew.

CAUTION: Feverfew should not be used during pregnancy because of the stimulant action on the womb. The fresh leaves may cause mouth ulcers in sensitive people.

Preparation and dosage: It is best to use the equivalent of one fresh leaf for 1–3 times a day. It is best used fresh or frozen.

Hyperactivity in Children

In this growing area of concern, it is clear that artificial food additives have a lot to answer for. It appears that young, developing nervous systems are particularly prone to the damage or irritation that many food additives can cause. The effect is one of excessive activity with only a few hours' sleep each night, and because of the over-activity such children are more prone to accidents. There is some association with eczema and asthma, both of which will be aggravated anyway by the over-activity. There may be difficulties with speech, balance and learning even if the child has a high IQ.

Anyone with a child that is suspected of having this problem will be under extreme stress themselves. So there are two things to look at, ways to help the child and ways for the parents to cope.

An excellent support and help group has been formed that is a mine of useful information in this problem. They can be contacted at the following address, but send an SAE:

Mrs Sally Bunday
Hyperactive Children's Support Group
59 Meadowside, Angmering
West Sussex, BN16 4BW, UK.

A treatment that can be quite effective is based on a diet by Dr Fiengold and cuts out all food and drink containing synthetic additives of any kind and certain natural chemicals. For more specific details contact the Group.

However, there are specific food additives to avoid, and these are by law marked on any package containing them. They are:

E102 Tartrazine
E104 Quinoline Yellow
E107 Yellow 2G
E110 Sunset Yellow
E120 Cochineal
E122 Carmoisine
E123 Amaranth
E124 Ponceau 4R
E127 Erythosine
E128 Red 2G
E132 Indigo Carmine
E133 Brilliant Blue
E150 Caramel
E151 Black PN
E154 Brown FK
E155 Brown HT
E210 Benzoic Acid
E211 Sodium Benzoate
E250 Sodium Nitrite
E251 Sodium Nitrate
E320 Butylated Hydroxyanisole
E321 Butylated Hydroxytoluene

These are additives that there is little doubt about, but the complete list of possible culprits is almost endless.

A combination of the diet and good herbal treatment for any bodily symptoms the child has developed should be able to clear the problem.

Herbal relaxants that may help include the following that may be best used as an infusion added to a bath. The way to do this is described in Chapter 8.

Red Clover: a gentle relaxing remedy that helps aid the liver and also clears the skin of minor eruptions.

Lime Blossom: a stronger, though still mild, relaxing herb.

Chamomile: an all-round relaxing plant for children.

Having said that, it is the parents who often need herbs for stress and tension, more than the children. Any parent supporting a hyperactive child would benefit from the advice given in the section on how to deal with long-term stress.

Pain and Neuralgia

It may come as a surprise, but pain is not an illness. It is a subjective sensation, and has been described as an emotion. It is usually an accompaniment to some bodily ill and often acts as an early warning sign. As such, pain plays a valuable role in health. Not that it should be welcomed but rather listened to. This is the most worrying aspect of the enormous consumption of pain killers today. Much is being masked and suppressed that should be listened to – not only physical ills but those of emotional pain as well. Much pain can have its roots in the subtleties of body language, with the pain acting as body semaphore for mental and emotional warning signs.

As with all other bodily manifestations, pain will be worse under all forms of stress. A good example would be backache worsened as a result of anxiety about a bank overdraft.

Different people will have varying degrees of pain tolerance and it is profoundly difficult to comprehend another's experience of pain. Pain can cause anxiety and depression, especially when associated with chronic illness.

Treatment of Pain

From what has been said, it should be clear that pain as such is not what the healer should focus on. Primarily it should be the roots of the pain that are seen to, and pain killers used only within a broader treatment of the pain's cause.

Appropriate treatment might lie in the hands of a chiropractor or osteopath for any pain related to structural problems. Acupuncture has a lot to offer. It is becoming increasingly clear that many headaches have their origin in jaw problems that good dentists may be able to help.

Herbal remedies are the basis of most of the pharmaceutical pain killing drugs used today. All the morphine and cocaine-type pain killers and anaesthetics come originally from plants. None of the strong anodynes is freely available, for obviously they must be used only under qualified observation. In the current state of medical monopoly this restricts properly qualified medical herbalists from using such herbs, an unfortunate state of affairs.

There are some gentle herbs that can relieve pain, but to underline the point, the cause of the pain must be sought. Safe herbs worth considering include the following:

St John's Wort: this is especially valuable for longstanding neuralgic pain used internally or the oil as an external application for at least three weeks. For details of how to make the oil see Chapter 8.

Jamaican Dogwood: also a mild sedative.

Valerian: it will aid in anxiety reactions that might accompany the pain.

Yellow Jasmine: this is a much stronger pain reliever that should be used only under skilled herbal advice.

Wild Lettuce: a good relaxing pain reliever, although the wild variety is now rather rare.

The above plants are for pain in general, but that is not very common! If pain is due to muscle spasms then try the antispasmodic herbs; if due to external problems use vulnerary ones. The complete list would be almost endless here, but bear in mind that anxiety will aggravate and be aggravated by pain.

THE MUSCULO-SKELETAL SYSTEM

Gravity is hard work, and it is our skeleton and musculature that carries the strain. Used well and treated with care the supporting structure of our bodies lasts as long as it is needed, but with misuse the door is opened to the miseries of arthritis, back problems and all the rest.

In the context of complementary medicine, the physical techniques such as osteopathy, chiropractic and Alexander therapy have most to offer as treatments. Herbal medicine is still of value, as we shall see, but prevention is always better than cure, so such approaches as yoga, massage, dance etc. should all be part of an approach that strengthens and supports the system in its work.

Here we shall focus on herbs and diet for the problems that so commonly plague the musculo-skeletal system, but to do the best possible it will often involve healing tools which are beyond herbs.

Herbs for the Musculo-skeletal System

A whole range of different actions can be indicated here, both for prevention and for treatment. As we shall see below, there are systemic problems such as rheumatoid arthritis that have diverse causes. Herbal treatment can thus involve many apparently unsuspected herbs for this system.

The anti-inflammatory remedies serve as alternatives to the usual drug treatments given in arthritis and rheumatism. They are best used in combination with remedies that work in a deeper way, but they can have a profound effect in easing pain and swelling. This is not treating the roots of the problem, however. Ones that are usually helpful include *Willow Bark, Wild Yam, Meadowsweet, Guaiacum, Celery* and *Angelica.*

These are all described elsewhere except *Guaiacum,* which follows.

GUAIACUM *Guaiacum officinale*
Part used: The heartwood.
Collection: The resin of the wood exudes naturally and is often collected and used as such, otherwise the heartwood itself is cut into small chips. The tree is found in South America and the Caribbean.
Constituents: Resin acids including guaiaconic, guaianetic and guaiacic acid; saponins; polyterpenoid; vanillin.
Actions: Anti-rheumatic, anti-inflammatory, laxative, diaphoretic, diuretic.
Indications: Guaiacum is a specific for rheumatic complaints. It is especially useful where there is much inflammation and pain present. It is thus used in chronic rheumatism and rheumatoid arthritis, particularly when an astringent is needed. It will aid in the treatment of gout and may be used as a preventative of recurrence in this disease.
Combinations: It may be used together with *Bogbean, Meadowsweet* or *Celery Seed.*
Preparation and dosage: Decoction: put 1 teaspoonful of the wood chip in a cup of water, bring to the boil and simmer for 15–20 minutes. This should be drunk three times a day.

CELERY SEED *Apium graveolens*
Part used: Dried ripe fruits.
Collection: The seeds should be collected when ripe in the autumn.
Constituents: 2–3 per cent volatile oil.
Actions: Anti-rheumatic, diuretic, carminative, sedative.

Indications: Celery Seeds find their main use in the treatment of rheumatism, arthritis and gout. They are especially useful in rheumatoid arthritis where there is an associated mental depression. Their diuretic action is obviously involved in rheumatic conditions, but they are also used as a urinary antiseptic, largely because of the volatile oil apiol.

Combinations: In rheumatic conditions they combine well with _Bogbean._

Preparation and dosage: Infusion: pour a cup of boiling water onto 1–2 teaspoonsful of freshly crushed seeds. Leave to infuse for 10–15 minutes. This should be drunk three times a day.

Tincture: take 2–4 ml of the tincture three times a day.

Many other herbs can act to reduce inflammation by helping the body in some indirect way that augments the natural healing power. Those described here all have a directly anti-inflammatory action.

A diverse collection of herbs have been described as anti-rheumatic. Strictly speaking, this is not an action but an observation of an effect. A large group of herbs can be described this way but have different primary actions. We can include _Angelica, Bearberry, Black Cohosh, Black Willow, Bladderwrack, Blue Flag, Bogbean, Boneset, Burdock, Cayenne, Celery Seed, Couchgrass, Dandelion, Devil's Claw, Guaiacum, Ginger, Juniper Berries, Mountain Grape, Mustard, Nettles, Poke Root, Prickly Ash, Sarsaparilla, White Poplar, Wild Yam, Wintergreen, Wormwood, Yarrow_ and _Yellow Dock._

From this list you will notice herbs that can be fitted into many catagories of action. All have a noticeable anti-rheumatic effect. Here we can discuss _Bogbean._

BOGBEAN   _Menyanthes trifoliata_
Part used: Leaves.
Collection: The leaves are best collected

between May and July. They may be dried in the sun or under moderate heat.

Constituents: Bitter glycosides, alkaloids, saponin, essential oil, flavonoids, pectin.

Actions: Bitter, diuretic, cholagogue, anti-rheumatic.

Indications: Bogbean is a most useful herb for the treatment of rheumatism, arthritis and rheumatoid arthritis. It has a stimulating effect upon the walls of the colon which will act as an aperient, but is should not be used to help rheumatism where there is any colitis or diarrhoea. It has a marked stimulating action on the digestive juices and on bile-flow and so will aid in debilitated states that are due to sluggish digestion, indigestion and problems of the liver and gallbladder.

Combinations: For the treatment of rheumatic conditions it will combine well with _Black Cohosh_ and _Celery Seed._

Preparation and dosage: Infusion: pour a cup of boiling water onto 1–2 teaspoonsful of the dried herb and leave to infuse for 10–15 minutes. This should be drunk three times a day.

Tincture: take 1–4 ml of the tincture three times a day.

DEVIL'S CLAW
          Harpagophytum procumbens
Part used: Rhizome.
Collection: It grows in Namibia in very arid conditions. The roots are collected at the end of the rainy season.

Constituents: Harpagoside, harpagide, procumbine.

Actions: Anti-inflammatory, anodyne, hepatic.

Indications: It is effective in some cases of arthritis. This is partially explained by the glycoside harpagoside which reduces inflammation in the joints. Its efficacy goes far beyond simple inflammation reduction though. Unfortunately, it does not always work, but is well worth considering where arthritis is accompanied by much swelling and pain. Devil's Claw can also be helpful for liver and gallbladder problems.

Combinations: Can be used with *Bogbean, Celery Seed* and *Meadowsweet* in arthritis.

Preparation and dosage: A decoction is made with ½–1 teaspoonful to a cup of water. Let simmer for 10–15 minutes and drink three times a day.

Tincture: take 1–2 ml three times a day.

WHITE POPLAR   *Populus tremuloides*
Part used: The bark.
Collection: The bark is collected in the spring.
Constituents: Glycosides, flavonoids, essential oil, tannin.
Actions: Anti-inflammatory, astringent, antiseptic, anodyne, cholagogue.
Indications: This herb can be used in arthritis and rheumatism where there is a lot of pain and swelling. It is especially useful in flare up phases of rheumatoid arthritis, but works best when used with other herbs to treat the whole body. Its action on the liver makes it widely usable and will stimulate appetite. It can be used in fevers and infections.
Preparation and dosage: Make a decoction with 1–2 teaspoonsful of the bark simmered in a cup of water for 10–15 minutes. This should be drunk three times a day, or use 2–4 ml of the tincture.

Many alteratives have a reputation for relieving rheumatic conditions. This highlights the broad way in which these problems can be helped. The alteratives work in a diverse collection of ways but all help return the body to health. This will help the body deal with the generalized systemic roots of the illness. Specific alteratives that come to mind here are *Black Cohosh, Burdock Root, Guaiacum* and *Sarsaparilla.*

Diuretics have a place in a broad treat-

ment of arthritis and rheumatic problems by the nature of their support of the cleansing processes of the kidneys. Of the many that could be used we can mention *Boneset, Celery Seed* and *Yarrow.*

Circulatory stimulants, of the kind mentioned in the section on the 'circulation system' will, help in improving the flow of blood through affected joints. This will speed the healing process and can reduce inflammation. Especially useful for internal use are *Cayenne* and *Prickly Ash.*

The rubefacients are widely used as lotions or liniments to ease pain, stiffness and inflammation. They are described in the section on them in Chapter 3. We can mention *Cayenne, Ginger, Mustard, Peppermint oil* and *Wintergreen.* All are described elsewhere except *Wintergreen,* which follows.

WINTERGREEN   *Gaultheria procumbens*
Part used: The leaves.
Collection: The leaves are gathered throughout the year but the summer is preferable. Dry in the shade to avoid oil loss.
Constituents: Volatile oil which has a large proportion of salicylate.
Actions: Anodyne, astringent, stimulant, diuretic, emmenagogue, galactogogue.
Indications: Its main use stems from the pain-reducing and anti-inflammatory effect of the oil. This explains its common use for reducing pain and swelling in acute arthritis and other joint problems. It is usually used as the liniment in muscular and skeletal problems of all kinds, including lumbago and sciatica. Internally it will have a diuretic effect because of irritation of the kidney, as well as a stimulating action on menstruation.
Preparation and dosage: An infusion can be made with 1 teaspoonful of the dried leaves to a cup of boiling water and left to

steep for 10 minutes. External use is described in Chapter 8.

The anodyne, or pain relieving, remedies can play a role where there is much discomfort, but it is no real treatment. The anti-rheumatics and anti-inflammatories can often help in this way, though they have a deeper action as well. Of especial help in this system are *Jamaican Dogwood, Valerian* and *St John's Wort.*

Bitters can often help in problems that afflict the muscles and bones through helping the whole process of digestion and assimilation. This helps general body wellbeing and so eases the rheumatic problem.

Problems of the Muscles and Bones

A plague in our society is the whole complex of rheumatic/arthritic/'lumbago' problems. The differential diagnosis is often complex and not relevant to a book like this. Herbal medicine has much to offer in the prevention and treatment of these problems but, as we shall see, there are limits to even the efficacy of our herbal remedies.

More than anywhere else, successful treatment will depend on treating the whole person, not just the joint or muscles. The problems are often a physical expression of a deep-seated physical problem, often exacerbated by diet and lifestyle. So three areas of approach can be identified – herbal, dietary and lifestyle re-evaluation. The last of these will be discussed below under rheumatoid arthritis, so we shall focus on diet and herbal medication here.

Rheumatism and Osteo-arthritis

While there are undoubted differences between rheumatism and osteo-arthritis, in terms of broad outlines of treatment we can consider them together. In most cases the basis of the development of these illnesses is either physical or dietary wear and tear building on an underlying tendency in this direction.

In some people certain dietary habits will lead over years to the development of rheumatic problems and possibly arthritis. Look at any good bookshop and you will see a whole range of 'arthritis diets' recommended. Here I shall suggest a very basic one that can be elaborated to suit the person concerned.

It can be divided into items to avoid, foods to cut down on and items to have:
AVOID
- Coffee: instant, decaffeinated or real ground coffee.
- Red Meat: beef, lamb, pork and pork products such as ham and bacon. Bovril, Oxo.
- Vinegar: except apple cider vinegar.
- Pickles.
- Tomatoes, Rhubarb, Gooseberries, Red and Black currants.
- Citrus Fruit.
- White sugar and sugar-containing products such as sweets.
- White bread and white flour products (cakes, biscuits and pastries).
- Artificial additives such as colouring, flavouring and preservatives.
- Processed and tinned food.
- Red Wine, port and sherry.
- Fizzy drinks.
- Smoking.
- Shell fish.
Anything that causes heartburn, indigestion or any allergy reaction should be avoided.
CUT DOWN ON
- Dairy products and eggs.
- Fried foods.
- Salt.
- Alcohol.

–Tea.
ENJOY
–Poultry.
–Fish.
–Green vegetables, especially celery (preferably organic).
–All other vegetables, not over-cooked.
–Salads and bean sprouts. Parsley.
–Sunflower oil.
–Apples, Pears, Bananas, Peaches, Green Grapes, ripe Plums, tropical fruit.
–Nuts and dried fruit (without preservatives or salt).
–Honey.
–Non-citrus fruit and vegetable juices.
–Herb Teas.
–Mineral water.

The diet provides the basis for recovery and prevention in people who suspect that they may be prone to such problems. However, it will not do much if the arthritis is due to physical wear and tear, for example, the farmer who develops the condition in the shoulder on which he has carried hay bales all his life.

With herbal medicine, as part of a broad approach, it is possible to cleanse the body and remove the source of arthritic development. Such treatments take time, but when the right approach is used the herbalist is often told 'I feel better in myself' long before the pain goes–a sign that bodily health and vitality is returning.

It must be pointed out again that successful healing depends on helping the unique situation, not in using stock mixtures. Having reiterated that, I shall discuss an example of how a broad approach might look. The mixture could be:

> *Bogbean* 2 parts
> *Willow Bark* 1 part
> *Black Cohosh* 1 part
> *Celery Seed* 1 part
> *Prickly Ash* 1 part
> *Yarrow* 1 part

Try an infusion of this mixture three times a day.

Why recommend a mixture of these herbs out of the range mentioned above, all of which may be helpful? The *Bogbean* is a primary anti-rheumatic remedy that is broadly applicable, as well as helping the liver and digestion as an hepatic. An alternative here might have been *Devil's Claw*. *Willow Bark* is a strong anti-inflammatory remedy that is safe to use even in high dosage. This will ease the pain and speed the reduction of any swelling and stiffness. Alternatives here would be *Meadowsweet* or *Guaiacum* if a more potent remedy is needed. *Black Cohosh* is an all-round anti-rheumatic with nervine relaxant properties that aid in soothing the whole person in the stress their bodies are under. *Celery Seed* is anti-inflammatory, anti-rheumatic and diuretic with very mild sedative properties. *Prickly Ash* is a stimulant to peripheral circulation and helps by increasing blood flow to the affected areas. *Yarrow* is a diuretic that helps the kidney remove waste from the body without forcing the process.

An equally effective combination could be put together with totally different herbs and the same result achieved. Herbalism is an art as much as a science, and the key to success is finding what suits each individual. You will see that the joints, muscles, liver, digestion, kidneys and nerves are all focused on in this mixture.

On the other hand, using herbs as 'simples' can be as effective. A 'simple' is a single herb used in larger amounts. For example, *Meadowsweet* can prove a most effective simple in rheumatism and the early stage of osteo-arthritis.

It is vital that the body gets a chance for enough healing sleep. Unfortunately, this is often stopped because of pain and discomfort at night. Herbs that are hypnotic and anodyne can be used at night quite safely. Examples would be *Jamaican Dogwood*,

Valerian and _Passion Flower_.

External liniments, rubs, poultices, etc., can prove beneficial in the relief of pain and the distress that accompanies it, but no real change in the underlying problem will occur. The rubefacient remedies are most relevant here through the stimulation of local blood flow. Details of how to make such preparations are found in Chapter 8. A warming, stimulant liniment for rheumatism can be made very simply by mixing equal parts of tincture of _Cayenne_ and glycerine. It should be rubbed into the affected area. Don't use it on broken or sensitive skin. Another useful pain-easing liniment is that of _St John's Wort_. The oil is rubbed into areas of sciatic or rheumatic pain as well as being used for neuralgia etc. The preparation is described in the appropriate chapter.

Rheumatoid Arthritis

Rheumatoid arthritis is characterized by swelling, pain and stiffness of joints in the body. However it is quite different in origin to the more common osteo-arthritis. In rheumatoid there is a proliferation of inflammatory tissue in the membranes that line some of the body's joints. The specific cause is unknown but is directly related to the body's immune system. It is the immune system that defends the body against disease organisms. For some reason in rheumatoid arthritis the defence process is started up against the body's own protein in the joint lining. This causes the painful inflammation and eventual destruction of tissue.

Amongst factors that disturb the immune system in prone people is the impact of stress, so any effective treatment of this difficult illness must include stress management that is relevant to the individual involved. An easing of tension and anxiety must be a priority. Relaxation techniques are invaluable, as can be insight counsell-

ing. In this context it is worth looking at the idea of 'friction'.

The changes in the joints that occur in arthritis cause a rubbing of the bones in such a way as to cause friction. However, there is often a long history of friction in the person's life before this pathological stage is reached. As already pointed out, the friction can be completely physical due to one's job. It can also be due to muscle tension holding the joints tighter together, which is often due to more psychological types of friction. This friction is caused by the daily toll of disagreement, conflict and general unease with others and ourselves. A lot can be done to change such problems. Herbal relaxants can help but fundamentally it is achieved by a change of attitudes or lifestyle. This is especially true for rheumatoid arthritis, but holds in osteo as well.

Diet plays a role in the aggravation and possibly even the origin of rheumatoid arthritis. The possible ramifications of this are complex, so advice should be sought from a skilled practitioner. The basics are those described above for osteo-arthritis with much emphasis laid on no dairy products with an avoidance of all artificial additives. The role of diet in the treatment of rheumatoid arthritis is a complex and contentious area.

Herbal medicine has a lot to offer, but as this is a deep-seated problem based in the immune system it is impossible to talk of specific remedies. A good herbalist will be of much help. The following plants have a role in any broad treatment, which must take into account the unique situation of the patient involved. Remember that to truly help, the whole person's condition must be treated, and they may suffer from more than just the named joint condition.

We can mention these remedies however: _Bogbean, Black Cohosh, Celery Seed, Wild Yam, Meadowsweet, Willow Bark, Bladderwrack, Bryony._

Gout

Gout can affect the whole body and not just the classic big toe; also it is not restricted to port drinkers! Herbs can help in promoting the removal of the build-up of uric acid in the body. The advice given above can help, but in addition diuretics and alteratives are especially indicated: _Boneset, Celery Seed, Wild Carrot, Yarrow, Gravel Root, Burdock, Birch._

Much water should be drunk and certain foods rich in purines are to be avoided. These include sardines, anchovies, fish roe, shellfish, liver, kidneys and beans. Coffee and tea should be avoided, as should alcohol.

Cramp

This is a problem that can have many causes. If it is recurring, the underlying cause must be identified. It can range from mineral deficiency to back and nerve problems. A symptomatic relief can usually be gained by using the anti-spasmodic _Cramp Bark._ For a more long-term treatment, combine this with circulatory stimulants such as _Prickly Ash_ and _Ginger._

Fibrositis

This is a problem that, strictly speaking, is a misnomer. However, when muscles, ligaments and tendons hurt, it does not really matter what you call it as long as the pain goes!

The general advice given above can help, but in addition the external use of a lotion that eases muscle tension and pain is invaluable:
Lobelia tincture
Cramp Bark tincture
Mix equal parts of each. This can be rubbed into the affected area as often as is helpful. Internal medication is as described for rheumatism.

Back Pain and Sciatica

For such problems it is almost always best to consult a good osteopath or chiropractor. The problem often has its origins in misalignment of the hips or vertebrae causing a pinching of nerves, and thus the pain and discomfort. Occasionally the problem may be due to lower abdominal congestion due to gynaecological or kidney problems. If this is the case they must be treated as a priority. Symptomatic relief through massage and aromatherapy can be valid. Please refer to Chapter 4.

Sprains

A common problem caused by accidental pulling of muscles, tendons and ligaments. A lotion, bath or compress of _Arnica_ will help reduce bruising and swelling. Distilled _Witch Hazel_ will ease the pain and swelling by using a compress moistened with this excellent herb. Stimulating baths with remedies such as _Ginger_ or _Thyme_ will improve circulation and so speed recovery.

THE SKIN

The skin is not simply a waterproof covering, it is a wonderful organ that has many functions. It is a vital part of the body's eliminative processes, regulation of the internal environment and a way in which we express who we are.

The skin often acts as a lightning conductor grounding dis-ease or stress through the body to express itself on the surface. It is as though it is a form of body semaphore. It often is a cry for help or attention, which the person will usually deny as such. It is this very denial that makes it necessary for the skin manifestation to appear. In this perception lies a powerful way of approaching skin disease. Through counselling and supportive psychotherapy much can be done to ease the impact of conditions such as psoriasis and so reverse the momentum of the illness and speed its clearing.

The skin is affected by many different things, from simple infections, through allergies to the more complex and obscure auto-immune problems. Any bodily problem will aggravate skin conditions, as will anxiety and tension, some of which may be actually brought on by stress itself. This is especially true of a form of eczema called atopic eczema and psoriasis. While psoriasis is not an emotional-based illness as many consider it to be it will of itself act as an emotional stress. In fact, this emotional stress caused by psoriasis is often one of the worst features of the condition.

Emotional factors and stress are important in the development, aggravation and perpetuation of many skin diseases, and the stress and misery caused by the skin disease may lead to a vicious circle. An awareness by friends, relatives and the general public that such conditions are not contagious, that it is not dirty, that it is not the sufferer's fault and that it causes them great embarrassment, would help to reduce stress caused by skin disease and make the treatment a lot easier.

Herbs for the Skin

All holistic approaches to medicine have a lot to offer in treating skin disease. Dietary approaches are especially indicated in skin problems, but this is an area that goes beyond the range of this book. Both used internally as systemic aids and externally as ointments and lotions, herbal remedies are particularly helpful.

The list of possible remedies is endless as by helping general bodily health, skin problems can be eased a lot. The identification of appropriate actions helps in the selection of remedies.

The alteratives are the remedies that come to mind primarily for internal treatment of the skin. Of the many that are known we can mention *Burdock Root, Cleavers, Figwort, Golden Seal, Poke Root, Yellow Dock, Sarsaparilla* and *Red Clover*.

You will see that we have a whole range of secondary actions here. For example *Yellow Dock* is a laxative, *Burdock* an hepatic and *Cleavers* is a lymphatic tonic.

Of those not already described let us look at *Figwort* and *Red Clover*.

FIGWORT   *Scrophularia nodosa*
Part used: Aerial parts.
Collection: The stalks and leaves are gathered during flowering between June and August.
Constituents: Saponins, cardioactive glycosides, flavonoids, resin, sugar, organic acids.
Actions: Alterative, diuretic, mild purgative, heart stimulant.
Indications: Figwort finds most use in the treatment of skin problems. It acts in a broad way to help the body function well, bringing about a state of inner cleanliness. It may be used for eczema, psoriasis and any skin condition where there is itching and irritation. Part of the cleansing occurs due to the purgative and diuretic actions. It may be used as a mild laxative in constipation. As a heart stimulant, it should be avoided where there is any abnormally rapid heartbeat.
Combinations: It combines well with *Wild*

Yam, Meadowsweet, Willow Bark, Yellow Dock, Bladderwrack, Bryony and Burdock Root in the treatment of skin problems.
Preparation and dosage: Infusion: pour a cup of boiling water onto 1–3 teaspoonful of the dried leaves and let infuse for 10–15 minutes. This should be drunk three times a day.
Tincture: take 2–4 ml of the tincture three times a day.

RED CLOVER   *Trifolium pratense*
Part used: Flowerheads.
Collection: The flowerheads are gathered between May and September.
Constituents: Phenolic glycosides, flavonoids, coumarins, cyanogenic glycosides.
Actions: Alterative, expectorant, antispasmodic.
Indications: Red Clover is one of the most useful remedies for children with skin problems. It may be used with complete safety in any case of childhood eczema. It may also be of value in other chronic skin conditions such as psoriasis. While being most useful with children it can also be of value for adults. The expectorant and antispasmodic action give this remedy a role in the treatment of coughs and bronchitis, but especially in whooping cough. As an alterative it is indicated in a wide range of problems when approached in a holistic sense. There is some evidence to suggest an anti-neoplastic action in animals.
Combinations: For skin problems it combines well with *Yellow Dock* and *Nettles.*
Preparation and dosage: Infusion: pour a cup of boiling water onto 1–3 teaspoonful of the dried herb and leave to infuse for 10–15 minutes. This should be drunk three times a day.
Tincture: take 2–6 ml of the tincture three times a day.

The diaphoretics can be helpful in increasing the amount of perspiration from the skin. This is not always sensed, but it helps in cleansing the skin and thus the whole body.

Tonics, hepatics and lymphatic herbs are all useful for the skin. You will notice that many of the alteratives mentioned could fit into these categories. Anti-microbial will often be indicated; *Echinacea* and *Garlic* are the most useful.

Vulneraries are, of course, used extensively for wound healing. These are explored below. Nervines are especially helpful for skin problems where there is irritation from the eruption or tension and anxiety within the person.

Oils, both the aromatic kind used in aromatherapy and bland medicinal ones, are used especially on the skin. They can be used for skin problems as shown below, but it is an excellent way to get such oils into the body for internal medication as they may be too strong to take internally as such.

Approaches to Skin Disease

For the majority of skin problems the most effective approach is to treat the body from within, rather than simply applying ointments. In this way the herbs will enable the body to regain a state of inner harmony and the skin problem will tend to clear up. Ointments, lotions and other external applications will ease symptoms and can do nothing but good. However, a real cure can only come from within. Let us first look at skin diseases that are a manifestation of internal problems.

Eczema

There are many distinct skin conditions which are called eczema. The term usually is applied to inflammatory reaction which can be in response to either internal or external irritants. It can take many forms, be dry and scaly or weeping. The most effective course of treatment is that which addresses itself to the cause. Identifying this cause can be extremely difficult and is best undertaken by a skilled practitioner.

Herbal medicines and dietary changes can prove most successful, especially in children. However for eczema of external origin it is usually sufficient to stop contact with the irritant. This may be detergents, nickel in jewellery or bra clasps, or cement. It is difficult to talk of a general approach to treating internally-based eczema as the causes are so diverse. Remedies that help in body cleansing and elimination are vital, and actions such as alteratives, lymphatic tonics and hepatics provide a sound foundation. If there is much irritation or associated anxiety or tension then the nervines can be most useful. Alteratives that may be used here include _Burdock Root, Cleavers, Figwort, Red Clover_ and _Nettles._

Notice that here we also have lymphatic and hepatic remedies. Herbs which in general are of secondary importance include _Fumitory, Dandelion, Golden Seal, Marigold_ and _Heartsease._

Of course, specific herbs can be the exact remedy required in some people, which makes herbalism such a challenge at times!

Dietary care is essential, with avoidance of dairy products being fundamental. The general guidelines for healthy, balanced eating, avoiding synthetic additives and any food allergens will speed the recovery from the condition. The replacement of cow's milk with that of goat's or soya beans can be helpful.

To soothe the skin and reduce itching, herbal ointments can prove quite effective. In some cases the eczema may even clear with external applications, but internal treatments are the key. Having said this, there is a wealth of knowledge on the formulation and value of herbal ointments, creams, lotion, poultices, etc. The details are discussed in Chapter 8. Certain oils will

be of value by themselves, such as _Avocado_ and _Almond._ Herbs applied directly or in any of the diverse extracts will at least ease the discomfort. A partial list would include _Chickweed, Marigold, Marshmallow Root_ and _St John's Wort._

In fact most of the demulcent or emollient herbs may be used. A specific for itching is _Chickweed._

CHICKWEED   _Stellaria media_
Part used: Dried aerial parts.
Collection: This very common weed of gardens and fields can be collected all year round, although it is not abundant during the winter.
Constituents: Saponins.
Actions: Anti-rheumatic, vulnerary, emollient.
Indications: Chickweed finds its most common use as an external remedy for cuts, wounds and especially for itching and irritation. If eczema or psoriasis causes this sort of irritation, Chickweed may be used with benefit. Internally it has a reputation as a remedy for rheumatism.
Combinations: Chickweed makes an excellent ointment when combined with _Marshmallow._
Preparation and dosage: Infusion: pour a cup of boiling water onto 2 teaspoonsful of the dried herb and leave to infuse for 5 minutes. This should be drunk three times a day. For external use Chickweed may be made into an ointment or can be used as a poultice. To ease itching, a strong infusion of the fresh plant makes a useful addition to bath water.

Psoriasis

This is one of the commonest conditions that affects white people with approximatly one in fifty people being affected at some time in their lives. It is of interest to note that the only racial type in the world that does not get it is the Native American.

Psoriasis can prove quite disabling for some people because it looks so unsightly and the general population can be so hurtful and uncaring simply through misunderstanding. It is not contagious and has nothing to do with uncleanliness.

It is little understood other than it appears to be an auto-immune problem. Please refer to that section (p.177). Treatment must take into account general health, family history and levels of stress. If there is a problem with the digestive system or other organs of elimination, such as the lungs, these must be treated and not simply the skin. The dietary suggestions described for auto-immune problems must be adhered to.

Herbs have a lot to offer, but still the condition can prove intransigent. The alteratives are primary, such as _Burdock Root, Yellow Dock, Cleavers_ and _Oregon Mountain Grape._

Tonics, diuretics and the whole range of eliminative remedies may have a role to play. The nervines can help if used in the context of stress management. It is a misconception that this is simply a nervous disease. Tension and anxiety will aggravate it, but only rarely cause it.

Ointments can help in easing discomfort and removing scales. This can often be done with simple ointment bases but herbs that may be added to reduce the inflammation as well include _Burdock, Golden Seal_ and _Marigold._

Acne

This tends to be a problem of adolescence and can be explained by hormonal changes, bad diet, stress and just about anything that is fashionable at the time! Herbal remedies that aid elimination and increase resistance can prove effective. Examples out of the whole range could be _Echinacea, Blue Flag,_

Nettles and _Dandelion Root._

If there is more of a suggestion of hormonal inbalance then consider the uterine tonics, hormonal normalizers or adaptogens, all of which are considered elsewhere.

Boils and Skin Infections

These can be a bothersome recurrent problem. They key is internal treatment with alteratives and anti-microbials combined with excellent diet, cleanliness and skin care. Herbs to consider amongst the range of eliminative remedies that fit in those two catagories are the following internal and external herbs: _Echinacea, Myrhh, Pasque Flower, Wild Indigo, Garlic, Nettles, Thyme_ and _Eucalyptus._

Allergies

The skin is a common site for allergies to manifest. They are discussed in a separate section (p.177).

The Hair and Scalp

A number of remedies are particularly good for the scalp and encouraging healthy hair growth. This does not mean that they will reverse the process of balding in men, but that the natural balance of oils and good circulation is maintained.

These remedies can be taken internally, used as a wash in the form of an infusion to rinse the hair, or of extracted essential oils. It is usually said that _Chamomile_ suits those with light hair while _Rosemary_ is good for dark hair. You will notice from the description of _Rosemary_ given below, that this herb has a wide range of activities in addition to being a hair tonic. The circulatory benefits it posseses may partially explain its role in helping hair, by helping scalp circulation.

ROSEMARY   *Rosemarinus officinalis*
Part used: Leaves and twigs.
Collection: The leaves may be gathered throughout the summer but are at their best during flowering time.
Constituents: 1 per cent volatile oil including borneol, linalol, camphene, cineole and camphor; tannins; bitter principle; resins.
Actions: Carminative, aromatic anti-spasmodic, anti-depressive, antiseptic, rubefacient, parasiticide.
Indications: Rosemary acts as a circulatory and nervine stimulant, which in addition to the toning and calming effect on the digestion makes it a remedy that is used where psychological tension is present. This may show, for instance, as flatulent dyspepsia, headache or depression associated with debility. Externally it may be used to ease muscular pain, sciatica and neuralgia. It acts as a stimulant to the hair folicles and may be used in premature baldness. The oil is most effective here.
Combinations: For depression it may be used with *Skullcap, Kola* and *Oats*.
Preparation and dosage: Infusion: pour a cup of boiling water onto 1–2 teaspoonsful of the dried herb and leave to infuse in a covered container for 10–15 minutes. This should be drunk three times a day.
Tincture: take 1–2 ml of the tincture three times a day. The oil is extracted in the way described in the Chapter 8.

ALLERGIES AND AUTO-IMMUNE PROBLEMS

There is an increasing prevalence in western society of the health problems that seem to be brought about by the body's inate immunity somehow going haywire. It is possible that this is because of the stresses put upon us all by our diets, by our society, by our inability to live in peace with our world.

In this section we shall look at allergies in general and auto-immune conditions.

Allergies

An allergy is an abnormally sensitive reaction to a substance in the environment. Often this thing will not of itself be harmful, but in sensitive people it will trigger the reaction. These so-called allergens can be almost anything, but the commonest are flower or tree pollen, some foodstuffs, household pets and even house dust.

There is a growing recognition that a whole range of conditions appear to be related to 'sub-clinical' allergies, especially to food additives. This is discussed under the section on hyperactivity (p.164).

The classic reaction that occurs can take different forms but commonly appears as hayfever, itching and a rash, a constantly runny nose, wheezing and joint pains. The symptoms are similar with different allergies because the body reacts in the same way with the release of a chemical called histamine into the blood-stream.

Times of stress or feelings of anxiety and tension will usually increase the severity or frequency of attacks. With some people, emotional upsets may even be the main factor involved.

Of course, the basis of any truly helpful treatment or management of allergic reactions is to stop the exposure to the 'thing' that is triggering it. This can be quite easy where the trigger has been identified as a certain food or animal, but often a simple avoidance is impossible. The commonest treatment is then to use drugs called anti-histamines which suppress the reaction in the body that the allergen is eliciting. For a holistic practitioner of any therapy this is a limited and possibly harmful approach.

The plant kingdom has been generous in herbs that aid the body in coping with allergies. There are three routes to the way a herbalist will combat any allergy:

1. Use remedies that help the person get well as a *whole* person. So not only are anti-allergy remedies used but also those that help any other specific problems unique to that person, all in the context of ensuring health is at a peak. The liver, lungs, kidneys and skin are especially important.

2. These herbs are used in conjunction with an individually worked-out diet (as each person's triggers are unique to them). Thus not only will it be based on sound ideas of good nutrition, but will take into account what must be avoided and compensate for any nutritional loss incurred.

3. The use of relevant relaxation methods to help the person deal with stress in their lives.

There are a multitude of plants that can help in allergic reactions, partially because of the individual nature of the reactions and symptoms. Herbs that ease the symptoms of hayfever, such as itching eyes, runny nose, and tight chest include the anti-catarrhal and anti-inflammatory remedies. Of major importance we can mention *Elder Flower* and *Berry, Eye Bright, Garlic, Golden Rod, Golden Seal, Nettles* and *Peppermint.*

A medical herbalist would also call into play herbs that have an action on a deeper level. These can be quite strong and are best used under professional advice. They include *Ephedra.*

EPHEDRA   *Ephedra sinica*
Common name: Ma Huang.
Part used: Aerial stems.
Collection: Gather the young branches in the autumn before the first frost, as the alkaloid content is then highest. They may be dried in the sun.
Constituents: More than 1¼ per cent alkaloids which include ephedrine and norephedrine; tannins; saponin; flavone; essential oil.
Actions: Vasodilator, hypertensive, circulatory stimulant, anti-allergic.
Indications: The alkaloids present in Ephedra have apparently opposite effects on the body. The overall action, however, is one of balance and benefit. It is used with great success in the treatment of asthma and associated conditions due to its power to relieve spasms in the bronchial tubes. It is thus used in bronchial asthma, bronchitis and whooping cough. It also reduces allergic reactions, giving it a role in the treatment of hayfever and other allergies. It may be used in the treatment of low blood pressure and circulatory insufficiency.
Preparation and dosage: Decoction: put 1–2 teaspoonful of the dried herb in one cup of water, bring it to the boil and simmer for 10–15 minutes. This should be drunk three times a day.
Tincture: take 1–4 ml of the tincture three times a day.

Auto-immune Disease

Many of the more intransigent and baffling of the medical scourges of today are being found to be auto-immune in nature. These conditions occur when the body attacks itself with its own defence system. This immune system is very effective and strong, so when misplaced it can cause much havoc.

The name and nature of the disease will

vary depending upon which part of the body is under attack. However, the basis of the problem will be similar in each case and mediated by the immune system. This system is still only slightly understood so I shall make no attempt at explaining it. The conditions that may fit in this category range from rheumatoid arthritis, multiple sclerosis, ulcerative colitis to psoriasis. There is some suggestion that cancer may have an auto-immune basis.

Holistic medicine has much to offer in these chronic problems in that it will help the body as a whole to be as well and integrated as possible. This will often be done by removing from the diet and environment things which act as stressors on the system. These things may be specific foods or inappropriate relationships.

From the evidence that research is rapidly building up, there can be no doubt that mental and emotional stress has much to answer for in auto-immune conditions. Whether it is as a cause or an aggravating factor is not really important. It is, however, vital that ease be brought into the person's life. This may be through relaxation or, perhaps more importantly, the finding of a purpose and meaning in their lives. Remember the old saying 'without vision, the people die'. Maybe this is the key to an understanding of the scourge of auto-immune disease.

Treatment of this whole range necessitates skilled help. This does not mean there is no place for self-help, but guidance and working with a holistic practitioner is far more likely to produce favourable results.

THE ENDOCRINE GLANDS

The endocrine glands are fundamental to all integration, coordination and communication within the body. The way they work and relate to each other and the rest of the body is a fascinating and almost endlessly complex subject. In conjunction with the nervous system they are at the interface of mind/emotion/body. In some of the spiritual traditions these glands were identified as the body's energy chakras, or power centres, before western science had identified their physical function. These are, by the way, quite different to the lymphatic glands that swell in the neck at times.

Many alternative therapies talk of treatments for glandular problems or as treatments for toning certain glands. I am not going to make any such claims here. It must be acknowledged that herbal activity on the endocrine glands, while real, is little understood. This makes it a grey area when the science is related to herbal experience. It is far too easy to make spurious psuedo-scientific claims for herbs, which masks their relevance in practice, even if we do not know what they may be doing to this or that gland.

Having made this apparent disclaimer, there is a certain amount that can be done with herbs for glandular problems. I will limit the discussion to generalities, as a more detailed examination will involve a degree of physiology and medicine that is beyond our scope here. For more specialized help, please consult a medical herbalist.

Admitting that this is a simplified

generalization, a good way to ensure glandular health is to ensure general health and well-being. This is ideally done through the use of herbal alteratives and bitters used in the context of good diet, healthy lifestyle and positive outlook on life. This should ensure health anyway! If any general illness or weakness is present this can be supported with appropriate herbal therapy.

Of all the integrated web of glands involved in endocrine balance we shall only mention a few here.

Adrenal Glands and Stress

Without going into the complex role of the adrenal glands in many bodily processes, it is important to note that one of the main sites of stress damage in the body are these glands. For someone under medium- to long-term stress it is most helpful to 'feed' these glands by using remedies that provide the precursors of the hormones. It enables the system to recover from stress faster and so avoid the greater potential problems. Some of this has been discussed in the section on the nervous system on p.153. Remedies that are quite specific are the adaptogens, and discussed under that heading are *Ginseng* and *Siberian Ginseng*.

In addition, bitters and general tonics can be helpful. Recent research has shown a role for the following two remedies, *Liquorice* and *Borage*.

LIQUORICE   *Glycyrrhiza glabra*
Part used: Dried root.
Collection: The roots are unearthed in the late autumn. Clean thoroughly and dry.
Constituents: Glycosides called glycyrrhizin and glycyrrhizinic acid; saponins; flavonoids; bitter; volatile oil; coumarins; asparagine; oestrogenic substances.
Actions: Expectorant, demulcent, anti-inflammatory, adrenal agent, anti-spasmodic,

mild laxative.
Indications: Liquorice is one of a group of plants that have a marked effect upon the endocrine system. The glycosides present have a structure that is similar to the natural steroids of the body. They partially explain the beneficial action that liquorice has in the treatment of adrenal gland problems such as Addison's disease. It has a wide usage in bronchial problems such as catarrh, bronchitis and coughs in general. Liquorice is used in allopathic medicine as a treatment for peptic ulceration, a similar use to its herbal use in gastritis and ulcers. It can be used in the relief of abdominal colic.
Combinations: For bronchitic conditions it is used with *Coltsfoot* or *White Horehound*. For gastric problems it may be combined with *Marshmallow, Comfrey* and *Meadowsweet*.
Preparation and dosage: Decoction: put ½–1 teaspoonful of the root in a cup of water, bring to the boil and simmer for 10–15 minutes. This should be drunk three times a day.
Tincture: take 1–3 ml of the tincture three times a day.

BORAGE   *Borago officinalis*
Part used: Dried leaves.
Collection: The leaves should be gathered when the plant is coming into flower in the early summer. Strip each leaf off singly and reject any that are marked in any way. Do not collect when wet with rain or dew.
Constituents: Saponins, mucilage, tannins, essential oil.
Actions: Diaphoretic, expectorant, tonic, anti-inflammatory, galactagogue.
Indications: Borage acts as restorative agent on the adrenal cortex, which means that it will revive and renew the adrenal glands after a medical treatment with cortisone or steroids. There is a growing need for remedies that will aid this gland with the

stress it is exposed to, both externally and internally. Borage may be used as a tonic for the adrenals over a period of time. It may be used during fevers and especially during convalescence. It has a reputation as an anti-inflammatory herb used in conditions such as pleurisy. The leaves and seeds stimulate the flow of milk in nursing mothers.

Preparation and dosage: Infusion: pour a cup of boiling water onto 2 teaspoonsful of the dried herb and leave to infuse for 10–15 minutes. This should be drunk three times a day.

Tincture: take 1–4 ml of the tincture three times a day.

Thyroid Gland

The thyroid gland has a central role in the control of metabolism and growth. Herbs can be helpful in controlling both over-activety and under-activity. Any treatment of such conditions will involve the use of appropriate nervines as well as general agents to augment that person's health. Again, this is a situation that needs skilled help.

For over-activity in this gland use *Bugleweed.*

BUGLEWEED   *Lycopus europaeus*
Part used: Aerial parts.
Collection: It should be collected just before the buds open.
Constituents: Flavone glycosides, volatile oil, tannins.
Actions: Cardioactive diuretic, peripheral vasoconstrictor, astringent, sedative, thryrocine antagonist, anti-tussive.
Indications: Bugleweed is a specific for over-active thyroid glands, especially where the symptoms include tightness of breathing, or where palpitations occur that are of nervous origin. Bugleweed will aid

the weak heart where there is associated build-up of water in the body. As a sedative cough reliever it will ease irritating coughs, especially when they are of nervous origin.
Combinations: Bugleweed may be used with nervines such as *Skullcap* or *Valerian.*
Preparation and dosage: Infusion: pour a cup of boiling water onto 1 teaspoonful of the dried herb and let infuse for 10–15 minutes. This should be drunk three times a day.
Tincture: take 1–2 ml of the tincture three times a day.

A herb that has a wide range of uses but can be specific for under-activity of the thyroid is *Bladderwrack.* It is an excellent source of minerals, including iodine.

BLADDERWRACK   *Fucus vesiculosus*
Part used: The whole plant, which is a common seaweed.
Constituents: It is rich in algin and mannitol, carotene and zeaxanthin. Iodine and bromine are present..
Actions: Anti-hypothyroid,   anti-rheumatic.
Indications: Bladderwrack may help in the treatment of underactive thyroid glands and goitre. Through the regulation of thyroid function there is an improvement in all the associated symptoms. Where obesity is associated with thyroid trouble, this herb may be very helpful in reducing the excess weight. It has a reputation in helping the relief of rheumatism and rheumatoid arthritis, both used internally and as an external application upon inflamed joints.
Preparation and dosage: It may usefully be taken in tablet form as a dietary supplement or as an infusion by pouring a cup of boiling water onto 2–3 teaspoonsful of the dried herb and leaving it to steep for 10 minutes. This should be drunk three times a day.

The Pancreas

Apart from the digestive role of the pancreas, it also contains endocrine glands called the Islets of Langerhans that produce insulin. Problems with insulin production or metabolism are integral in the disease Diabetes Mellitus. There are many claims for herbal 'cures' for this problem; they tend to be spurious. However, there is no doubt that herbs can help pancreatic function in some cases. This is a job for an expert, though, and not self-

help. The bitters have a reputation for 'kick starting' the glands as well as the herb *Goat's Rue,* which is described under 'Galactagogues'.

Sex Hormones

Sexual functioning and reproduction is integrally involved with hormones. The herbs that can help here are described in some depth in the section on reproduction (p.144).

FEVERS AND INFECTIONS

It is the common wisdom of our society that we 'catch' colds. In other societies and other times infections and fevers were considered to be possession by evil spirits. Our science tells us one truth, their beliefs told them something different. Who is to say what is truly so?

To a medical herbalist and most practitioners of holistic medicine, we do not catch infections; rather we let them in. By this I mean that the body's innate defence systems are for some reason lowered and so the infective organisms take the opportunity offered them. The result is a cold, cystitis or whatever.

This perception of the problem dictates the therapeutic approach. Rather than simply killing the organism, attention is placed upon raising the defences of the immune system. This does not negate using life-saving antibiotics or herbal anti-microbials, but puts their use in a broader holistic context.

Throughout our discussion of bodily systems specific infections have been mentioned. Here we shall look at the process itself and how to manage it.

Fevers and Fever Management

A fever is simply the symptom of raised body temperature, usually caused in response to infection by some disease-causing organism. They are no longer as common as in the past, largely due to the successful use of antibiotics and hygiene. The list of fevers and fever-causing organisms would fill a book – but not this one! It is worth noting and celebrating the success of the World Health Organisation in eradicating smallpox; this is a great achievement.

Fever control with herbal remedies is possible and quite effective when done by a skilled practitioner. However, it is not simply a case of using a remedy for a fever. A whole series of complex factors must be addressed. The key is to help the body through the fever, aiding its own innate recuperative powers, and treat the whole person. Such advice cannot be repeated enough. Antibiotic drugs may be necessary within this process, but used by themselves a whole range of longer-term problems can be invoked. This is the basis of repeated childhood infections, as we shall discuss below. But again such drugs are lifesavers in some situations; there is no clear-cut right or wrong here.

The antibiotics will kill the organism and anti-inflammatory drugs such as aspirin will inhibit the fever response, but with herbs we have the possibility of strengthening the body to help it through the battle. The aim is to shorten the fever through improvement of the immune response and at the same time use appropriate remedies to reduce excessive suffering from the symptoms.

Bear in mind that not all fevers are infectious in origin and may be due to 'auto-immune' conditions, which are discussed on p.177.

The fever can be seen as a manifestation of the body mobilizing its armoury of defences. The physiology of the fever process is complex, being mediated by the hypothalamus in the brain as well as centres around the body. We shall bypass the details, but a conservative approach of allowing the body to do the work itself is the best course. The problem here is our conditioning and lack of trust in the body's wisdom. If in doubt at all get professional advice. Remedies that can be used to help the body control the process are the diaphoretic, circulatory stimulants and anti-microbials. If the temperature continues to rise, however, the use of drugs may be necessary.

In the recuperative phase of infections and fevers it is often appropriate to consider bitters and tonics. We shall look at specific examples below.

Herbs for Fevers and Infections

As already pointed out, it is best not to think in terms of specific remedies for specific infections but look at ways to raise resistance to the onslaught once it has started. Of course it is always preferable to prevent the infective organism getting a hold in the first place. This can be done through ensuring adequate hygiene, a good and balanced diet and the use of herbs described below as prophylactics if there is suspicion of a potential problem.

Diaphoretics

These are remedies that in their simplest form promote sweating. However, they work on a much deeper level to help the bodily response of a fever to be effective. A large number are available to us, but perhaps the most relevant here are _Boneset, Yarrow, Vervain, Elder Flower, Hyssop, Lime Flower, Peppermint, Rosemary, Ginger_ and _Cayenne._

Circulatory Stimulants

Herbs that increase the flow of blood to the periphery of the body will help in the process of cleansing and support the diaphoretics mentioned above. In fact, some will fit into both categories: _Ginger, Cayenne, Mustard, Horseradish, Prickly Ash._

Anti-microbials

These remedies described in depth elsewhere in the book are a good basis for any herbal treatment of infection. Some of them work through a direct effect upon invasive organisms while others beef up bodily defences. But to be honest, not enough is known to say how they truly work, but work they do. A widely applicable list would include _Echinacea, Wild Indigo, Garlic_ and _Myrrh._

A range of secondary actions will be appropriate either in the recuperative phase or in specific conditions or personal constitutions.

Diuretics

The use of these remedies to aid and

support kidney function will help the cleansing process. Many of the diaphoretic remedies are also diuretics and this is no co-incidence.

Alteratives and tonics

These 'blood cleansers' will help the whole system deal with the infection or fever, but more importantly will speed recuperation from the rigours the body will have gone through.

Nervines

The nervine tonics are especially helpful in dealing with post infection depression or with extremes of delirium during a fever. A herb renowned for such use is *Vervain*.

Infections and the Systems

Rather than focus on the specific syndromes and organisms, here we shall discuss which remedies will be specifically useful for infections system by system. A professional herbalist would, of course, take note of disease syndromes and infective organisms but in the present context it would confuse the picture unnecessarily.

Ear, Nose and Throat

A common site for infection in children, this is where the whole picture is commonly compounded by repeated over-use of antibiotics. The specific herbs to use will depend on the guidelines given in the section about this system on p.132, but herbs that can prove specifically relevant for a multitude of infections are *Garlic, Echinacea, Wild Indigo, Golden Seal, Eucalyptus, Thyme* and *Balm of Gilead*.

The Lungs

This is considered in depth elsewhere but we can mention the following for infections of the lungs: *Garlic, Echinacea, Elecampane,* *Blood Root, White Horehound, Aniseed Oil, Eucalyptus Oil* and *Coltsfoot*.

The Digestive System

By far the best remedies here for general problems are *Garlic, Meadowsweet* and *Golden Seal*.

For more specific problems please see the appropriate section on p.105. If the problem is one of worm infestation, herbs have much to offer. However, in Britain the Medicines Act has limited the availability of some of the most useful remedies. Consider: *Wormwood, Tansy, Garlic Rue* and *Southernwood*.

The Urinary System

A number of herbs are quite specific for urinary infections because of the excretion of their antiseptic oils. Care must be taken with the stronger ones where there is any history of kidney disease as the oils may aggravate it. These are discussed in the section on that system on p.139 but let us mention *Bearberry, Juniper, Yarrow, Couch Grass, Buchu* and *Echinacea*.

The Reproductive System

Infections here must be diagnosed with skilled and proper attention as a number of problems in later life are avoidable though correct holistic treatment initially. Herbs with anti-infective affinity for this system if used in conjunction with uterine tonics would include the remedies mentioned for the urinary system plus *Echinacea, Wild Indigo, Nasturtium* and *Blue Cohosh*.

The Musculoskeletal System

Myalgia and bone problems are always best treated in as broad a way as possible. It is worth mentioning the following in addition to the basic anti-microbials: *Black Willow, Bogbean* and *Devil's Claw*.

The Nervous System

If infections occur in the nerves it will usually be because the whole being is over stressed and so stress management is essential. This is described in the chapter on that system. With problems such as neuritis and shingles, although occasionally very intransigent, we can mention *St John's Wort, Echinacea, Pasque Flower* and *Peppermint Oil*.

The Skin

Skin infections can usually be avoided by cleanliness and attention to hygiene. If an infection does get a hold it may be coming from within, in which case internal medication is essential, or it might be an external attack allowed because of lowered resistance. In such cases a combination of internal and external use of herbal remedies will usually prove effective. Some to consider include *Pasque Flower, Garlic, Echinacea, Eucalyptus Oil* and *Myrrh*.

7
HERB GARDENS AND CULTIVATION

The Healing Garden

We in the west are starting to regain the recognition of connection with nature, of the profound links between all aspects of life. The use of herbs in healing is but one aspect of the oneness of life that is planet Earth. The growing of healing plants or their collection from the wild is another expression of relationship and ecological rapport that is open to us.

The garden as an expression of nature's perfection and harmony is a rich and potent image. In the mythology of many countries and peoples, the image of the garden as a wellspring of spiritual and physical healing emerges often. Realizing that herbal and healing gardens have always been with us lends richness and depth to our connection with gardens and healing plants today.

The garden of Eden described in the Bible is at the core of western culture. Like all of the archetypal gardens, Eden is represented as a place where boundless peace prevailed. Sweet smells filled the air and brilliant flowers shone like precious gems. The great tree at the very centre of the garden prevailed as the nourisher of all life. This tree was the source of the four great rivers which went out into the four directions. These rivers, in turn, spread the tree's nourishment throughout the garden, or world.

So herbs and the garden as the wellspring of life and healing is central to the very roots of our culture and spirituality. The use of herbs today, whether for health or cooking, links us into a tradition straight from the heart of God – a divine gift for us all. However, the divide between cultivated garden and the wilds of nature is a purely artificial one, a product of human creativity and control. When considering healing plants, we can see the whole of the plant kingdom as our garden.

Ideally, herbs are best for healing purposes when collected from the wild. However, that is often impossible because the habitat has been destroyed or the person lives in the middle of an enormous city. So, in addition to the spiritual and aesthetic role of herb gardens, we can add their convenience for the herbalist!

The design and layout of the herb garden has evolved as society has changed. Many ideas have been developed about the relationship of plants, shape of beds, etc. Some wonderful books have been written on this fascinating subject. Please refer to the Bibliography for books about herb garden layout and construction.

A simple idea that is well worth resurrecting from our horticultural past is the wonderful Elizabethan practice of creating a herb lawn. We shall use this as an example of the possibilities for herb gardening in general.

Herb Lawns

Certain low-growing herbs will make a good dense turf which can be walked on without damage and will stand up well to dry conditions. When the turf consists exclusively of herb plants it is generally sufficient to mow only two or three times in a season, as soon as the flowers appear, to keep it green. The one exception to this is the creeping thyme, which is not mown until the flowers have faded. Where herbs and grass are mixed, however, weekly mowing will be necessary to keep the grass in check.

A fertile soil is not right for a herb turf as it will encourage the growth of weeds and make the herbs too lush, so sand must be added to impoverish the soil. This will also ensure good drainage. In the first year a good deal of hand weeding will be needed, but in following years the growth will be so dense that weeds will be suppressed.

There are three creeping herbs which are commonly used for making turfs:

● *Creeping Thyme – Thymus serpyllum,* obtainable with flowers in various shades of pink and purple, and also white.
● *Roman Chamomile – Chamaemelum nobile,* preferably either the double form or the flowerless form 'Treneague'. The double-flowered chamomile is

sturdier in growth than 'Treneague', which is only suitable for paths which will not be used a great deal, or for making the turf seats which were a feature of Tudor herb gardens.
● *Pennyroyal – Mentha pulegium,* which makes a very close turf but needs a more fertile, moisture retaining soil.

These should be planted in the spring, after accumulating a stock of small plants the previous year. *Chamomile* and *Pennyroyal* can be propagated by dividing the stock plants and growing the small rooted shoots in a nursery bed, Thyme must be grown individually. The prepared site is planted at 10 – 15 cm intervals in spring and by early autumn there will be a good cover. If the weather is dry, occasional water is needed. If a mixed grass/herb lawn is wanted then use Chamomile. After the grass has become established, the Chamomile can be inserted at 15 – 20 cm intervals in the spring.

Cultivation of Specific Herbs

Many excellent books have been written about the cultivation of herbs. The techniques are no different to those of any gardener, whether in window boxes, small gardens or acres. There is such a wealth of practical wisdom available that I shall leave gardening to the experts. A small selection is referred to in the Bibliography. There is no substitute for direct experience, the books can only at best offer advice and guidance. You have to make your own mistakes!

Below are some very basic cultivation guidelines for a small range of commonly grown herbs.

Angelica
Angelica is a short-lived plant, dying back to ground level each year. It may not flower

and seed for two or three years, but once seed has formed the plant will die. However, if the flower heads are removed before the seed is set, its life can be prolonged for a further one or two years.

Allow some of the seed to fall to the ground and germinate naturally, because seed harvested and later sown is often unsuccessful. In the following spring thin out and transplant the seedlings. Angelica must be grown in moist soil in a position where there is shade during the hottest part of the day. In full sun the growth will be poor and the leaf stems tough and stringy. Plenty of room is needed for the wide-spreading leaves.

Bearberry

This is a creeping shrub with shining evergreen leaves that make it an attractive ground cover plant for the front of a border on lime-free soils. Plenty of decayed leaf mould or peat should be worked into the surface layer of the bed, with it being planted in partial shade and watered freely in periods of drought. The plant can be increased very easily by carefully detaching rooted stems from the parent plant; avoid too frequent disturbance of the whole plant however.

Borage

The seed is normally sown where the plants are to grow, but they can be transplanted if this is more convenient. Seedlings are thinned or transplanted 30 cm apart. The plants grow quickly, and often two or three generations can come from one spring sowing or from self-sown seeds in one year on light soils. The last seedlings to germinate will over-winter and provide plants which flower early the following spring. These plants and those from an early spring sowing may grow so rapidly that by midsummer they may become top-heavy with too great a profusion of flowering shoots. By this time much seed will have been scattered around, so that the large old plants may be discarded and young plants grown on in their place. On heavy soils, however, seedlings are unlikely to survive the winter and some seed must be harvested each autumn and stored for sowing the following spring. On light soils this beautiful plant, if not kept in check, will take your garden over with unwanted seedlings that will appear everywhere.

Caraway

Caraway requires a well-drained, friable soil in an open, sunny position. The seed is sown in early summer in the position where the plants are to grow and the seedlings are thinned out to 10 cm apart as soon as they are large enough to handle. The plants will flower the next year in early summer, and the fruits will begin to ripen about eight weeks later. When the main umbels are ripe the plants should be cut to the ground, tied in small bunches, and hung up in an airy shed over a cloth to catch the seed. This is then dried before being stored in an airtight container.

Coriander

Growing conditions must promote rapid growth to ensure that fully ripened seed is obtained. This means a well-drained soil and a sunny position. Sow the seeds where they are to grow, in late spring when the soil has warmed up, thinning to 10 – 15 cm apart as soon as the seedlings are large enough to handle. However, if only a few plants are wanted, a pinch of seed could be sown in a few pots, thinning to one seedling per pot and planting them out in late May without breaking the ball of roots. Flowering takes place in July and August, and when fully ripened the seed is harvested as for Dill. It should be stored in an airtight container, where the flavour will improve still further with keeping.

Cowslip

Although rarely seen in cultivation, cowslips can be raised from seed, but as this must be sown immediately it is ripe it would usually be necessary to gather it from the wild. The seeds are now available, thankfully, from specialist seed merchants. Cowslips grow best on light well-drained soil, both in sun or partial shade. Once the seedlings are fully grown, frequent division of the clumps will keep the plants growing strongly.

Dill

Dill must be grown on light, well-drained soil, in a place where it will be sheltered from wind. When growing for the seed, sowing should be done early, as soon as the soil is warm and friable, to allow plenty of time for growth and thus ensure that the seeds will ripen before the weather becomes cool. If leaves and flower stems only are wanted, sowing need not take place until early summer. The seed must be sown where the plants are to grow. Water freely in dry weather. On late cold soils growth may be too slow to allow time for the seed to ripen. If only a limited number of plants are required, seed could be sown in a seed pan and protected from the cold, and the individual seedlings transplanted while still very young into small pots. When well rooted these should be planted out without further root disturbance. Fresh young growth can be cut for use as required throughout the summer, and the plants harvested when they develop a reddish-purple flush. Cut the entire plant to ground level and hang up in small bunches in an airy place to ripen, placing a cloth underneath to catch the falling seed.

Fennel

Fennel grows rapidly and in three or four years becomes somewhat woody. A supply of young plants should be maintained by re-placement with self-sown seedlings or by division of old plants. Once fennel is established in the garden many self-sown seedlings will be found. Any not required should be removed immediately as they will become difficult to eradicate later. Florence fennel is cultivated mostly in southern Europe and Israel; it tends to run to seed when attempts are made to grow it in cooler climates. Seed is sown annually in summer in a moist sunny position in rich soil, and if it is sown in June it is less likely to run to seed. In a dry summer it must be kept well watered.

Garlic

The single cloves only are needed for planting, as well as for use in the kitchen, and these are obtained by removing the skins of the main bulb and separating the single segments. These often vary greatly in size and the larger should be selected. A fertile soil is necessary for good growth, but not one that has recently been manured. Late autumn planting in the open is possible in southern England, but it is best to delay this until the early spring in regions where the winters are harsh; e.g. in northern England. Plant the cloves in a trench or separately with a trowel; they should be placed 5 cm deep and 20 cm apart. No attention will be required apart from weeding. The bulbs should be harvested in late summer when the leaves are just beginning to turn yellow. Lift with a fork, tie in small bunches, and hang up in a dry, airy place to finish ripening. The bulbs may appear to be entire at first but will divide into cloves as they dry. For storage the bulbs can be made into ropes, as is done with onions, or put into small nets, and stored in a completely dry and frost-proof place.

Hyssop

Hyssop has a long flowering period which continues late into the autumn, and as it is rather tender it should not be cut back until the following year when new growth is evident. Then trim with shears to remove all the previous year's dead flowering stems, cutting lightly into growing wood. As old plants are generally less winter-hardy than young ones they should be replaced as soon as they become woody. Often small-rooted shoots can be separated from the parent plant and kept in a shady place until well established; the separation should be carried out in spring with the aid of a hand fork. An alternative method is to make cuttings of well-ripened shoots of the current year's growth. These can be stripped from the bush, inserted in a cold frame and treated as half-ripe cuttings. If well rooted they can be planted in the open the following spring.

Insect Powder Plant

This plant is hardy in the south of England and grows best on calcareous soils and sandy, well-drained sites. It is perfectly hardy on lime-free clays but becomes somewhat unkempt in appearance. The silvery mounds persist through most winters. From midsummer for several weeks the pure white flowers are produced in abundance, making the plant a highly decorative addition to the herb border. The densely packed plants need to be divided frequently if free flowering is to be maintained. This should be done in spring during damp weather, as soon as active growth becomes apparent. If the plants are disturbed in the autumn and the following winter is very wet and cold they may not survive. The flowers last well in water and are very useful for small flower arrangements.

Uses

The use of several species of pyrethrum as insecticides originated in Iran, and in the nineteenth century *Crysanthemum cinera-* *riifolium* was selected as the most effective. The plant is now grown commercially in a number of countries, the most important of these being Japan and Yugoslavia. For commercial crops the plants are raised from seed and the flowers are gathered in the third, fourth and fifth years; after this period the yield declines and the old plants are replaced by seedlings. The flowers are picked without stems when they are three-quarters open, and are then dried and crumbled. Dusts and also sprays containing the essential oil are used as insecticides, especially where it is necessary to use non-poisonous deterrents on food crops. It will kill all cold-blooded creatures and must not be used near pools containing fish. Prolonged handling of pyrethrum dust can cause dermatitis and asthma.

Lavender

L. angustifolia grows best and produces the finest fragrance when grown on well-drained but moisture-retaining soil in a sunny place. There are several varieties of this common lavender: 'Grappenhall', a robust plant with deep lavender blue flowers; 'Old English', highly scented; and 'Dutch Lavender' with remarkably grey leaves. When compact, low-growing bushes are required 'Hidcote', with violet-coloured flowers, or 'Munstead', with lavender blue flowers could be chosen, both with narrow leaves; neither of these varieties, however, is so fragrant as the first-mentioned varieties. The species *L. latifolia* has a sweet and enjoyable scent although the oil, known commercially as 'spike lavender' oil, is inferior to that of *L. angustifolia*.

To keep lavender bushes compact and shapely they must be clipped over with shears to the base of the flowering stems as soon as the flowers have been gathered or have faded. If this is not done in late autumn it can be done just as the new growth starts in spring. Lavender is a short lived plant and needs to be replaced after five to seven years. It is readily propagated by tearing small slips of ripened shoots from a healthy plant and inserting these in sandy soil in the open ground in late summer. One year later they can be planted finally.

Lemon Balm

There is no comparison between lemon balms grown on light soils in the sun and those which are grown on moist soils shaded in the hottest part of the day. The latter have fresh green foliage with a fresh lemony fragrance, whereas the former have yellowish green leaves and a harsh aroma. Young plants are preferable for the same reason, and after three or four years the old and by now large, overcrowded bushes should be replaced. Propagation is by division of the old plants, i.e. by splitting off pieces of the outer growth with surface runners attached, or by selecting young seedlings invariably to be found in the vicinity of the parent plants. As a garden feature the fresh green, free-growing new plants are so much more attractive in appearance. Lemon balm is very attractive to bees and for this reason is also known as bee balm.

Lemon Verbena

On thin and well-drained soils, and if planted where it will receive maximum sunshine, this shrub withstands most cold winters. In severe winters the top growth will be killed to ground level, but normally new shoots will eventually grow from the crown late in the next year. No tender shrub should ever be cut back late in the summer as this would encourage new growth which will not ripen before the onset of winter. Also the previous season's twiggy growth acts as a protection for the crown of the plant, shielding it from frost damage. Old plants are always more vulnerable in

adverse conditions, and it is wise as a precaution to propagate lemon verbena at intervals of five to six years. Both soft- and hard-wood cuttings root easily during the summer. The rooted cuttings should be kept indoors during the first winter and not planted out until the spring.

Lovage

When grown on heavy soils lovage easily attains its full height; on light free-draining soils it may be far shorter unless plenty of humus is added for the retention of moisture. Waterlogging in winter is fatal, causing the fleshy roots to rot. Shelter and sun are essential for successful growth. For a continuous supply of good growth, division will probably be needed every three to four years. This is carried out in early spring just as new growth is emerging; don't disturb the roots in the autumn as this may cause rotting during the winter when growth is dormant. Division is carried out with a sharp spade or knife as the prongs of a fork may damage the tough fleshy roots and cause decay.

Nasturtium

A light soil in a sunny place is best for nasturtiums, but they will tolerate a shady place provided the drainage is good. They are very useful for maintaining a continuous supply of gaily coloured flowers throughout the summer. The seed is sown in late spring where the plants are to grow. Dwarf forms will be suitable for the front of the herb border but climbing forms are useful to make a colourful display on a trellis at the back.

Garden Parsley

This should be grown on fertile, moist, well-cultivated soil and is best in positions which are shaded during the hottest part of the day. It is propagated by seed sown in spring, but as cold soil inhibits germination sowing should be delayed until the soil has warmed. If the drills are sown and then partially covered with soil, and boiling water is poured over them before they are completely filled in, germination will be accelerated. Transplanting seedlings can be done successfully provided they are very small. If the roots of the seedlings are well developed they may be damaged by transplantation, and this will make them likely to bolt. Thinning is essential to obtain strong plants which will come through the winter. Crowded plants are more liable to damage during cold wet spells. In cold areas it may be advisable to cover the plants with well-ventilated cloches during frosty periods, or to maintain a winter supply by keeping a pot on a windowsill. As with many biennial plants, the life of parsley can be lengthened by one or two years if it is not allowed to flower and seed. On the other hand, self-sown seedlings will keep up the supply and thus make further planned sowing unnecessary unless the winter is unusually wet and cold.

Peppermint

A friable, moist soil is essential, with the addition of well-decayed compost or manure, and an open situation without too much shade is required. As the plants are hybrids they must be propagated by vegetative means, and strong healthy stolons should be planted 5 cm deep and 30 cm apart in autumn. After three to four years plants will need to be dug up, divided and replanted.

Rosemary

This shrub, requiring sun and good drainage, is best grown in the shelter of a wall. When grown in the open garden it may be damaged by the winter gales. Young and vigorous plants will withstand severe winter conditions better than woody bushes, and once the plants have become straggling they should be replaced. This is usually necessary after five to six years. Careful pruning will help to keep the growth compact, but branches should never be cut back into bare wood. Propagation is simple as short woody shoots removed from the parent plant in summer will root easily in sandy soil in the open.

Rue

On well-drained soils this evergreen shrub is generally unharmed by low temperatures, and thus is particularly valuable in the winter garden. It should be grown in a sunny open place to encourage robust and hardy growth. To maintain the dense cushion-like habit the plant should be lightly clipped with shears just as growth commences in spring. Rue is easy to propagate. A well-ripened shoot with a heel removed from the shrub in late summer and inserted in sandy soil in a sunny place in the open will usually form roots by the following spring.

Sage

Full sun and good drainage are essential for this strongly aromatic herb. Unless it is closely trimmed after flowering the bush will become leggy and open, liable to be damaged by wind and heavy snowfalls. The 15 cm long flower spikes terminate the annual growth, and as the flowers fade these spikes must be clipped hard back. Where a high yield of sage is important the flowerless form known as 'English broad leaf' is grown. Sage must never be cut back below the young growth as the bare old wood will not produce new buds, even with careful pruning. After four to five years sage bushes become sprawling and untidy and are usually replaced. Cuttings with woody ends will root easily if put into sandy soil in a shady place during the summer months.

Southernwood

Southernwood needs light soil and sun. Its ultimate height is controlled by yearly clipping. As new growth appears in spring the last year's growth should be cut back to 5 – 6 cm above its base; the numerous fresh shoots will quickly make an attractive dome-shaped hummock of new foliage. Unless this cutting back is done each year the untrimmed bush will become straggling and open.

Sweet Cicely

It is one of the earliest herb plants to come into growth in the spring, but in a very hot summer the growth may almost cease. It is easily grown and spreads rapidly both by small root tubers and by seeding, and on the heavier soils it will become very invasive unless kept in check by removing the seed before it is shed. The spreading plants are restrained by frequent dividing and re-planting, or by replacing old plants with some of the small plants from root tubers which will be found in the vicinity.

Sweet Basil

Basil is not an easy plant to maintain in good condition. Its growth is very tender and easily damaged by careless handling or exposure to wind, and it must be grown in a sheltered position where it will be pro-tected from hot sun. Bush basil, however, will tolerate adverse conditions better than sweet basil. The seed should be sown in a frost-free place in spring, and as root distur-bance causes a check to growth it is usual to sow a few seeds in small pots to avoid having to prick out. Thin the seedlings and pot on as necessary and, finally, when all danger of frost has passed, plant them in the open without any root disturbance, into well-drained soil with plenty of humus. In dry weather water freely. It is possible to maintain a winter supply of basil by grow-ing either type in containers on a window-sill in a warm room.

Common Thyme

This is the thyme most commonly grown in gardens. An ideal position for it is a sloping bank of well-drained soil in full sun, but if this is not available a bed of stony soil should be prepared. As the leafy shoots fade the bushes should be clipped over with shears; this will encourage a new growth of shoots for the remainder of the summer. After this second crop has been gathered in early September the plants should again be trimmed with shears. After four to five years the plants become increasingly woody and less productive of young shoots for kitchen use and will need to be replaced by newly propagated stock. Young plants can be obtained from the original stock by filling the plant with well-drained soil up to the base of the young wood. New roots will form on this wood and the plant can be lifted the following spring and the rooted growths separated and transplanted.

After reviewing this small selection of plants let us now consider how all plant material may be harvested, dried, stored and prepared for use.

General Guidelines for Harvesting

The specific details for parts of plants do not vary whether collecting from the wild or from a cultivated garden. However, there are a number of points to bear in mind when collecting from the wild:

- Collect away from main roads because the exhaust fumes settle on the leaves.
- Avoid field borders where crop spray-ing has been going on.
- Collect only from places where there is a concentration of the plant you are after. Such concentration suggests that it is a good ecological site for the plant and so will be healthiest there.

- Bear in mind the conservation needs of our environment and do not over-collect. Never strip a site. If collecting foliage, try not to damage the rest of the plant.

Leaves, Stems and Flowers

For any aerial part, whether leaves, stems or flowers, always gather them on a sunny day after the dew has evaporated off the plants, but before the full heat of the day has filled the garden. For plants with volatile oil, such as _Mint_ and _Thyme,_ just before noon is a good time to harvest. By then the oils have had a chance to reach the leaves, but have not yet been drawn off by the day's heat. Rain washes away some of the aromatic oils, so after a rainstorm wait a day or two before harvesting in order to let the plants' oils collect again.

Unless it is time to harvest the entire plant, think of your harvesting as a pruning of the plant or the herb patch. To allow most plants to survive after selective harvesting, never pick more than half of their available harvest, or even a quarter to be safe. And if you are at all uncertain about how much selective harvesting the plants can tolerate, start out by taking only one-tenth. Be sure to observe the herbs during that season and the next, noting the effects of the harvest.

Gather plants that are healthy, and do not pick them from places exposed to noxious fumes from cars or chemicals used in agriculture. You have more control over this aspect of harvesting if you have grown your plants at home than if you are collecting from the wild. Foragers must not only be careful of trespassing on private property and disturbing the habitat when collecting wild plants, they must also be very skilled at avoiding wild places that have been sprayed with herbicides or pesticides. Avoid picking herbs at roadsides, next to farm fields (unless you know the farm is organic), and

even close to your neighbour's fence if they use herbicides.

With tender, non-woody stemmed herbs, gathering of leaves, stems, or flowers can be easily done with scissors or a sharp knife. Tough or woody stems will require pruning shears at gathering time. Generally speaking, it is better for the plant you are harvesting, as well as for the final dried herb, if you harvest whole branches or stems, rather than stripping off leaves and leaving the stripped stems and branches on the plant. Herbs with flexible stems such as _Mint, Pennyroyal,_ and _Lavender_ can be picked whole. When stripping the dried herb from its stem or branch, keep the leaves as whole as possible. This helps preserve their healing properties longer. When harvesting hairy or prickly plants like _Comfrey, Borage_ or _Mullein,_ wearing gloves will ease the whole experience!

Woody Stems

Harvesting material from plants with more woody stems, and parts of trees, is possible as long as you are careful to harvest the parts as if pruning the plant. Some plant parts, such as _Oak leaves_ or _Elderberry leaves,_ may be easier to harvest by picking each leaf separately, but as a general rule, the harvesting-by-branch method works best. If only the herb's leaves are to be used, hang the harvested stems or branches upside down in bunches for a few days. This will bring the sap present in the stems or branches into the leaves. Then, spread the leaves on screens in thin layers until dry, as described below.

Harvesting Roots and Bark

Digging up the roots of plants such as _Dandelion_ is relatively easy if you have properly prepared their growing bed. In cultivating long-rooted plants, a deep bed that is porous and well-aerated is necessary, so that the roots can be harvested by hand. For uncultivated plants growing in soil that is compacted, digging up roots is more of a challenge. A shovel with a long, thin blade is helpful. Dig a hole straight down and to one side of the root. Gradually remove soil on the side of the hole towards the root. Then pull the root sideways into the hole. This method will damage the root less than the common practice of digging down all around the root and then pulling it up, and especially when the root is deeper than one shovel-length.

Therapeutic parts of trees often come from the inner bark of their roots, trunks, or branches. This presents more of a problem to the conscientious harvester, because removing the bark from standing trees disfigures and injures them, while digging up roots can be equally traumatic. Taking sections of trunk bark from living trees is to be avoided. An obvious solution is to use the bark of branches that may need pruning anyway, rather than ruining a strong living tree.

The bark from the trunk is usually more potent than the bark from branches, and the bark from roots is more potent still. This poses problems for the environmentalist! A way to avoid cutting down healthy trees is to find trees that are being cut down anyway; select trees that need thinning or removing. Likely candidates for root or trunk bark include orchard trees that are too old and are being removed; young trees that need thinning; trees that must be removed because they are in the way of a road, house, power line, or scenic view; and trees that have been injured by lightning, cars, animals, or weather.

A safe way to gather root bark from healthy trees is as if it is being given a gentle root pruning. To collect roots from a living tree, dig down at the outermost edge of the tree's root range. The roots' circumference will fall roughly parallel with the circumference of the tree's branches. Root bark,

like trunk bark, gets thicker as trees get older, so very young trees will not provide much. When harvesting for root bark, be very careful to avoid cutting main roots. Find a moderate-sized root (the smaller the root, the less potent it is) and cut it out cleanly with pruning clippers, an axe, or a saw.

Twigs and small branches of any tree whose bark is used for healing purposes can be used instead of the trunk bark. These are cut in the spring when the sap rises. Strip off the small branches' inner bark and cut it into small pieces before drying. Chop and dry the tiny twigs (see p.197).

It is the living cambium layer of roots, trunks, and branches that is used in herbal medicine. The methods used to expose this soft inner bark can vary with each tree. Initially scrape, chop, cut, or pry off the coarse outer bark. Several implements come in handy for this task. A knife with a strong, sharp blade and point is good for scraping bark off roots that are not very thick and hard. A small, sharp hatchet can separate chips of inner bark from the heartwood of the branch you have harvested. A broad chisel and a hammer can also be used to chip off inner bark. A crowbar or small spade is useful for prying off outer bark or strips of inner bark.

Whatever tool is used, be sure it is not only sharp, but easy to handle, and comfortable to hold. After removing sections of the outer bark, cut down through the cambium layer with a knife or chisel, depending how hard and thick the wood is. Then remove this inner bark in strips, squares, or chips, whichever is easiest. Cut the bark into small pieces before drying it in the shade or in a warm place for several weeks.

Gathering

Whether gathering plants in your herb garden or backyard, in the woods, or on a neighbour's land, consider the carrying containers for your harvest. They should be large enough and should allow plenty of air-flow through them. Flexible baskets with handles or shoulder straps, double canvas bags that hang over the shoulder, and clean drawstring bags made of burlap or other cloth are all good choices.

After harvesting plant parts, limit their exposure to sunlight and prepare them for drying as soon as possible. If using a vehicle to transport the harvest, protect the herbs from wind, dust, or heat. If they are piled in a car, keep the windows open to keep the temperature down and prevent premature drying, but cover the herbs with a light cloth to shade them from the sun.

Details about the main medicinal plants are found under the entry for the plant throughout the book.

Drying Herbs

Correctly dried herbs will retain much of their original colour, aroma, and healing qualities. Drying herbs correctly is not too difficult, but it does demand some careful attention to each plant's attributes. The first step is to take the plants out of direct sunlight as soon as they have been gathered.

Try to make sure that leafy herbs are kept clean of soil when you harvest them. A layer of mulch in the garden helps keep plants clean and free of mud from splashing rain. Wash herbs only if they really need it, because washing may affect their quality. If you do need to wash your herbs, wash them quickly under cold running water. Allow washed herbs to dry well before placing them on a drying rack or hanging them. Gently pat them dry and place them in a cool, airy place to rid them of all moisture before beginning the drying process. If it is not possible to let your herbs air-dry naturally outdoors or in a warm attic, a

heater can be used to maintain a steady, even temperature between 35° and 38° C.

Leafy Parts

The leafy parts of most herbs with volatile oils dry best at temperatures between 35° and 38° C. Commercial herb processors often use much higher temperatures, but the home gardener can afford to dry herbs the way they should be dried: slowly and steadily. When herbs are drying, the flow of air over and around them is possibly more important than the heat. Greater air circulation makes a lower drying temperature possible. Herbs containing volatile oils should be dried in the shade, not in the sun, as their oil would vaporize.

Flowers

Flowers are more delicate and fragile than other plant parts and are especially vulnerable to damage from water. Protect from water after gathering and dry them in a drying room or dryer with a temperature around 32° C. If it is too hot or too cool or not airy enough in the drying room, flowers will discolour and lose their subtle qualities completely.

Roots and Barks

Roots and barks should be carefully washed and cleaned of soil. Chop before drying into pieces 2.5 cm thick or less with a small axe or knife, depending on how tough the root is. It is easiest to chop bark before drying. Most roots can be dried in the sun, but sometimes, depending on the herb's properties, this is not desirable or possible. For example, if a root is gathered in October, there may not be enough sunlight to dry it properly. In this case, dry the roots indoors in an airing room or dryer. Another case for care is if the root is rich in volatile oil, such as _Valerian_.

If drying seeds such as caraway or fennel, place the whole herb branches or stems in large paper bags. Hung upside down with their umbels toward the bottom of the bag, the herbs will drop their seeds into the bag. Another way to dry herbs in paper bags is to cut a hole in the bag's bottom and stick the herbs' stems through. Cut a few ventilation holes in the sides of the bag before placing the bunch of herbs in it. Then, hang the bag of herbs from the ceiling. This ensures a well-aerated set-up that will keep the herbs clean as they dry.

Drying Racks

A good drying rack is essential for the gardener who plans to dry quantities of herbs for medicinal use. You can construct a simple herb-drying rack with several levels. Window screening can be used both to maximize airflow and to support the herbs drying on racks. Avoid metal screens. You can also make screens from broad mesh cloth, such as muslin. Benches similar to those used in saunas, but made from thin strips of hardwood 2.5 cm wide, are also good drying platforms if whole branches or large herbs are being dried. Leave 2.5 cm of space between each slat. Do not finish the wood with any stains, varnishes, or oils. Whether you use racks, screens, or benches, be sure to lay out the herbs in thin layers so they dry evenly.

Drying Rooms

Try to determine beforehand how much drying space you will need, based on quantities of herbs and the cycle of harvest times for each herb. To dry about one-quarter acre's worth of fresh herb materials, a drying room with about 185 sq m of flat drying space is needed. A clean attic is a good place to put the drying rack of herbs. The entire wall of a shed can be converted to a herb-drying area by building drying racks onto its walls.

Barns or sheds can be good herb-drying

places, but they have a few potential drawbacks. The usually loose construction intended to allow plenty of air circulation may also allow dirt and insects to enter. This also makes it difficult to keep out moisture. A more sophisticated drying set-up involves construction of, or conversion into, a forced-air drying room or shed. You can use rafters, screens, or racks in the drying shed or spread the herbs on a raised 'floor', a framework of beams covered with permeable sisal cloth. Air is forced into the shed with a centrifugal fan mounted on an outside wall of the building, near floor level. Place a screen and filter over the fan intake to prevent insects and dust from entering. The room also needs an open-and-close exhaust vent near the ceiling. For this you can use a window screen, a hatch, or a circulating vent.

This fan can also contain heating elements to provide warm air. For large rooms, a propane or natural gas heater is more efficient than an electric fan-heater. A solar hot air collector on the south side of the drying shed is a good idea, although this does not always ensure heat in our climate! There are many ways to do this, ranging from an actual greenhouse-type construction to simply supporting some black plastic over the ground and ducting the airflow into the fan.

How Long to Dry?

Drying time for herbs varies with the particular plant and the part of the plant being dried. Flowers should be light and well-dried, but not so dry that they crumble into powder with any handling. In general, leaves should be brittle enough to break between the fingers, but not so dry that they crumble. Stems and stalks should be breakable between the fingers but not flexible. Bark and roots should be dry enough to snap if they are thin, or chip easily with the blow of a hammer if they are thick. With a little experience, it is easy to know when herbs are dried properly. The result should smell, taste, and look much like the original fresh plant, except that it is dry. A herb that is green and fragrant when fresh should also be green and fragrant when dried. Don't judge your dried herbs by the appearance of shop-bought herbs. The latter are usually several shades lighter, browner or yellower than properly dried herbs should be.

Storing Home-dried Herbs

Heat, light, air, and bacteria can all reduce the healing properties of herbs, as can plastics and metal. Dried herbs must be protected from these factors with proper storage. For short periods of several weeks or so, you can store herbs in a wax paper bag that is in turn placed inside a brown paper bag. For longer storage, use a tightly capped glass jar, preferably made of dark glass to protect herbs from deterioration caused by light. Preserving jars that have glass lids that close with metal clamps to form an airtight seal are best. If metal lids are used, place a piece of wax paper over the jar before screwing down the lid. Do not use soft plastic jars or bags to store medicinal herbs because not all plastic is approved for food use, and the container you choose may have a residue that will taint the herbs. Even if it is approved for food, plastic encourages condensation inside the container that will hasten decomposition. You can also store herbs in fibre drum barrels (such as the kind that hold bulk dried goods in natural foods stores), air-tight wooden boxes or bins, and wooden barrels.

Try to approximate the amount of herbs to be dried before making the first harvest, thus enabling storage space needed to be worked out. If too much is dried at once, you will soon run out of cabinet space. Plan to keep small jars of dried herbs in the kitchen or medicine chest for regular use, but find a convenient larger space for the bulk storage jars or containers that hold the entire harvest. This not only saves cabinet space in the kitchen, but it also ensures the freshness of the stored herbs. Opening and closing a big container of herbs all the time only hastens spoilage.

The best places for long-term storage of herbs are dry, dark, and cool.

It is essential to label the herbs carefully with the name of the plant and the date of harvesting. You may wish to include other details of cultivation of harvest, such as phases of the moon and weather conditions at the time of harvesting, seed or stock source, type of fertilizer or growing methods used, location of the growing plant, and methods and duration of drying. If this is not done it is very easy to end up with lots of dried green leaves, not knowing what any of them are!

Using Wild Plants

The value of fresh herbs over dried, and even wild over cultivated, has been stressed repeatedly in this book. Wild plants can make an excellent source of food and, of course, medicine. The Bibliography has good references for wild plant identification, wild food plants etc. Nature is bountiful in plants that we can use.

There is a problem here, and that is an environmental one. The wild places of the world are being desicrated and raped at a speed that staggers the mind. Five thousand acres of the Amazon rain forest are cleared _every day!_ Hedgerows in Britain are going, wet meadows are being drained and our agricultural land is being turned into a biological desert. Britain is already the least forested country in Europe. If we add to this the threat from pollution the picture for a wild-plant collector is worrying indeed.

In the face of this it can be argued that

wild plants should not be picked at all but conserved and their habitat protected. It is largely because of overpicking that the _Cowslip_ is now relatively uncommon in Britain.

In the last section guidelines have been given for how to collect wild plants. Please adhere to them and only ever collect if it will not disrupt the environment.

If in doubt, DON'T.

8
HERBAL PHARMACY

Herbal pharmacy is an art as well as a science. Knowing how to prepare the remedies is as much part of the skill of a herbalist as which ones to use. Various methods of using plants have developed over the centuries to enable their healing properties to be released and become active. After the right choice of herbs has been made, the best way to prepare them must be selected.

No doubt the first way in which our ancestors used herbs was by eating the fresh plant. Since then, over the thousands of years that herbs have been used, other methods of preparing the plants have been developed. With our modern knowledge of pharmacology we can make conscious choices as to which process we use to release the biochemical constituents needed for healing.

It should be clear by now that the property of any herb is not just the sum of all the actions of various chemicals present. There is a synergy at work that acts to create a therapeutic whole that is more than the sum of its parts. If the method of preparation destroys or loses part of the whole, much of the healing power is lost. The preparation must be done carefully and consciously.

Preparations for Internal Use

Undoubtedly the best way of using herbs is to take them internally since it is from within that healing takes place. There are three kinds of preparations for taking internally:

- Water-based,
- Alcohol-based,
- Fresh or dried herbs.

Let's consider each of these in turn.

Water-based Preparations

This is quite simply a tea, though some people prefer to use the word tisane. The two basic ways to prepare such water-based extracts (teas) are infusions and decoctions. When the herb to be used contains any hard, woody material, decoctions are used, otherwise infusions are used.

Infusions

If you know how to make tea, you know

how to make an infusion. It is the simplest and most commonly used method, and both fresh or dried herbs can be used to prepare one.

Where one part of dried herb is needed in a tea or medicine, it can be replaced by three parts of the fresh herb, the difference being due to the higher water content of the fresh herb. If the preparations call for one teaspoonful of dried herb, it can be substituted by three teaspoonsful of fresh herb.

To make an infusion:

1. Take a china or glass teapot which has been warmed and put one teaspoonful of the dried herb or herb mixture into it for each cup of tea.
2. Pour a cup of boiling water in for each teaspoonful of herb that is already in the pot and then put the lid on. Leave to steep for ten to fifteen minutes.

This is a general guideline and the quantities will vary depending on which herb is being used.

Infusions may be drunk hot – which is normally best for a medicinal herb tea – or cold. They may be sweetened with _Liquorice Root,_ honey or brown sugar.

Herbal teabags can be made by filling little muslin bags with herbal mixtures; use them in the same way as ordinary teabags.

To make larger quantities to last for a while, the proportion should be 30 grams of herb to half a litre of water. The best way to store it is in a well-stoppered bottle in the refrigerator. However, the life of such an infusion is not very long, as it is so full of lifeforce that any micro-organism that enters the infusion will multiply and thrive in it. If there is any sign of fermentation or spoiling, the infusion must be discarded. Whenever possible, infusions should be prepared only when needed.

Infusions are usually prepared from plant parts such as leaves, flowers or green stems, where the substances wanted are easily accessible. If infusion of bark, root, seeds or resin is wanted, it is best to powder them first to break down some of their cell walls and make them more accessible to the water.

Seeds, for instance, like _Fennel_ and _Aniseed,_ should be slightly bruised before being used in an infusion to release the volatile oils from the cells. Any aromatic herb should be infused in a pot that has a well-sealing lid, to ensure that only a minimum of the volatile oil is lost through evaporation.

When working with herbs that are sensitive to heat, either because they contain highly volatile oils or because their constituents break down at high temperature, a cold infusion is best. The proportion of herbs to water is the same, but in this case the infusion should be left for six to twelve hours in a well-sealed earthenware pot. When the liquid is ready, strain and use it.

Milk may be used as a base for a cold infusion. Milk contains fats and oils which aid in the dissolving of the oily constituents of plants. These milk infusions can also be used for compresses and poultices, adding the soothing action of milk to that of the herbs. There is, however, one contraindication for the use of milk in an infusion, that is, if there is any evidence of an internal reaction to milk in the form of oversensitivity or allergy, or if the skin becomes irritated when it is applied externally, then avoid such infusions.

The infusions made as directed will be the base for many other preparations described later.

Apart from their purely medicinal use herbs can make an exquisite addition to one's lifestyle and can open a whole world of subtle delights and pleasures. They are not only medicines or alternatives to coffee, but can by their own right make excellent teas. While everyone will have their own favourite herbs, here is a list that make delicious teas, either singly or in combination. From this list you can select those which you like the taste of most, or those that also augment your health:

Flowers: *Chamomile, Elder Flower, Hibiscus, Lime Blossom, Red Clover.*
Leaves: *Peppermint, Spearmint, Lemon Balm, Rosemary, Sage, Thyme, Hyssop, Vervain.*
Berries: *Hawthorn, Rose Hips.*
Seeds: *Aniseed, Caraway, Celery, Dill, Fennel.*
Roots: *Liquorice.*

Decoctions

Whenever the herb to be used is hard and woody, it is better to make a decoction rather than an infusion to ensure that the soluble contents of the herb actually reach the water. Roots, rhizomes, wood, bark, nuts and some seeds are hard and their cell walls are very strong, so to ensure that the active constituents are transferred to the water, more heat is needed than for infusions and the herb has to be boiled in the water.

To make a decoction:

1. Put one teaspoonful of dried herb or three teaspoonsful of fresh material for each cup of water into a pot or saucepan. Dried herbs should be powdered or broken into small pieces, while fresh material should be cut into small pieces. If large quantities are made, use 30 grams of dried herb for each half litre of water. (These are general guidelines; more specific dosages for each herb are given in the herbal section). The container should be glass, ceramic or earthenware. If using metal it should

be enamelled. *Never use aluminium.*
2. Add the appropriate amount of water to the herbs.
3. Bring to the boil and simmer for the time given for the mixture or specific herb, usually ten to fifteen minutes. If the herb contains volatile oils, put a lid on.
4. Strain the tea while still hot.

A decoction can be used in the same way as an infusion.

When preparing a mixture containing soft and woody herbs, it is best to prepare an infusion and a decoction separately to insure that the more sensitive herbs are treated accordingly.

When using a woody herb which contains a lot of volatile oils, it is best to make sure that it is powdered as finely as possible and then used in an infusion, to ensure that the oils do not boil away.

Alcohol-based Preparations

In general, alcohol is a better solvent than water for most plant constituents. Mixtures of alcohol and water dissolve nearly all the relevant ingredients of a herb and at the same time act as a preservative. Alcohol-based preparations are called tinctures, a description that is occasionally also used for preparations based on glycerine or vinegar, as described below.

The methods given here for the preparation of tinctures show a simple and general approach; when tinctures are prepared professionally according to descriptions in a pharmacopoeia, specific water/alcohol proportions are used for each herb, but for general use such details are unnecessary.

For home use it is best to take an alcohol of at least 30 per cent (60° proof), vodka for instance, as this is about the weakest alcohol/water mixture with a long-term preservative action.

To make an alcoholic tincture:

1. Put 120 grams of finely chopped or ground dried herb into a container that can be tightly closed. If fresh herbs are used, twice the amount should be taken.
2. Pour half a litre of 30 per cent (60° proof) vodka on the herbs and close tightly.
3. Keep the container in a warm place for two weeks and shake it well twice every day.
4. After decanting the bulk of the liquid, pour the residue into a muslin cloth suspended in a bowl.
5. Wring out all the liquid. The residue makes excellent compost.
6. Pour the tincture into a dark bottle. It should be kept well stoppered.

As tinctures are much stronger, volume for volume, than infusions or decoctions, the dosage to be taken is much smaller, between 5 to 15 drops, depending on the herb taken.

Tinctures can be used in a variety of ways. They can be taken straight or mixed with a little water, or they can be added to a cup of hot water. If this is done, the alcohol will partly evaporate and leave most of the extract in the water, which with some herbs will make the water cloudy, as resins and other constituents not soluble in water will precipitate. Some drops of the tincture can be added to a bath or footbath, or used in a compressor mixed with oil and fat to make an ointment. Suppositories and lozenges can be made in this way too.

Another way of making a kind of alcohol infusion is to infuse herbs in wine. Even though these wine-based preparations do not have the shelf-life of tinctures and are not as concentrated, they can be very pleasant to take and most effective in some conditions. There is a long history of using wine in this way, and in fact most aperitifs and liqueurs were originally herbal remedies, based on herbs such as *Wormwood, Mugworth* and *Aniseed* as aids to the digestive process.

In her book *Herbal Medicine,* Dian Dincin Buchman gives the following excellent recipe for a tonic wine with a very nice taste:

1 pint Madeira
1 sprig of *Wormwood*
1 sprig of *Rosemary*
1 small bruised *Nutmeg*
2.5 cm of bruised *Ginger*
2.5 cm of bruised *Cinnamon Bark*
12 large organic raisins

Pour off about an ounce of the wine. Place herbs in the wine. Cork the bottle tight. Place the bottle in a dark, cool place for a week or two. Strain off the herbs. Combine this medicated wine with a fresh bottle of Madeira and mix thoroughly. Sip a small amount whenever needed. It helps settle the stomach, gives energy and makes you feel better.

A herbal wine can be made simply by steeping the herbs in a wine. Another commonly used kind is *Rosemary* wine:

1 bottle white wine
1 handful of fresh *Rosemary leaves*

Steep the leaves for about a week in the wine and then filter the herbs off. You can use it whenever needed and it will help to settle the digestion and act as a mild relaxing nervine.

You can also ferment the herbs themselves; after all, even grapes are herbs. All the aromatic herbs make good wines; also *Elderberry* and *Dandelion* are especially useful as medicinal wines.

To make a good *Dandelion* wine you will need:

2 litres of *Dandelion Flowers*

1 tablespoonful of bruised *Ginger Root*
The peel of one orange, finely cut
The peel of one lemon, finely cut
700 grams of demerara sugar
The juice of one lemon
1 teaspoonful of wine yeast

Bring the 2 litres of water to the boil and then leave to cool. Separate the flowers of *Dandelion* from the bitter stalks and put them in a large bowl. Pour the cooled water over the flowers and leave for a day, stirring occasionally. Pour the whole into a large pot, add the *Ginger* and the rinds of orange and lemon, then boil for 30 minutes. Strain the liquid and pour it back into the rinsed bowl. Mix the sugar and the lemon juice into the bowl and allow the mixture to cool. Then cream the wine yeast with some of the liquid and add it to the bowl. Cover the bowl with a cloth and leave it to ferment in a warm place for two days, keeping a dish under the bowl to catch any liquid that may froth over the brim. After two days, pour the liquid into a cask which you have to bung with cotton wool to allow any gas to escape, or pour it into a jar that has an air lock (these bottles with airlocks are commonly available from chemists' shops in the UK or from home-brewing suppliers in other countries). Leave the mixture in the cask until all the fermentation has ceased, when gas bubbles no longer form. Then close the cask tightly for about two months. Finally, siphon the clear liquid into bottles, which have to be kept for another six months before they are ready for drinking.

Vinegar-based tincture
Tinctures can also be made using vinegar, which contains acetic acid that acts as a solvent and preservative in a way similar to alcohol. Whenever you make a vinegar tincture, it is best to use apple cider or wine vinegar, as it has in itself excellent health-augmenting properties. Synthetic chemical vinegar should not be used. The method is the same as for alcoholic tinctures and if you steep spices or aromatic herbs in vinegar, the resulting fragrant vinegar will be excellent for culinary use.

To make a herb vinegar, wash and slightly bruise the freshly picked plant and steep in wine or cider vinegar for 2 – 6 weeks. Strain through muslin and then use. The proportions in such vinegars are very approximate. Usually it is based on filling a container with the herb and filling to the top with vinegar.

Good herbs for such vinegars include: *Garlic, Tarragon, Mint, Basil, Thyme, Dill* etc.

Glycerine-based tincture
Tinctures based on glycerine have the advantage of being milder on the digestive tract than alcoholic tinctures, but they have the disadvantage of not dissolving resinous or oily materials quite as well. As a solvent it is stronger than water but weaker than alcohol.

To make a glycerine tincture, make up half a litre of a mixture consisting of one part glycerine and one part water, add 110 grams of the dried, ground herb and leave it in a well-stoppered container for two weeks, shaking it daily. After two weeks, strain and press or wring the residue, as with alcoholic tinctures. For fresh herbs, due to water content, put 220 grams into 25 per cent water plus 75 per cent glycerine (½ litre).

Syrups
In the case of fluid medicine – be it infusion, decoction or tincture – that has a particularly unpleasant taste, it is sometimes advisable to mask the taste by combining the fluid with a sweetener. One way to do this is to use a syrup, which is the traditional way to make cough mixtures more palatable for children, or any herbal preparation more

'toothsome', as Culpepper used to call it!

A simple syrup base is made as follows: pour half a litre of boiling water onto 1.1 kilograms of sugar, place over heat and stir until the sugar dissolves and the liquid begins to boil. Then take off the heat immediately.

This simple syrup can best be used together with a tincture: mix one part of the tincture with three parts of syrup and store for future use.

For use with an infusion or decoction, it is simpler to add the sugar directly to the liquid: for every half litre of liquid add 350 grams of sugar and heat gently until the sugar is dissolved. This again can be stored for future use and will keep quite well in a refrigerator. Since normally sugar is not a 'health food', syrups are best for gargles and cough mixtures only.

Dry Preparations

Occasionally it is better to take herbs in a dry form, with the advantage that you do not taste the herb and also that you can take in the whole herb, including the woody material. The main drawback lies in the fact that the dry herbs are unprocessed, and therefore the plant constituents are not always as readily available for easy absorption. In a process like infusion, heat and water help to break down the walls of the plant cells and to dissolve the constituents, something which is not always guaranteed during the digestive process in the stomach and the small intestines. Also, when the constituents are already dissolved in liquid form, they are available a lot faster and begin their action sooner.

A second drawback for taking some of the herbs dry, as in capsules, lies in the very fact that you do not taste the herb. For various reasons – even though they taste unpleasant – the bitter herbs work much better when they are tasted, as their effectiveness depends on the neurological sensation of bitterness. When you put bitters into a capsule or a pill, their action may well be lost or diminished.

Taking all these considerations into account, there are still a number of ways to use herbs in dry form. The main thing we have to pay attention to is that the herbs be powdered as finely as possible. This guarantees that the cell walls are largely broken down, and helps in the digestion and absorption of the herb.

Capsules

The easiest way to use dry powdered herbs internally is to use gelatine capsules. (These come in various sizes and can be obtained from most chemists. Capsules not made of animal products are also produced. Ask in your area for suppliers.) The size you need depends on the amount of herbs prescribed per dose and on the volume of the material. A capsule size 00 for instance will hold about 0.5 grams of finely powdered herb.

Filling capsules is done like this:

1. Place the powdered herbs in a flat dish and take the halves of the capsule apart.
2. Move the halves of the capsules through the powder, filling them in the process.
3. Push the halves together.

Pills

The simplest way to take an unpleasant remedy is to roll the powder into a small pill with fresh bread, which works most effectively with herbs such as *Golden Seal* or *Cayenne*. Instead of using bread, the powder can be combined with cream cheese.

You can make a more storable pill by making lozenges, which can be swallowed whole if you cut them to the appropriate size.

Lozenges

The method of making lozenges is based on combining a powdered herb with sugar and a mucilage to produce the characteristic texture. Lozenges are the ideal preparation for remedies to help the mouth, throat and upper respiratory tract as in this way they can work where they are most needed.

The mucilage may be obtained from *Marshmallow Root, Slippery Elm Bark, Comfrey Root* or from one of the gums such as *Tragacanth* or *Acacia*.

This is how to make lozenges using *Tragacanth:*

Bring half a litre of water to the boil and then mix it with 30 grams of *Tragacanth,* which has been soaked in water for 24 hours and stirred as often as possible. Then beat the mixture to obtain a uniform consistency and afterwards force the mixture through a muslin strainer. When the mucilage is ready, mix it with the powdered herb to form a paste, and if you feel you need to, add sugar for the taste. Roll the paste on a slab, preferably on marble, which has been spread with cornstarch or sugar to avoid the paste sticking to the slab. Cut into any shape and size you like and leave the lozenges exposed to the air until they are dry. Then store them in an airtight container.

Instead of using dry herbs, you can also use essential oils. A good example would be *Peppermint* oil. Mix 12 drops of pure *Peppermint* oil with 60 grams of sugar and then combine this with enough of the mucilage of *Tragacanth* to make a paste. Then proceed as above and store the product in an airtight container for later use.

External Remedies

As the body can absorb herbal compounds through the skin, a wide range of methods and formulations has been developed that takes advantage of this fact. Douches and suppositories, though they might appear to be internal remedies, have traditionally been categorized as external remedies.

Baths

The best way of absorbing herbal compounds through the skin is by bathing in a full body bath with half a litre of infusion or decoction added to the water. Alternatively, you can also take a foot- or hand-bath, in which case you would use the preparations in undiluted form.

Any herb that can be taken internally can also be used in a bath. Herbs can, of course, also be used to give the bath an excellent fragrance.

To give some idea of herbs that are particularly good to use: for a bath that is relaxing and at the same time exquisitely scented, infusions can be made of *Lavender Flowers, Lemon Balm, Elder Flowers* or *Rosemary Leaves*. For a bath that will bring about a restful and healing sleep, add an infusion of either *Valerian, Lime Blossom* or *Hops* to the bath water. For children with sleep problems or when babies are teething, try either *Chamomile* or *Lime Blossom,* as the herbs mentioned above may be too strong. In feverish conditions or to help the circulation, stimulating and diaphoretic herbs can be used, such as *Cayenne, Boneset, Ginger* or *Yarrow*.

These are just some of the possibilities. Try out others for yourself. Chapter 4 on aromatherapy, a healing system based on the external application of herbs in the form of essential oils, discusses other ideas. These oils can also be used in baths by putting a few drops of oil into the bathwater.

Instead of preparing an infusion of the

herb beforehand, a handful of it can also be placed in a muslin bag which is suspended from the hot water tap so that the water flows through it. In this way a very fresh infusion can be made.

Douches

Another possibility of using herbs externally is the use of a douche, the application of herbs to the vagina, which is particularly indicated for local infections. Whenever possible, prepare a new infusion or decoction for each douche. Allow the tea to cool to a temperature that will be comfortable internally. Pour it into the container of a douche bag and insert the applicator vaginally. Allow the liquid to rinse the inside of the vagina. Note that the liquid will run out of the vagina, so it is easiest to douche sitting on the toilet. It is not necessary actively to hold the liquid in. In most conditions indicating a need for douching it is advisable to use the tea undiluted for a number of days three times daily. If, however, a three to seven day course of douching (along with the appropriate internal herb remedies) has not noticeably improved a vaginal infection, see a qualified practitioner for a diagnosis.

Ointments

Ointments are semi-solid preparations that can be applied to the skin. Depending on the purpose for which they are designed, there are innumerable ways of making ointments; they can very in texture from very greasy ones to those made into a thick paste, depending on what base is used and on what compounds are mixed together.

Any herb can be used for making ointments, but *Arnica Flower* (note that *Arnica* is not advisable on open wounds), *Chickweed, Comfrey Root, Cucumber, Elder Flower,* *Eucalyptus, Golden Seal, Lady's Mantle, Marigold Flower, Marshmallow Root, Plantain, Slippery Elm Bark, Yarrow* and *Woundwort* are particularly good for use in external healing mixtures.

The simplest way to prepare an ointment is by using vaseline or a similar petroleum jelly as a base. While this has the disadvantage of being an inorganic base, it has a number of advantages that make it very useful. Vaseline is easy to handle so a simple ointment can be made very quickly. Besides this it has the advantage of not being absorbed itself by the skin, making it useful for instance as the base for the anti-catarrhal balm described later. Here the vaseline just acts as a carrier for the volatile oils which can thus evaporate and enter the nasal cavities, without being absorbed through the skin.

The basic method for a vaseline ointment is to simmer 2 tablespoonsful of a herb in 220 grams of vaseline for about 10 minutes. A single herb, a mixture, fresh or dried herbs, roots, leaves or flowers can be used.

As an example, here is a recipe for a simple *Marigold* ointment, which is excellent for cuts, sores and minor burns.

Take 60 grams (about a handful) of freshly picked *Marigold Flowers* and 200 grams of vaseline. Melt the vaseline over low heat, add the *Marigold Flowers* and bring the mixture to the boil. Simmer it very gently for about 10 minutes, stirring well. Then sift it through fine gauze and press out all the liquid from the flowers. Pour the liquid into a container and seal it after it has cooled.

In more traditional ointments, instead of using vaseline a combination of oils were used that act as a vehicle for the remedies and help them to be absorbed through the skin, plus hardening agents to create the texture desired. The following example is the prescription for a simple ointment from the British Pharmacopoeia from 1867 for 'Unguentum Simplex':

White wax 60 grams – beeswax can be used)
Lard 90 grams – Vegetable fat, i.e. cooking fat, can be used)
Sweet Almond oil 90 ml
Melt the wax and lard in the oil on a water bath, remove from heat when melted, add almond oil and stir until cool.

In this basic recipe, the lard and the almond oil facilitate the easy absorption of the herbal remedies through the skin. Instead of these carriers we can also use one or more of lanolin, cocoa butter, wheatgerm oil, olive oil and vitamin E. The wax thickens the final product, and for this effect we could also use lanolin, cocoa butter, or most ideally beeswax, depending on the consistency we want to achieve.

To make a herbal ointment from a simple base like the one described above involves a number of steps:

1. Make the appropriate water extract, either an infusion or decoction, and strain off the liquid to be used in step 4.
2. Measure out the fat and oil for the base.
3. Mix the fat and oil together.
4. Add the strained herbal extract and stir it into the base.
5. Simmer until the water has completely evaporated and the extract has become incorporated into the oil. Be careful not to overheat the mixture and watch particularly for the point when all the water has evaporated and the bubbling stops. If additional thickeners (like beeswax) need to be incorporated, they can be added at this point and melted with the base, heating slowly and stirring until completely blended.
6. If a perishable base is used (such as lard), a drop of tincture of benzoin should be added for each 30 grams of base.
7. Pour the mixture into a container.

Suppositories

Suppositories are designed to enable the insertion of remedies into the orifices of the body. While they can be shaped to be used in the nose or the ears, they are most commonly used for rectal or vaginal problems. They act as carriers for any herb that it is appropriate to use, and there are three general categories of these. First, there are herbs acting to soothe the mucous membranes, reduce inflammations and aid the healing process. Such as the root and the leaf of *Comfrey*, the root of *Marshmallow* and of *Golden Seal*, and the bark of *Slippery Elm*. Secondly, there are the astringent herbs that can help in the reduction of discharge or in the treatment of haemorrhoids, such as *Periwinkle*, *Pilewort*, *Witch Hazel* and *Yellow Dock*. And thirdly, there are remedies to stimulate the peristalsis of the intestines to overcome chronic constipation; in other words, the laxatives. It will often be appropriate in any of these three categories to include with the above one of the antimicrobial herbs.

As with ointments, we can choose from different bases, keeping in mind that it has to be firm enough to be inserted into the orifice and at the same time can melt at body temperature, once inserted, to liberate the herbs it contains. The herbs should be distributed uniformly in the base, which is particularly important when using a powdered herb, which is the easiest form of herb to use for this purpose. To prepare a suppository: Mix the finely powdered herb with a good base, perferably cocoa butter, and mould it in the way described below.

A more complex method has to be used when we want to avoid the introduction of powdered plant material into the body. The simplest form of preparing suppositories in this way uses gelatin and glycerine – both animal products – and either an infusion, a decoction or a tincture, in the following proportions:

Gelatin	10 parts
Water (or infusion, decoction, tincture)	40 parts
Glycerine	15 parts

The gelatin is soaked for a while in the water-based material and then dissolved with the aid of gentle heating. Then the glycerine is added and the whole mixture is heated on a water bath to evaporate the water, as the final consistency desired depends on how much water is removed. If it is removed completely, a very firm consistency will be achieved.

The easiest way to prepare a mould – for both kinds of bases – is to use aluminium foil which you can shape to the length and shape you need. The best shape is a torpedo-like, 2.5 cm long suppository. Pour the molten base into the mould and let it cool; you can then store the suppositories in the moulds in a refrigerator for a while, though it is always preferable to make them when they are needed.

Compresses

A compress or fermentation is an excellent way to apply a remedy to the skin to accelerate the healing process. To make a compress, use a clean cloth – made either of linen, gauze, cotton wool or cotton – and soak it in a hot infusion or decoction. Place this as hot as possible upon the affected area and either change it when it cools down or cover the cloth with plastic or waxed paper and place a hot water bottle on this, which you can change when it cools, as the heat will enhance the activity of the herb.

All the vulnerary herbs make good compresses, as do stimulants and diaphoretics in many situations.

Poultices

The action of a poultice is very similar to that of a compress, but instead of using a liquid extract, the solid plant material is used for a poultice.

Either fresh or dried herbs can be used to make a poultice. With the fresh plant you apply the bruised leaves or root material either directly to the skin or place it between thin gauze. With the dried herb, they must be made into a paste by adding either hot water or apple cider vinegar until the right consistency is obtained. To keep the poultice warm, you can use the same method as for the compress and place a hot water bottle on it.

When you are applying the herb directly to the skin, it is often helpful first to cover the skin with a small amount of oil, as this will protect the skin and make removal easier.

Poultices can be made from warming and stimulating herbs, from vulneraries, astringents and also from emollients, which are demulcents that are soothing and softening on the skin, such as *Comfrey Root, Flaxseed, Marshmallow Root, Oatmeal, Quince Seed,* and *Slippery Elm Bark.*

Poultices are often used to draw pus out of the skin and there are a multitude of old recipes. Some of them use *Cabbage*, which is excellent, others use bread and milk, some even soap or sugar. An old recipe for a *Flaxseed* meal poultice was as follows:

Mix a sufficient portion of the meal with hot water to make a mushy mass. Spread this with a tablespoon on a piece of thin flannel or old muslin. Then double in a half inch of the edge all round to keep the poultice from oozing out. When it is on, cover it at once with a piece of oiled silk, oiled paper, or thin rubber cloth, to keep the moisture in.

Liniments

Liniments are specifically formulated to be easily absorbed through the skin, as they are used in massages that aim at the stimulation of muscles and ligaments. They are not for internal use. To reach these areas and to carry the herbal components there, liniments are usually made of a mixture of the herb with alcohol or occasionally with apple cider vinegar, sometimes with an addition of herbal oils. The main ingredient of a liniment is usually *Cayenne*, which may be combined with *Lobelia* or other remedies. The following liniment is described by Jethro Kloss: (imperial measurements!)

Combine two ounces powdered *Myrrh*, one ounce powdered *Golden Seal*, one-half ounce *Cayenne Pepper*, one quart rubbing alcohol (70 percent): Mix together and let stand seven days; shake well every day, decant off, and bottle in corked bottles. If you do not have *Golden Seal*, make it without.

Perhaps an even better one to use is: *Lobelia* and *Cramp Bark* equal parts, plus *Cayenne*, a pinch; all in vodka for a compound tincture liniment or in rubbing alcohol as above.

Oils

Many herbs are rich in essential oils. There are herbs like *Peppermint*, whose oils are volatile and aromatic, and others with very little aroma, such as *St John's Wort*.

Herbal oils come in two forms, depending on the mode of extraction. First of all there are the pure essential oils, which are extracted from the herb by a complex and careful process of distillation. Only an expert can make these at home. These oils are best obtained from specialist suppliers, who distil them as the basis for aromatherapy and take care that they are as pure as possible. Synthetic oils are sold as 'pure', so always buy from reputable dealers.

The second way of extracting oils is much simpler and resembles the method of cold infusion. Instead of infusing the herb in water it is put into an oil, whereby a solution of the essential oil in the oil-base is obtained. The best oils to use are vegetable oils such as Olive, Sunflower or Almond oil, but any good pressed vegetable oil can be used and these are preferable to mineral oils.

To make a herbal oil, first cut the herb finely, cover it with oil and put in a clear glass container. Place this in the sun or leave in a warm place for two to three weeks, shaking the container daily. After that time, filter the liquid into a dark glass container and store the extracted oil.

A typical and very nice example of such an oil is *St John's Wort* oil, which makes a very red oil that can be used externally for massages and to help sunburns and heal wounds. It can also be taken internally in very small doses to ease stomach pains. To make it, pick the flowers when they are just opened and crush them in a teaspoonful of olive oil. Cover them with more oil, mix well and put in a glass container in the sun or a warm place for three to six weeks, at the end of which the oil will be bright red. Press the mixture through a cloth to remove all the oil and leave it to stand for a while, as there will be some water in the liquid which will settle on the bottom so that the oil can be decanted off. Then store the oil in a well-sealed, dark container.

9
HERBS AND COOKING

Perhaps the most widely used plants are those that augment cookery with their aroma or spice. Many excellent books have been written by cooks who know their herbs and spices. Here we shall just mention a few that can be used and some suggestions for their use. The Bibliography has references for more detailed exploration.

There are no rules in the use of herbs and spices in cooking. It is all a matter of taste. Take chances and experiment with combinations and quantities. It is always best to start with a small amount of the herb to sample its delights, because you might find that you thoroughly dislike one particular herb that the books say is wonderful. After all they are your taste buds!

With most leafy herbs it is best to add them to the cooking near the end to ensure that a minimum of aroma is lost.

There is no real difference between herbs and spices, other than that culinary herbs are usually dried leaf and spices are powders.

The details of storage and drying given elsewhere are of great importance here as these plants are the very ones rich in oils. So take care in maintaining the quality of your culinary herbs and spices to ensure you get the most out of them.

There are a number of ways to use the herbs in addition to simply sprinkling them on the dish. It is possible to concoct your own mixed herbs, herb pepper, herb spice and herb vinegar. Some suggestions are given here but it is fun to experiment!

Mixed Herbs

Mix well the following herbs, store and label. Small amounts may be put into muslin sachets and used as bouquet garni.

Parsley	2 parts
Marjoram	1 part
Winter Savory	1 part
Thyme	1 part

Other combinations or specific varieties of each herb can be tried in various combinations.

Herb Pepper
Mix equal parts of powdered
  Marjoram
  Rosemary

Thyme
Mace
Black Pepper
Sift and store in a well stoppered bottle.

Herb Spice
Mix equal parts of powdered
  Basil
  Bay Leaves
  Marjoram
  Thyme
with a tablespoon of
  Black Pepper
  Powdered Cinnamon
  Powdered Mace
  Powdered Nutmeg
Remember that this is just a suggestion, please try other combinations of your own liking.

Here we shall review a small range of common herbs and spices.

Angelica

The young leaves may be added to salads, and fresh leaf stems may be cooked with acid fruits such as blackcurrants, gooseberries and rhubarb to counteract tartness, using 60g of angelica to 500g of fruit. The flavour is distinctively mild and sweet. Candied angelica can be prepared from the young, fleshy leaf stems. The selected stems are cut into 10 cm lengths and steeped in cold salted water – 8 g to l litre of water – for ten minutes to retain the green colour, then rinsed well and simmered until tender. The outer skin and stringy fibres should be removed, and the pieces candied. Beware of too much sugar in your diet though!

Allspice

This is rather like a blend between cloves, cinnamon and nutmeg. It is used in cakes and biscuits and as a general spice.

Aniseed

Has a liquorice-like taste with good medicinal properties described elsewhere in the book. The leaves may be used in salads or cooking and the slightly bruised seeds as a general spice.

Basil

A strong-tasting herb that should be used with moderation as it can become too all-pervasive. It has a wide range of uses in cooking, adding a delicious flavour to whatever it is used with.

Bay Leaf

A beautiful culinary tree for any garden, providing the dish with an aromatic and slightly bitter flavour that can be widely used.

Borage

The leaves can be cooked with other green vegetables, in soups, and very young leaves and tips of growth added to salads. Leaves and flowers are put into wine and like cucumber have a cooling effect. The flowers can be crystallized and used for cake decoration or used fresh in salads.

Caraway

The seed has a distinctive spicy flavour and is often added to rye bread, cakes, meat and fish dishes. It is excellent cooked with cabbage, and is also used in certain cheeses and pickles. If surplus plants are grown, some roots may be dug in the first year and cooked as a vegetable. Young foliage may be chopped for use with a green salad.

Cardamon

A seed that has good carminative properties. A slightly ginger-like spice.

Cayenne

This is hot chilli pepper, whose excellent medicinal properties are discussed in the book. It is used wherever a hot spice is desired.

Coriander

The seed should be crushed or pounded to release the aroma. It is an essential ingredient in the making of curry powder and mixed spice. It can be added to bread, spiced cakes, also to soups and casseroles. The young roots can be eaten as a vegetable and chopped leaves added to salads.

Dill

It has a pleasant, mild caraway-like flavour. The leaves can be cooked with a wide range of meat, fish and savoury dishes, or used freshly chopped in all kinds of salads. The flowering stems are added to pickled gherkins and cucumber; whole or ground seeds are used to flavour fish dishes, cream cheese, herb butter and salad dressings, are cooked with vegetables, and sprinkled on bread.

Fennel

The flavour of fennel is strong and the young leaves are best in cookery. As a carminative, it is used to counteract the richness of oily fish such as herrings or mackerel. A few sprigs can be placed inside the fish. Chopped leaves can be added to a sauce or stuffing. It may be chopped and sprinkled over meat before cooking, added to soups, egg dishes, sandwich fillings and salads and to vegetables such as beans or cabbage. The crushed ripe seeds are used to flavour savoury dishes and herb bread and biscuits.

Fenugreek

A useful medicinal remedy that makes a good addition to curry powders and as a general spice.

Garlic

The common prejudice some people have against garlic is probably due to over-use, but when added sparingly it is a valuable seasoning and can be used in a great variety of savoury dishes. According to taste one or two whole cloves or small slivers can be inserted into meat for roasting or grilling or pounded and added to sauces, casseroles etc. A garlic press is best for extracting the juice or pulp. If only a very mild flavour is required, a cut clove should be rubbed round the inside of the casserole or salad bowl.

Hyssop

This useful medicinal herb can be added to salads, fruit cocktails, soups etc. It has a slightly bitter, minty taste.

Lemon Balm

The fresh leaves have a delicate lemon flavour as well as the gentle relaxing effects of the herb, described elsewhere. It makes a good tea and is a widely-applicable herb if you like the taste. As a source of lemon flavouring it has been superseded by the introduction of real lemons, but the herb can be used in the majority of dishes where a lemon flavour is needed. More of this herb will be needed than is usual with most herbs because of the delicate flavour. Freshly picked young leaves may be added to green salads and fruit salads. A few sprigs cooked with stewed apples or rhubarb impart a flavour which is pleasantly lemony without being acid. A few sprigs can be added to a cup of milkless tea in place of the more usual slice of lemon. They are a useful addition to pot pourri or to a mixture of herbs for sachets or pillows. The essential oil is used commercially as a constituent of various liqueurs.

Lemon Verbena

The strongly lemon-scented leaves can be used as a substitute for lemons when these are scarce or expensive, although they lack the acidity. They can be used to flavour cakes and stewed fruit and in drinks, and in any dish where lemon is used purely as a flavouring. Fresh or dried leaves are used to make a fragrant and refreshing tea.

Lovage

Lovage has a distinctive rich flavour which adds body to any savoury dish. Leaves, stems, roots and seeds are all used. If a few can be spared, the emerging shoots, when 10 – 12 cm long, may be eaten like celery. Young leaves may be added to salads or cooked with chicken, and two or three short lengths of the succulent leaf stalks can be added to casseroles and soups. Any tender roots left over after division can be boiled and served with French dressing. The young stems can be candied. The dried seeds store well for winter use and can be put into muslin bags for use in soups or stews and added to herb breads and biscuits. The leaves also dry well and retain a pleasant green colour and a good flavour. Unlike most herbs, Lovage is put into the dish at the commencement of cooking, but as it is strongly flavoured only small amounts are required.

Marigold

The medically-valuable petals can be used as an alternative to saffron in cooking, and the leaves may be added to salads.

Marjoram

One of the few herbs almost everyone has heard of and probably tasted – a must in all kitchens.

Mints

There are many different kinds of this genus of flowers. Personal taste will dictate which is more often used. They all make pleasant teas for general drinking and make good additions to salads.

Nasturtium

Leaves, flowers and seeds can be used in the kitchen. They have a hot peppery taste and contain vitamin C. Young flowers add colour to a green salad, and the unripe seeds can be pickled in vinegar as a substitute for capers. The leaves dry well for winter use, and the ripened seeds can be dried and ground in a pepper mill for use as a seasoning.

Oregano

This is in fact a wild species of Marjoram – a wonderful herb that is a must for pizzas!

Garden Parsley

Parsley is a mineral-and vitamin-rich herb that should be freely eaten and not used merely as a garnish. The stems are always included in a bouquet garni. When parsley is used it should always be added towards the end of the cooking period to preserve the vitamin content and colour. Chopped leaves are added to soups, sauces, omelettes and scrambled eggs and sprinkled over salads and cooked vegetables. It is the main ingredient of dried mixed herbs.

Rosemary

Rosemary is a useful kitchen herb, but only young leaves should be used and these are usually removed before serving. Soft young sprigs laced into the skin of a joint of lamb or of a chicken before roasting impart a good flavour, and sachets of rosemary leaves can be cooked with casseroles, old potatoes or spinach. It features largely in Greek and Italian cookery. It is one of the most strongly flavoured herbs, and care should be taken not to use it to excess.

Sage

Like most of the highly aromatic herbs sage has long been used to flavour food and wine, and is used commercially in the processing of foods. Although its strong flavour is not popular with everyone it is widely used in stuffing for rich meat and poultry, and in pork sausages, meat loaves and certain hard and soft cheeses; e.g. sage Derby cheese with its flecks of green. As an alternative, whole leaves may be placed on roasting joints or grills of pork or veal or on liver for braising, and when treated in this way only a little of the pungent oil is released from the leaf.

Sweet Cicely

Sweet Cicely has a sweet, mildly aniseed aroma. It may be used as a sugar substitute by sufferers from diabetes. Finely chopped young leaves may be added to lettuce and vegetable salads, mixed into cream cheese, or sprinkled over omelettes, strawberries and trifles. The acidity of certain fruits such as black or red currants, gooseberries, plums or rhubarb is reduced by adding a few pieces of leaf stem or leaves, or by using dried leaves (2 – 3 teaspoonsful to 454 g of fruit). As well as lessening the quantity of sugar required this herb gives an attractive flavour to the fruit. If the herb is used in highly seasoned dishes, however, the delicate flavour is lost.

Tarragon

A subtle herb that will enhance any dish it is used in. Widely used in French cooking, it is also a common ingredient in herb vinegars.

Common Thyme

Common thyme is strongly flavoured and should be used sparingly. It is one of the herbs included in a bouquet garni, and also in dried mixed herbs. It can be used in any savoury dish and sprinkled over salads and vegetables. A delicious marinade for chicken portions consists of chopped fresh or dried thyme with olive oil, grated lemon rind and juice, a little garlic and freshly ground black pepper and salt. It must be stressed, however, that if thyme is used too lavishly its flavour will be overwhelming and will destroy the natural flavour of the food.

Vegetables as Medicine

Herbs are quite simply vegetables, maybe unusual vegetables, but still vegetables! The foods we eat from the plant kingdom can in the same way act as medicines. If you have studied the material so far it has been made clear where this is especially so. In this section common items of food are considered as potential healing agents. The naturopaths would use such dietary aids as the foundation of their healing work, for after all we are what we eat.

Grains

Oats

This is what a traditional herbalist would call a nervine trophorestorative or tonic. It is described in depth in the section on 'Nervines' in Chapter 3. Organic or home-grown oats are best, thus ensuring the best quality. Only a small patch need be planted and cropped in midsummer when in seed. The whole plant is used to make the tincture.

Barley

A body-building tissue-healing grain that is good in all wasting or debility. It contains an alkaloid called hordenine which is diuretic, mildly relaxing for the chest. It is renowned as barley water for kidney problems where it can be combined with *Corn*

Silk or *Couch Grass* for urinary stones, infection or irritation.

Rice-water

This is full of the B vitamins and is traditionally used as first aid in diarrhoea in the third world.

Wheat-grass

A generally cleansing vegetable as salad or tea. Widely used in drastic cleansing programmes.

Vegetables

Artichokes

This is a gently supportive and stimulating liver remedy that encourages balanced digestion and the avoidance of constipation.

Asparagus

The flowering tops and shoots are diuretic because of the asparagine present. They can help in removal or possibly breaking up kidney stones.

Avocados

A wonderful vegetable, now freely available in Britain, that is rich in vitamin E and Selenium, providing a solid foundation for a low allergen diet. The oil makes a good cosmetic base and is used in face creams etc.

Beetroot

This valuable vegetable will tend to colour both stools and urine pink, but this is quite safe. The juice is reputedly anti-inflammatory and blood cleansing. This is the basis of its use in cancer raw juice therapy.

Cabbage

A staple green vegetable in much of the world. Whole books have been written on the medicinal value of this green leaf! Due to a small amount of an isothiocyamate present it is contra-indicated in thyroid disease. It makes a wonderful poultice using the raw leaves, for joint and muscle problems, skin wounds etc. It is absorbing so may be used on ulcers, wounds, boils, acne, varicose ulcers and neuralgias because it is counter-irritant.

Carrot

This common vegetable contains carotene, the precursor of vitamin A, so it does help you see in the dark! It is a beneficial cleansing vegetable. It is most useful for those on a limited diet. It is the most non-allergenic of the root vegetables and is an alterative, especially aiding liver function. It is the main vegetable in raw juice therapy. Carrots improve resistance to infection, and healing internal ulcers. They increase the red blood cell count and so may be used in anaemia. The whole vegetable provides bulk in bowel disorders. Wild carrot seeds are a herbal diuretic, and wild root is specific for urinary stones.

Celery

This is described elsewhere in the book as an anti-inflammatory and anti-rheumatic remedy when used as the seed. The stems and leaves are rich in calcium and will also help in easing the intensity of arthritis.

Leek

Like its relatives the onion and garlic, it lowers cholesterol levels in the blood, normalizes clotting time, and is effective against kidney stones. It can guard against infections, act as a diuretic, soothe gut inflammations, and chest complaints. This was why it made the basis of stew for tuberculosis sufferers and other convalescences. As a herb, it is used as a decoction for the kidneys.

Lettuce

Lettuce is a herbal sedative whose milky latex has an opiate-like action. Wild lettuce is described in another section of the book. The freshly made juice of *Wild Lettuce* drunk may have the sedative opiate action, although this varies with climate and soil conditions. With a good sample even a salad serving may make one drowsy. It can be safely used as a medicinal vegetable in nervous bowel, colic, etc.

Olives

While technically a fruit, olives are usually considered vegetables in use. Olives are rich in unsaturated fats, but not the kind that are vital for health. The oil has been used as a temporary relief for gallbladder stones, although the evidence is equivocal. Although a health food used as a staple in the Mediterranean, the oil content makes it inadvisable for people with cardiovascular problems. Medicinally, it is used by practitioners for kidney and bile duct problems. The leaf of the olive tree dilates peripheral blood vessels and is used in Yugoslavia traditionally to lower blood pressure.

Onion

The health properties of this amazing vegetables are legion. As with its close relatives garlic and leeks, onions reduce the clotting of platelets and can be anti-thrombitic. It is good for bronchial complaints and is reputed to lower raised blood-sugar levels. As an antiseptic and anthelmintic, it is sterilizing to both mouth and throat, urinary infections such as cystitis and works as a diuretic. Raw it may be used as a poultice with vulnerary and rubefacient actions, being most helpful for burns, and chilblains. Unfortunately, much of its benefit is lost during cooking.

Potato

In much of the world this is the most nutritious, cheapest, and most productive food staple. It contains up to only 6 per cent protein but it is of good biological value. The skin is rich in vitamin C at the beginning of its storage life but slowly fades and can be easily cooked out. The green parts of the tuber are high in potentially dangerous alkaloids so avoid, especially in pregnancy. It is used raw as a medicine: the juice is vulnerary for ulcers, wounds etc. and anti-inflammatory internally. Slices may be used as poultices for chilblains, wounds, cuts (not really antiseptic). Potatoes should stay in the kitchen for first aid.

Radishes

This hot remedy is a circulatory stimulant. It will help to increase resistance and phlegm expectoration. It is also a diuretic and liver stimulant.

Fruit

Apple

One of the most effective non-cereal bulk laxatives, high in pectin, which appears to lower cholesterol uptake from the diet. This makes them indicated in cardio-vascular problems, along with other fruits. They are indicated for rheumatism and gout, congestive bronchitis, kidney and urinary tract problems as a soothing diuretic. It may help in liver disease. This makes apples an advisable food for most people; they are almost Britain's best health asset. Although they give an acid feeling to teeth, there is a stimulation of alkaline saliva and washing, so are preventative to decay. Raw apples are cleansing to teeth and of all fruits, cause the least problems.

Apricot

Rich in iron and minerals and so is used in anaemia, the apricot is a bulk laxative and gentle alterative. It may be used fresh or dried. Chinese apricots are considered better because less chemicals are used.

Fig

This is a laxative, gentle enough for children; good as food, or in chemist shops as the syrup for adults. All syrups are teeth-rotting. It can be used as poultice for wounds or piles (haemorrhoids). All this applies to dried figs, but especially to wild. They are least acid when dried longest; usually there is not much pesticide residue. Like prunes, there is no acid when dried well.

Grapes

These are often considered the most cleansing of fruits but those for sale in British shops are all coated with pesticides so it is better to grow your own.

Orange

This generally wonderful fruit gives problems to an appreciable minority of people. Oranges should not be eaten by migraine sufferers, along with chocolate, cheese and red wine. They are one of the few fruits contra-indicated in arthritis. For most people they are fine. Satsumas and tangerines act in similar ways, although grapefruit are usually alright and lemons almost never give trouble. Orange-flower water was used in the past for 'hysteria' because of a slightly relaxing effect. The leaves are anti-spasmodic and may be used in insomnia and epilepsy.

Pear

The large storage cells make the pear an in-appropriate fruit in conditions such as diverticulitis, because it worsens any bowel inflammation, acting like sandpaper. Otherwise it is an excellent fruit.

Strawberry

This delicious fruit is rich in salicylates, which may help to explain its traditional use in rheumatism. A fresh extract lowers raised blood pressure, is high in iron, acts as a diuretic and aids liver function. The outer seeds may disturb diverticulitis, and some sensitive people develop skin allergies.

Others

Beans and Pulses

They are all high in protein, some of high biological value. This is especially so when used in combinations. High levels of iron and other minerals are present. They are body-building without making demands on the digestive system and are thus good for convalesence.

Tea

Good tea is a wonderful herb, but we should be concerned when large amounts are regularly consumed. The plant contains xanthenes, theophylline and caffeine. These can all act as heart and nervous system stimulants. It is also rich in tannins which reduce the digestive system's ability to absorb food, leading to constipation. It should only be drunk in moderation. Tea is not advisable in any arthritic condition. It is also very rich in fluoride, which makes the debate about fluoridation of water in the UK rather a joke, as most people take far more fluoride from their cups of tea than from the water in the tea. This herb was introduced into Europe as a medicinally relaxing, cooling, and anti-asthmatic remedy. Green tea is much to be preferred, as most British black tea has dye in it.

Coffee

This herb is described in the section on nervine stimulants. Due to its relatively high content of the alkaloids caffeine and theobromine, it has a direct stimulating action on the central nervous system and a secondary diuretic effect. It is greatly abused in this country as a source of easy stimulation, which makes it a major aggravator of all stress-related problems. It should be avoided in arthritis of all kinds.

Cocoa Beans

A number of rather active plant drugs are found in cocoa, the basis of chocolate. Without exploring its chemistry, it contains a whole range of chemicals similar to caffeine that have neurological and capillary effects. This is the fundamental reason why it should be avoided in migraine. Of course it must also be avoided in any condition where there is raised blood-sugar such as diabetes. The carob bean makes an excellent substitute.

10
_____ USING DYE PLANTS _____

Plants offer a whole range of colours that soothe the senses and in an aesthetic sense connect us with the Earth. It might be easier to use chemical dyes, and the results might be far brighter, but there is a place for subtlety in today's garish world.

Here we shall briefly consider some of the plant dyes and how to use them. It is an art and science in itself, so please follow up the references in the Bibiography.

Apart from knowing about the herbs and their colours, the effect and need for mordants must be considered. Some natural dyes are not 'fast' and will fade or wash out if not bound to the material in some way. This is usually done with some sort of chemical mordant. These include commonly available chemicals such as:

acetic acid, alum, ammonia, caustic soda, copper sulphate, ferrous sulphate, lime , potassium bitartrate, potassium dichromate, tannic acid, tartaric acid.

The directions for using each plant, which mordant to use and the possible variations needs a comprehensive book or guide. As general guidelines, however, the following will usually do:

- wash the material with a mild soap to remove any natural wax.
- plant fibres as a rule take longer to mordant.
- to mordant, the clean material is simmered (wool), boiled (cotton, linen), or soaked in hot water (silk) in which the chemical has been dissolved.
- after the correct length of time, rinse the material and allow to dry.
- prepare dye bath by soaking the herb in water overnight and then boiling until the colour has been extracted.
- strain and use 18 litres of dye bath to a pound dry weight of material.
- for wool, cotton or linen, simmer in the dye bath for as long as necessary to achieve desired colour. For silk keep the temperature below 71°C.
- rinse a number of times, each one a little cooler than the last, until the rinse water remains clear.
- After drying, the material is ready for use!

Below are some examples of common plants used as dyes. A comprehensive list would be much longer. Notice that some need a mordant, and some will produce different colours with different mordants.

You can create your own blends producing quite unique, and usually unrecreatable colours, by experimenting. Have fun!

Plant	Part used	Colour	Material	Mordant
Alder	Bark	Grey/brown to black	Wool, cotton	Ferrous sulphate
	Leaves	Brown/yellow	cotton	Alum
		Green/yellow	Wool, cotton	Alum
Alder Buckthorn	Bark	Bronze/brown	Wool	
Alkanet	Root	Red	Wool	
Almond	Leaves	Yellow	Wool	
Cranberry	Stems/leaves	Yellow	Wool	Alum
		Yellow/red	Wool, linen, cotton	Alum
Apple Tree	Bark	Yellow	Wool	
Barberry	Leaves	Black	Wool	Ferrous sulphate
	Roots	Yellow	Wool	
	Twigs and young leaves	Red/yellow	Wool	
Blackberry	Young shoots	Grey	Wool	Alum
Blackthorn	Bark	Red/brown/ black	Wool	Ferrous sulphate
Bloodroot	Rootstock	Red/orange	Wool	Alum
Bracken	Roots	Yellow	Wool	Chrome
	Young shoots	Yellow/green	Silk	Alum
		Grey	Silk	Ferrous sulphate
Coltsfoot	Herb	Yellow/green	Wool	Alum
		Green	Wool	Ferrous sulphate
Cornflower	Flowers	Blue	Wool	
Dandelion	Root	Magenta	Wool	
Dog's Mercury	Herb	Green/yellow to blue	Wool	
Dyer's Bedstraw	Roots	Red	Wool	
Dyer's Broom	Flowering tops	Yellow	Wool	
		Green	Wool	Alum dye over indigo

Plant	Part used	Colour	Material	Mordant
Elder	Fruit	Violet	Wool	Alum
		Lilac	Wool	Alum and salt
	Leaves	Lemon yellow	Wool	Alum
Elecampane	Roots	Blue	Wool	
Fumitory	Herb	Yellow/green	Wool	
Golden Rod	Flowers	Yellow	Wool	Alum
		Gold	Wool	Chrome
Heather	Young tips	Green	Wool	Alum
	Flowering Plant	Yellow	Wool	None
	Tops	Purple	Wool	Alum
	Plant after flowering	Brown	Wool	None
Iceland Moss	Lichen	Brown	Wool	
Juniper	Berries	Brown	Wool	
Lady's Mantle	Green parts	Green	Wool	
Larch	Needles	Brown	Wool	
Larkspur	Flowers	Green	Wool	Alum
Madder	Roots	'Laquer red'	Wool	Alum
		'Garnet red'	Wool	Chrome
		Red	Silk	Alum
		Red	Leather	
Marigold	Petals	Yellow	Wool/silk	Alum
Meadowsweet	Tops	Green/yellow	Wool	Alum
	Roots	Black	Wool	None
Nettle	Herb	Green	Wool	Alum
Onion	Outside skin	Burnt orange	Wool	Alum
		Brass	Wool	Chrome
		Green	Wool	Ferrous sulphate
Oak (Quecus robur)	Bark	Black	Wool	Ferrous sulphate
Ragwort	Herb	Yellow	Wool	Alum
Rowan	Bark	Grey	Wool	
St John's Wort	Tops	Yellow	Wool	Alum
Sorrel	Leaves	Green/yellow	Wool	
Tansy	Leaves	Yellow/green	Wool	
Tea	Leaves	Rose–tan	Wool	
Walnut	Green hulls of nuts	Dark brown	Wool	Alum
Wild Crab Apple	Bark	Yellow	Wool	
Yellow Dock	Roots	Black	Wool	Chrome

11
POT-POURRIS

Another non-medical but still life-enhancing use of plants is the creation of pot-pourris. These are mixtures of flowers, oils and other aromatic material that are usually kept in a decorative container. Whenever the uplifting aroma is desired, just take the lid off. They are usually very beautiful to look at as well because of the flower petals used.

If you are using your own herbs, dry them in the way described in Chapter 8. If you are going to use ready dried material, it is worth searching out a good source of well-dried, colourful and aroma-rich herbs. This is not always easy. It is usual to add some sort of fixative material to hold the aroma for a long time. A range of such fixers is listed below.

Here is a guide to making a potpourri:

- Mix your flower petals to the colour combination desired.
- Put into a large bowl, and for each quart of petals add a tablespoon of powdered or crushed fixative material.
- Carefully stir, with any oils or other components.
- Store in a sealed container for about six weeks to let the whole fragrance become a oneness.
- Don't fill completely so that the mixture can be stirred every few days.
- After six weeks divide the whole into smaller containers or sachets.

There are countless combinations that could be tried. Be adventurous and use your nose and your eyes to help decide. The following are suggestions that can be selected from.

Flowers
Aster, Chamomile, Carnation, Cornflower, Elder, Elecampane, Heliotrope, Jasmine, Jonquil, Lavender, Lemon Verbena, Lily of the Valley, Lime, Marigold, Mullein, Orange, Pansy, Peppermint, Rose, Rose Geranium, Sweet Violet, Violet.

Leaves
Balm, Basil, Bay, Lavender, Lovage, Patchouli, Rose, Rose Geranium, Sage, Sweet Cicely, Sweet Vernal Grass, Thyme, Woodruff.

Spices
Allspice, Caraway, Cardamom, Cinnamon, Cloves, Ginger, Mace, Nutmeg.

Fixatives
Gum Benzoin oil, Gum Mastic, Myrrh, Oakmoss, Orris Root, Sandalwood, Sweet Flag Root.

Oil
Any you like! Refer to Chapter 4 on 'Aromatherapy'.

Others
Aniseed, Cedar Wood, Angelica Root, Lemon peel, Orange peel, Rose buds, Tonka Beans, Vanilla pods.

12
BECOMING A
MEDICAL HERBALIST

All that has gone before may have stimulated you to study medical herbalism in more professional depth. On the other hand the book may have dispelled your illusions and blown away any interest that was there. If that is the case, well thank you for looking at the book!

Herbalism in the United States is in a paradoxical position. Interest in all aspects of herbalism is growing and flourishing; yet, educational avenues are scarce. Because this is one of the very few developed countries where medical herbalism in some form is not legally recognized, acquiring professional training is a challenge.

As there is no licensing body, no degree-giving schools of herbalism currently exist. Naturopathic medicine covers the basics within the context of its broad approach, as do the acupuncture colleges for oriental herbalism. Some chiropractic schools briefly cover herbalism. Considering the inherent constraints of these colleges, the National College of Naturopathic Medicine in Portland, Oregon, and John Bastyr College in Seattle, Washington, have the best "botanic" medicine courses.

Plants as sources of medicine are still extensively studied in the pharmacy schools, especially those with pharmacognosy departments. However, this study alone does not create a herbalist!

The best education in herbalism is offered by schools that are currently outside the educationally orthodox. Such places have developed where there are herbalists, rather than where the demand is. They are small in scale and, on the whole, excellent at what they do. As they are expressions of the vision, skills, and wisdom of the herbalists involved, they each have their own strengths and weaknesses. Some offer full-time training; others are based on workshop formats or correspondence courses. A comprehensive listing of such schools can be obtained from:

California School of Herbal Studies
P.O. Box 39
Forestville, CA 95436
(707) 887-7457

The California School of Herbal Studies is perhaps the best known school of its kind and offers courses that range from the practical skills of gardening, wildcrafting, and medicine-making to herbal therapeutics for both the beginner and health care professionals.

BIBLIOGRAPHY

There is a bewildering array of books about herbs and their uses, cultivation, preparation, and folk lore. This partial bibliography focuses on medical herbalism rather than trying to cover all aspects of this vast field.

Herbals

Grieve, Mrs. M., *A Modern Herbal*, Volumes I and II, Dover Publications.

Griggs, Barbara, *Green Pharmacy*, Norman and Hobhouse, 1981.

Hoffmann, David, *The Holistic Herbal*, Element Books, 1983.

Hoffmann, David, *Successful Stress Control*, Healing Arts Press, 1987.

Mabey, Richard, *The New Age Herbalist*, Collier Books, 1988.

Mills, Simon, *Dictionary of Modern Herbalism*, Healing Arts Press, 1988.

Moore, Michael, *Medicinal Plants of the Mountain West*, Museum of New Mexico Press, 1979.

Priest and Priest, *Herbal Medications*, L.N. Fowler & Co., Ltd., 1982.

Schauenberg and Paris, *Guide to Medicinal Plants*, Keats Publishing, Inc., 1977.

Stuart, Malcom, ed., *Color Dictionary of Herbs and Herbalism*, Van Nostrand, 1979.

Thomson, William, *Medicines From the Earth*, McGraw-Hill, 1978.

Tierra, Michael, *The Way of Herbs*, Orenda/ Unity Press, 1980.

Pharmacognosy and Eclectic Medicine

Brinker, F., *An Introduction to the Toxicology of Common Botanical Medicines*, National College of Naturopathic Medicine, 1983.

Ellingwood, F., *American Materia Medica, Therapeutics and Pharmacognosy*, 1898, Eclectic Medical Pub., 1983.

Felter, H. W., *The Eclectic Materia Medica, Pharmacology and Therapeutics*, 1922, Eclectic Medical Pub., 1983.

Felter and Lloyd, *King's American Dispensatory*, Eclectic Medical Pub., 1983.

Robinson, T., *The Organic Constituents of Higher Plants*, Cordus Press, 1983.

Ross and Brian, *An Introduction to Phytopharmacy*, Pitman Medical Publishing, 1977.

Trease and Evans, *Pharmacognosy*, 12th Edition, Baillere Tindall, 1983.

Tyler, Brady, and Robbers, *Pharmacognosy*, 8th Edition, Lea & Febiger, 1981.

British Herbal Pharmacopoeia, British Herbal Medicine Association, 1979.

231

Newsletters

American Herb Association quarterly newsletter, PO Box 353, Rescue, CA 95672.
The Business of Herbs, PO Box 559, Madison, VA 22727.
Herbalgram, PO Box 12602, Austin, TX 78711.
Lawrence River of Natural Products, PO Box 186, Collegeville, PA 19426-0186.

Professional Journals

Economic Botany
Journal of Ethnopharmacology
Journal of Natural Products
Planta Medica

METRIC CONVERSION

Length
1 centimetre = 0.39 inch
1 metre = 3.28 feet

Area
1 square metre = 10.76 square feet (=1.2 square yards)

Capacity
1 litre (=1,000 millilitres) = 1.76 pint

Weight
1 gram (= 1,000 milligrams) = 0.03 ounce
1 kilogram (= 1,000 grams) = 2.21 pounds

Temperature

0°C =	32°F
5°C =	41°F
15°C =	59°F
20°C =	68°F
30°C =	86°F
40°C =	104°F
50°C =	122°F
60°C =	140°F
70°C =	158°F
80°C =	176°F
90°C =	194°F
100°C =	212°F

Conversion formula: $F = \dfrac{9 \times C}{5} + 32$

INDEX

235